Clinical Simulations for Nursing Education

Learner Volume

Clinical Simulations for Nursing Education

Learner Volume

Marcia L. Gasper, EdD, RNC
Associate Professor of Nursing
East Stroudsburg University School of Nursing
East Stroudsburg, PA

Patricia M. Dillon, PhD, RN
Associate Professor of Nursing
LaSalle University School of Nursing and Health Sciences
Philadelphia, PA

Clinical Consultant
Andrew Storer, DNP, ACNP, FNP-c, RN
Director of Performance Improvement
Department of Emergency Medicine
Thomas Jefferson University
Philadelphia, PA

F.A. Davis Company • Philadelphia

F. A. Davis Company
1915 Arch Street
Philadelphia, PA 19103
www.fadavis.com

Printed in the United States of America

Last digit indicates print number: 10 9 8 7 6 5 4 3 2 1

Publisher, Nursing: Lisa B. Houck
Developmental Editors: William F. Welsh and Niki R. Chester
Director of Content Development: Darlene D. Pedersen
Senior Project Editor: Christina C. Burns
Design and Illustration Manager: Carolyn O'Brien

As new scientific information becomes available through basic and clinical research, recommended treatments and drug therapies undergo changes. The author(s) and publisher have done everything possible to make this book accurate, up to date, and in accord with accepted standards at the time of publication. The author(s), editors, and publisher are not responsible for errors or omissions or for consequences from application of the book, and make no warranty, expressed or implied, in regard to the contents of the book. Any practice described in this book should be applied by the reader in accordance with professional standards of care used in regard to the unique circumstances that may apply in each situation. The reader is advised always to check product information (package inserts) for changes and new information regarding dose and contraindications before administering any drug. Caution is especially urged when using new or infrequently ordered drugs.

Library of Congress Cataloging-in-Publication Data

Gasper, Marcia L.
Clinical simulations for nursing education: learner volume/Marcia L. Gasper, Patricia M. Dillon.
p. ; cm.
Includes bibliographical references and index.
ISBN 978-0-8036-2180-0 (alk. Paper)
I. Dillon, Patricia M. II. Title.
[DNLM: 1. Education, Nursing–methods. 2. Patient Simulation. 3. Problem-Based Learning–methods. WY 18]

610.73076–dc23

2011042069

Preface

Dear Learner:

We developed this book of simulated patient care experiences to help you attain the knowledge, skills, and attitudes you will need to deliver safe, holistic, evidenced-based, and competent care to your patients.

Your instructor(s) have chosen this book to provide you with opportunities to practice critical assessment, monitoring, and nursing care management skills in a controlled, safe, risk-free environment.

These simulations will promote your development of communication and collaboration skills, as well as self-awareness and insight into your strengths and areas for improvement in patient care delivery through the process of debriefing. Preparing for and participating in these simulated structured patient encounters will allow you to master multiple objectives and demonstrate critical thinking in a multidimensional environment which can foster increased confidence and lead to the development of competence.

This book contains all the information necessary for your successful preparation for and participation in the simulation scenarios. The scenario format is designed to allow you to apply the nursing process in a realistic patient care situation, requiring you to consider the complexity of factors that influence a patient's condition and the care you need to provide. You receive the benefit of moving from theory to application in a controlled setting, while your instructor(s) can help you to transition safely from the classroom to the nursing practice setting.

Contributors to this text are experienced clinicians and/or nurse educators who have been chosen for their individual expertise. The scenarios are based on real-life patient care situations, and incorporate built-in decision points where you, assuming the registered nurse role, must make assessments in real time, respond to changes in patient condition, and take appropriate action. The hope is that you will immerse yourself in the experience, focus on the "patient" as a unique, whole person, and not simply attend to environmental or physiological factors.

Each scenario is based on a client with a specific problem (excluding the assessment simulations), formatted in the same way to promote ease of use, and contains the following:

Title: The title identifies what situation, disease, or patient condition the scenario addresses.

Learning Outcomes: Cognitive, psychomotor, affective, communication, safety, and leadership and management/delegation outcomes are included in all scenarios. Additional outcomes are included as appropriate to the specific patient care situation.

Overview of the Problem: A brief overview of the client problem for each scenario is provided unless the scenario does not focus on a particular patient problem. We also provide a list of pertinent topics so that you can review and prepare for the simulation experience. Your instructor(s) may use this list to make an individualized assignment for you in your required texts or other resources. This must be completed prior to your participation in the simulation experience.

Review Questions: Your instructor(s) will use these questions to evaluate your presimulation knowledge.

Related Evidenced-Based Practice Guidelines: A list of relevant guidelines has been included as appropriate in each simulation scenario and contributors have made every effort to incorporate current evidenced-based practice into the simulations themselves. As a life-long learner, you are encouraged to stay abreast of nursing research and new guidelines as they become available in order to provide the highest quality of nursing care.

Simulation

Client Background: This section introduces the patient and his or her history to you. The more complex the scenario, the more patient information we have provided. You will need to use and apply the information we have provided to complete the presimulation student assignments.

Admission Sheet: This section provides demographic data similar to that found on a hospital admission sheet.

Provider's Orders: We have provided current provider's orders as they stand at the start of each scenario. Additional orders may be provided to you by the simulation facilitator(s) during the course of the simulation as it unfolds.

Nursing Report: When appropriate to the situation, the nursing report updates you with the patient's current condition at the start of the scenario. In some scenarios, you will be the first nurse encountering the patient, and no report is provided.

Student Simulation Prep Assignments: This section provides specific assignments for you to complete prior to participation in the simulation experience. These assignments address important areas of nursing knowledge including roles and equipment for provision of care, critical thinking to identify relevant data, focused health assessment, diagnostic tests, medications, nursing process, and delegation.

References: Each scenario is based on current evidence-based practice and includes a list of references.

The Simulation Experience

Your instructor(s) will provide direction for your participation and role in the simulated patient care encounter. If a patient care simulator is used, you should assess and interact with the simulator as you would a real patient.

Debriefing: Your instructor(s) may choose to use the standard debriefing form we have provided with you and your peers following the simulated patient care encounter. These and other forms needed to create a realistic scenario are provided in the Appendix. Since these forms will most likely be needed more than once, you will want to avoid writing directly in the book in the event that you will want to copy the forms for repeated use.

We hope you approach these simulated patient care experiences wholeheartedly, with enthusiasm, and with the goal of developing the knowledge, skills, and attitudes you will need to deliver safe, holistic, evidenced-based, and competent care to your patients.

Patricia M. Dillon, PhD, RN

Marcia L. Gasper, EdD, RNC

Contributors

Claire Basset, RN, MSN
Assistant Professor of Nursing
Coordinator of Clinical Simulation Lab
Georgia Perimeter College
Clarkston, Georgia
Elder Abuse / Thoracic Trauma
Paranoid Schizophrenia with Judy Myers

Elaine Benedict, MS, RN
The Ohio State University Medical Center
Senior Reimbursement Analysis
Columbus, Ohio
COPD / CHF with Patricia M. Dillon and Virginia Hallenbeck

Maryjane Cerrone, MSN, RN-BC
Advanced Practice Nurse
Team Leader, Pain Education & Research
Lehigh Valley Health Network
Allentown, Pennsylvania
Intractable Pain

LeAnn Chisholm, MSN, RN, CCRN, CEN
High-Fidelity Simulation Coordinator and Instructor
Dishman Department of Nursing
Lamar University
Beaumont, Texas
ARDS with Eileen Curl and Sheila Smith

Eileen Deges Curl, PhD, RN
Chairperson and Professor
Dishman Department of Nursing
Lamar University
Beaumont, Texas
ARDS with LeAnn Chisolm and Sheila Smith

Patricia M. Dillon, PhD, RN
Associate Professor of Nursing
LaSalle University School of Nursing and Health Sciences
Philadelphia, Pennsylvania
Respiratory Assessment
Cardiac Assessment
Abdominal Assessment
Head-to-Toe Assessment
Patient Safety
Admission and Care of a Patient with Unstable Angina with Elaine Gross
Abdominal Pain
Aspiration Pneumonia
Perioperative Care with Elaine Gross
Pediatric Asthma with Andrew Storer
Head Injury
Meningitis
Uncontrolled Atrial Fibrillation
Cardiac Arrest
Cardiac Arrhythmia / Rapid Response
CHF / COPD with Virginia Hallenbeck and Elaine Benedict
Spinal Cord Injury
Syncopal Attack
Delirium vs. Dementia
Shock
DKA

Carol Egan, RN, BSN
Staff Educator
Samaritan Health Services
Lebanon, Oregon
Placental Abruption with Marcia L. Gasper

Marcia L. Gasper, EdD, RNC
Associate Professor of Nursing
East Stroudsburg University School of Nursing
East Stroudsburg, Pennsylvania
Postpartum Hemorrhage
Dystocia
Placental Abruption with Carol Egan
Assessment of the School-aged Child with Marjorie Maine-Nyarko

Donna Gibson, RN, MSN
Curriculum Manager
School of Nursing
Kaplan University
Chicago, Illinois
Postoperative Assessment Following Laparoscopic Cholecystectomy with Wendy Thompson

Donna Grather, RN, BSN, CEN, PHRN
Pediatric Trauma Coordinator
Lehigh Valley Health Network
Allentown, Pennsylvainia
Fracture/Suspected Child Abuse
Spleen Injury

Elaine Gross, RN, MSN
Education Coordinator
The Montgomery County Education Center
Royersford, Pennsylvania
Admission and Care of a Patient with Unstable Angina with Patricia M. Dillon
Perioperative Care

Virginia J. Hallenbeck, DNP(c), RN, ACNS-BC
Clinical Nurse Specialist
The Ohio State University Medical Center
University Hospital East
Columbus, Ohio
COPD/CHF with Patricia M. Dillon and Elaine Benedict

Mary E. Holtschneider, RN-BC, BSN, MPA, NREMT-P
Nurse Educator
U.S. Department of Veterans Affairs
Durham VA Medical Center
Durham, North Carolina
Pulseless Electrical Activity

Pasquale V. Iemma, MSN, RN-BC
Academic Chair
School of Nursing at Pembroke Pines, Florida
Kaplan University
Precipitous Delivery with Wendy Thompson

Lorretta Krautscheid, RN, MS
Director, Learning Resource Center, School of Nursing
University of Portland
Portland, Oregon
Immediate Newborn Care
Postoperative Cesarean Section
Postoperative Hip

Karen S. Lotz, RN, MSN Ed.
Nursing Instructor (PN)
Pasco-Hernando Community College
Brooksville, Florida
Lithium Overdose with Daryle Wane

Marjorie Maine-Nyarko, RN, MSN, CPNP
Adjunct Clinical Instructor, Pediatric Nursing
Cedar Crest College
Allentown, Pennsylvania
Assessment of the School-Aged Child with Marcia L. Gasper

Anne Martin, RN, MScN, Post MSN (ACNP)
Project Manager, NCSBN Simulation Study
Indiana University School of Nursing
Carmel, Indiana
Atypical Chest Pain
Subdural Hematoma/Alcohol Withdrawal

Claranne Mathiesen, RN, MSN, CNRN
Stroke Program Manager
Lehigh Valley Hospital
Allentown, Pennsylvania
Stroke

Judy L. Myers, MS, RN, CNS-BC
Program Coordinator
Center for Excellence in Children's Mental Health
University of Minnesota
Minneapolis, Minnesota
Paranoid Schizophrenia with Claire Basset

Cynthia Peterson, MS, RN
Assistant Professor
Department of Nursing
Husson University
Bangor, Maine
HHNK

Lori Pierangeli, PhD, RN
Associate Professor of Nursing
East Stroudsburg University
East Stroudsburg, Pennsylvania
Unresponsive Patient at Home

Cynthia L. Pins, MS, RN
Nursing Faculty
North Hennepin Community College
Brooklyn Park, Minnesota
Intestinal Obstruction

Diane Saleska, MSN, RN
Associate Teaching Professor
College of Nursing
University of Missouri
St. Louis, Missouri
Postoperative Complication
Blood Transfusion Reaction

Sheila Smith, PhD, RN, CNE
Associate Professor
Director, Edna Horn Gay Learning Center
Lamar University
Dishman Department of Nursing
Beaumont, Texas
ARDS with LeAnn Chisolm and Eilene Curl

Andrew Storer, DNP, ACNP, FNP-c, RN
Director of Performance Improvement
Department of Emergency Medicine
Thomas Jefferson University
Philadelphia, Pennsylvania
Gunshot Wound
Adult Asthma with Patricia M. Dillon
Pediatric Asthma with Patricia M. Dillon

Paula Stubbings, RN, BSN, MN
Nursing Instructor
University of the Fraser Valley
Chilliwack, British Columbia, Canada
Care of the Patient with a Colostomy
Narcotic Overdose/Bipolar Disorder

Natalie "Lu" Sweeney, MSN RN CNS
Simulation Program Director
Department of Nursing
Dominican University of California
San Rafael, California
Thermoregulation and Hypoglycemia

Wendy Thomson, EdD(c), MSN, BSBA, RN, CNE
Director of Curriculum
Kaplan Higher Education
School of Nursing
Chicago, Illinois
Precipitous Delivery with Pasquale Iemma
Postoperative Assessment Following Laparoscopic Cholecystectomy with Donna Gibson

Daryle Wane, PhD, ARNP, FNP-BC
Professor of Nursing
Pasco-Hernando Community College
Generic Program Track Coordinator ADN Program
New Port Richey, Florida
Lithium Toxicity with Karen Lotz

Elizabethe Westgard, RN, MSN
Staff Nurse
Albert Einstein Medical Center
Nursing Quality and Patient Safety Specialist, Penn Presbyterian Medical Center
Philadelphia, Pennsylvania
Complications of Vascular Access

Reviewers

Wonda Lou Brown, RN, MSN
Nursing Instructor
Connors State College of Nursing
Muskogee, Oklahoma

Kelley Connor, MS, RNC
Instructor
Boise State University
Boise, Idaho

Louise S. Frantz, BSN, RN
Adjunct Faculty
Pennsylvania State University
Lehigh Carbon Community College
Schnecksville, Pennsylvania
Northampton Community College
Bethlehem, Pennsylvania

Julia Gogle, RNC, BSN
Patient Care Specialist
Labor & Delivery, Perinatal Unit
Lehigh Valley Health Network
Allentown, Pennsylvannia

Anne Hautamaki, MSN, RN
Adjunct Faculty
Oakland Community College
Waterford, Michigan

Aprille L. Haynie, MSN, RN
Faculty
Huron School of Nursing
Cleveland, Ohio

Deborah L. Heckler, RN, MS, BSN, Postgraduate Certificate in Education
RN Quality Coordinator
Union Memorial Hospital
Baltimore, Maryland

Karie Ruekert Kobiske, RN, MSN, Cs-ANP, APNP
Assistant Professor of Nursing
Carroll College
Waukesha, Wisconsin

Rosemary Macy, PhD, RN
Associate Professor
Boise State University
Boise, Idaho

Barbara Maxwell, MSN, MS, BSN, RN
Associate Professor of Nursing
Program Coordinator
State University of New York Ulster County Community College
Stone Ridge, New York

Sharon M. Nowak, RN, MSN
Associate Professor of Nursing
Jackson Community College
Jackson, Michigan

Mendy Stanford, RN, MSN
Skills Laboratory Coordinator and Simulation Specialist
Treasure Valley Community College
Ontario, Oregon

Ramesh C. Upadhyaya, RN, CRRN, MSN, MBA
Clinical Instructor
University of North Carolina at Greensboro
Greensboro, North Carolina

Deborah L. Weaver, RN, PhD
Associate Professor
Valdosta State University
Valdosta, Georgia

Contents

Appendix 427

Index 469

Assessment 1

1-1 Abdominal Assessment/Appendicitis

ASSESSMENT

STANDARD FORMS

These templates are included in the Appendix; copy before each use.

LEARNING OUTCOMES

Cognitive

The student will be able to:

1. Identify pertinent history questions relevant to an abdominal assessment.
2. Describe the techniques of physical assessment as applied to the abdominal assessment.
3. Differentiate normal from abnormal findings.
4. Describe the signs and symptoms of appendicitis.
5. Correlate the signs and symptoms with the pathophysiology of appendicitis.
6. Identify appropriate nursing interventions for a patient with appendicitis.

Psychomotor

The student will be able to:

1. Perform an abdominal assessment.
2. Implement appropriate nursing interventions for a patient with appendicitis.

Affective

The student will be able to:

1. Reflect upon performance in the simulation of abdominal assessment.
2. Identify areas that worked well in the simulation of abdominal assessment.
3. Identify areas that needed improvement in the simulation of abdominal assessment.

Communication

The student will be able to:

1. Communicate effectively with the patient.
2. Communicate effectively with members of healthcare team.
3. Document assessment findings accurately and succinctly.
4. Practice transparent thinking (thinking outloud) to facilitate group problem solving.
5. Use Directed Communication (directing a message to specific individual) when delegating tasks.
6. Employ Closed-Loop Communication (acknowledgment of receipt of the message and status) to acknowledge communications from others.

Safety

The student will be able to:

Administer and maintain specific protecting interventions with attention to safety of the client and healthcare professional.

1. Demonstrate a safe environment with attention to hazards to healthcare providers, visitors, and the client. Includes body mechanics, tripping hazards, equipment issues.
2. Demonstrate attention to national patient safety goals. Includes patient identification standards, effective communication among healthcare providers, and safe medication administration.
3. Demonstrate attention to standard precautions. Includes hand washing, infection control measures, and use of personal protective equipment (PPE) as needed.

OVERVIEW OF THE PROBLEM

History Questions

- Reason for seeking care: perform symptom analysis
- Health history: review current, past, family, review of symptoms, and psychosocial history

Physical Exam

- Inspection
  - Size, shape, symmetry, condition of skin
- Auscultation
  - Bowel sounds, vascular sounds
- Percussion
  - Abdomen and organs
- Palpation
  - Light: surface characteristics
  - Deep: organs, masses
- Special maneuvers

Appendicitis

Definition

Obstruction of the appendiceal lumen and subsequent acute bacterial invasion of the appendiceal wall; constitutes an acute emergency.

Pathophysiology

Appendicitis occurs with obstruction of the appendiceal lumen which can lead to subsequent infection. The process begins with inflammation and edema causing periumbilical pain. As the inflammatory process progresses, pain localizes to the RLQ. There is a danger that the inflamed appendix may rupture and result in peritonitis.

Risk Factors

- Occurs more frequently in men than women.
- Most frequently occurs between the ages of 10 and 30 years.

Assessment

Subjective

- Generalized abdominal pain progresses to RLQ pain at McBurney's point, with positive rebound tenderness
- Anorexia and nausea

Objective

- Vital signs: elevated temperature, shallow respirations
- Diarrhea or constipation
- Vomiting, fetid breath odor
- Splinting of the abdomen, flexion at the knees

Diagnostic Tests

Lab data

- Elevated WBC >10,000
- Elevated neutriphils >75%
- Elevated CRP

Diagnostic studies

- Ultrasound
- CT scan

Treatment

- Surgical emergency

Nursing Management

Goals: Promote comfort

- Preoperative
  - Explain procedures
  - Assist with diagnostic workup
- Postoperative
  - Relieve pain related to surgical incision
  - Prevent infection
    - Wound care, dressing technique
  - Prevent dehydration
    - IV therapy, I&O, fluids by mouth, increase to solids as tolerated
    - Prevent complications
    - Promote ambulation

Evaluation/Outcome Criteria

- No infection
- Tolerates fluids and food by mouth
- Heals without complications

REVIEW QUESTIONS

1. Name five common abdominal complaints.
   Answer:

2. Dividing the abdomen into four quadrants and then into nine areas, identify the underlying structures.
   Answer:

Quadrants

RUQ	LUQ

Quadrants—cont'd

RUQ	LUQ

RLQ	LLQ

Areas

Right Hypochondriac	Epigastric	Left Hypochondriac

Right Lumbar	Umbilical	Left Lumbar

Right Inguinal	Hypogastric	Left Inguinal

Continued

Right Inguinal	Hypogastric	Left Inguinal

3. Identify five specific surface characteristics obtained through inspection of the abdomen.
Answer:

4. Describe three types of movements that may be seen upon inspection of the abdomen.
Answer:

5. What is the rationale for auscultating the abdomen prior to palpation?
Answer:

Related Evidence-Based Practice Guidelines

The Joint Commission National Patient Safety Goals Hospital Program. Retrieved from http://www.jointcommission.org/GeneralPublic/NPSG10_npsgs.htm

SBAR Technique for Communication: A situational briefing model. The Institute for Healthcare Improvement was downloaded on December 19, 2008, from http://www.ihi.org/IHI/Topics/PatientSafety/SafetyGeneral/Tools/SBARTechniqueforCommunicationASituationalBriefingModel.htm

Clinical Practice Guidelines: Right Lower Quadrant Pain.http://www.guideline.gov/appendicitis

Assessment and management of acute pain. Institute for Clinical Systems Improvement—Private Nonprofit Organization. 2000 Oct (revised 2008 Mar). 58 pages. NGC:006371

Topics to Review Prior to Simulation

- Adult abdominal assessment.
- Nursing care of a patient with appendicitis.
- Perioperative nursing care for a patient undergoing laporoscopic surgery.
- IV medication administration and IV therapy.

SIMULATION

Client Background

Biographical data

- Age: 25
- Gender: male
- Height: 6 ft
- Weight: 220 lb

Cultural considerations

- Language: English
- Ethnicity: Italian
- Nationality: American
- Culture: no significant cultural implications identified

Demographic

- Marital status: single
- Educational level: college
- Religion: Catholic
- Occupation: sales

Current health status

- Abdominal pain

History

- Psychosocial history
  - Social support: family and girlfriend
- Past health history
  - Medical: good health, no major health problems
  - Surgical: none
- Family history: negative

Admission Sheet

Name:	Tim Rossetti
Age:	25
Gender:	Male
Marital Status:	Single

Admission Sheet—cont'd

Educational Level:	College
Religion:	Catholic
Ethnicity:	Italian
Nationality:	American
Language:	English
Occupation:	Sales

Hospital
Provider's Orders

Patient's Name: Tim Rossetti
Allergies: NKDA

Diagnosis: r/o appendicitis

Date	Time	Order	Signature
8/12/08	3 PM	Vital signs: q 4 hr	
		Diet: NPO	
		Activity: bed rest	
		IV therapy: 1,000 mL 5% D/NSS q 8 hr	
		Medications: Morphine 4 mg IV now Flagyl 500 mg IVPB now Cipro 400 mg IVPB now Diagnostic studies: CBC, BMP, UA CT with contrast of abdomen	
8/12/08	6 PM	For laproscopic appendectomy Flagyl 500 mg IVPB now Cipro 400 mg IVPB now	
		Type and screen	Dr. Drayton

Nursing Report

Mr. Tim Rossetti is a 25-year-old white male who presents in the Emergency Room with the chief complaint of abdominal pain. The pain started around lunch time. The patient is holding his RLQ and is bent over.

(You are the emergency nurse who has the first encounter with patient.)

Student Simulation Prep Assignments

1. Identify items and their purpose in the care of a patient with appendicitis.

Item	Purpose
IV pump	
Oxygen and cannula	

2. *Identify team members and their specific roles in the care of a patient with appendicitis.*

Team Member	Role
Primary nurse (ER)	
Primary nurse (medical-surgical unit)	
Secondary nurse (medical-surgical unit)	
Physician	

3. *Relevant Data Exercise: Fill in the columns below.*

(The triage nurse was first to see patient.)

Relevant Data from Report	Relevant Data from Other Sources	Data Missing	Sources for Missing Data	Data Requiring Follow-up

4. *Initial Focused Assessment*

After reviewing the client background and nursing report, you are ready to assess your client's current status. Under each category, identify how you would target your assessment and what you would expect to find for the patient with appendicitis.

History

Are there any questions you need to ask the patient or family to obtain additional relevant data?

Physical Exam

- General appearance:
- Integumentary:
- HEENT:
- Respiratory:
- CV:
- Breasts:
- Abdominal:
- Neuro:
- Musculoskeletal:
- Reproductive:
- Additional:
- Developmental:

What are the nursing implications considering the developmental stage of your patient?

Answer:

5. Diagnostic Tests

What diagnostic test results relevant to the patient's current problem are needed to plan care?

Complete the table using Van Leeuwen et al, *Davis's Comprehensive Handbook of Laboratory and Diagnositc Testing with Nursing Implications* 4e, or other diagnostic test reference.

Diagnostic Test	Significance to This Patient's Problem
CBC	
BMP	
CT abdomen	
Urinalysis	
Type and screen	
C-reactive protein?	

6. Treatment

Identify drugs that are used to treat a patient with appendicitis.

Complete the table using Deglin et al, *Davis's Drug Guide for Nurses* 12e, or other drug reference.

Medication	Dose, Route, Frequency	Indications	Side Effect	Nursing Implications
Flagyl	500 mg IV q 6hr			
Cipro	400 mg IV q 12 hr			
Morphine	2 mg, IV stat			
Percocet	2 tabs po q 4 hr prn			

7. Nursing Problems/Diagnoses

Identify three priority nursing problems/diagnoses.

Assessment Data	Priority Problem	Intervention	Expected Patient Outcome	Which Interventions Could Be Delegated to Unlicensed Personnel?
1.				
2.				
3.				

References

Deglin, J. H., & Vallerand, A. H. (2009). *Davis's drug guide for nurses* (11th ed.). Philadelphia: F. A. Davis.

Dillon, P. (2007). *Nursing health assessment: A critical thinking and case studies approach* (2nd ed.). Philadelphia: F. A. Davis.

Erikson, E. H. (1950). *Childhood and society*. New York: Norton.

Goolsby, M., & Grubbs, L. (2006). *Advanced assessment interpreting findings and formulating differential diagnoses* Philadelphia: F. A. Davis.

Lagerquist, S. (2006). *Davis's NCLEX-RN success*. Philadelphia: F. A. Davis.

Mahadevan, M., & Graff, L. (2000). Prospective randomized study of analgesic use for ED patients with right lower quadrant pain. *American Journal of Emergency Medicine, 18*(7), 753-6.

Paulson, E. K., Kalady, M. F., & Pappas, T. N. (2003). Clinical practice. Suspected appendicitis. *New England Journal of Medicine, 16*:348(3), 236-42.

Van Leeuwen, A. M., Poelhuis-Leth, D. J., & Bladh, M. L. (2011). *Davis's comprehensive handbook of laboratory and diagnostic tests with nursing implications.* (4th ed.). Philadelphia: F. A. Davis

1-2 Head-to-Toe Assessment

ADULT/MEDICAL SURGICAL

STANDARD FORMS

These templates are included in the Appendix; copy before each use.

LEARNING OUTCOMES

Cognitive

The student will be able to:

1. Identify pertinent history questions relevant to the hospitalized patient.
2. Differentiate between a regional and a system approach in performing a head-to-toe assessment on the hospitalized patient.
3. Identify patient safety goals specific to the hospitalized patient.

Psychomotor

The student will be able to:

1. Obtain a pertinent health history on a hospitalized patient.
2. Perform a head-to-toe physical assessment on a hospitalized patient.
3. Implement patient safety standards.

Affective

The student will be able to:

1. Reflect upon performance in performing head-to-toe assessment of a patient.
2. Identify factors that worked well during the simulation of head-to-toe assessment.
3. Identify factors that needed improvement during the simulation of head-to-toe assessment.
4. Develop self-confidence in performing a head-to-toe assessment on a hospitalized patient.

Communication

The student will be able to:

1. Communicate effectively with the patient while performing a head-to-toe assessment on a hospitalized patient.
2. Use SBAR when communication assessment findings.
3. Accurately and succinctly document assessment findings.
4. Practice Transparent Thinking (thinking out loud) to facilitate group problem solving.
5. Use Directed Communication (directing a message to specific individual) when delegating tasks.
6. Employ Closed-Loop Communication (acknowledgment of receipt of the message and status) to acknowledge communications from others.

Safety

The student will be able to:

Administer and maintain specific protecting interventions with attention to safety of the client and healthcare professional.

1. Demonstrate a safe environment with attention to hazards to healthcare providers, visitors, and the client. Includes body mechanics, tripping hazards, and equipment issues.
2. Demonstrate attention to national patient safety goals. Includes patient identification standards, effective communication among healthcare providers, and safe medication administration.
3. Demonstrate attention to standard precautions. Includes hand washing, infection control measures, and use of personal protective equipment (PPE) as needed.

Leadership and Management/Delegation

The student will be able to:

1. Identify tasks that can be legally, ethically, and safely delegated to unlicensed assistive personnel (UAP) or licensed practical nurse (LPN) in the care of a patient when performing a head-to-toe assessment.
2. Identify and prioritize patient's needs in care of a patient when performing a head-to-toe assessment.
3. Prioritize multiple patient assignment.

OVERVIEW OF THE PROBLEM

Head-to-Toe Assessment

Preparation

- Assemble all equipment needed for the examination
- Explain to patient what you are going to do
- Provide privacy for patient
- Use at least two patient identifiers when providing care
- Assess/reconcile medications
- Involve patient in care
- Communicate clearly to patient and all members of healthcare team

Performing the Assessment

- Maintain standard precautions
- Work from the right side of patient
- Maintain body mechanics
- Assess fall risk
- Properly position patient
- Perform assessment in systematic manner, work head-to-toe, compare side-to-side
- Perform assessment in an organized and timely fashion
- Provide the patient with explanations throughout the assessment process

History

You will obtain a patient history. This provides you with:

- Biographical data
- Current health problems/reason for admission
- Past health problems
- Family history
- Medications/allergies
- Psychosocial history

Ask questions as you perform the physical exam.

Physical Exam

Approach

- System
  - Best for focused assessment
- Regional/head-to-toe
  - Best for complete assessments
  - Minimizes position change

Additional Data

Check diagnostic tests

Documentation

Document by systems

Charting:

- Check list/flow sheet
- Chart by exception, only positive findings
- Pertinent negatives

REVIEW QUESTIONS

1. What equipment would you need to perform your head-to-toe assessment?
   Answer:

2. Name four patient safety goals that should be considered when performing a head-to-toe exam?
   Answer:

3. What is the advantage of performing a head-to-toe assessment by region rather than system?
   Answer:

4. A combination stethoscope is best for auscultation. What is the purpose of a bell and diaphragm?
   Answer:

5. When performing palpation, which part of the hand is best for detecting temperature changes? Vibrations? Pulsations?
   Answer:

Related Evidence-Based Practice Guidelines

The Joint Commission National Patient Safety Goals Hospital Program. Retrieved from http://www.jointcommission.org/GeneralPublic/NPSG10_npsgs.htm

SBAR Technique for Communication: A situational briefing modelpublished by The Institute for Healthcare Improvement was downloaded on December 19, 2008, from http://www.ihi.org/IHI/Topics/PatientSafety/SafetyGeneral/Tools/SBARTechniqueforCommunicationASituationalBriefingModel.htm

Topics to Review Prior to the Simulation

- Complete health assessment
- Health history
- Physical exam of the adult
- Cardiac disease
- Cardiac medications

SIMULATION

Client Background

Biographical Data

- Age: 73
- Gender: female
- Height: 5 ft 3 in
- Weight: 155 lb

Cultural considerations

- Language: English
- Ethnicity: African American
- Nationality: American
- Culture: no significant cultural considerations identified

Demographic

- Marital status: married
- Educational level: college
- Religion: Methodist
- Occupation: retired

Current health status

- Felt dizzy last night, passed out. Husband prevented fall

History

- Psychosocial history
  - Social support: family
- Past health history
  - Medical: + HTN, CAD, DJD
  - Surgical: no surgeries
- Family history: + CVD, HTN

Admission Sheet

Name:	Donna Turner
Age:	73
Gender:	Female
Marital Status:	Married
Educational Level:	College
Religion:	Methodist
Ethnicity:	African American
Nationality:	American
Language:	English
Occupation:	Retired

Hospital
Provider's Orders

Patient's Name: Donna Turner
Allergies: NKDA

Diagnosis: Syncope

Date	Time	Order	Signature
		Admit to Telemetry	
		Cardiac monitor	
		Vital signs: q 4 hr with neuro check	
		BP supine, sitting, standing	
		Diet: Low sodium	
		Activity: BRP	
		IV therapy: Intermittent transfusion device (INT) with routine NSS flush	

Continued

Diagnosis: Syncope—cont'd

Date	Time	Order	Signature
		Medications: Lisinopril 10 mg po daily Cardizem 30 mg po daily Hydrochlorothiazide (HCTZ) 25 mg po daily Tylenol 650 mg q 4–6 hr prn for pain	
		Diagnostic studies: ECG CT scan head done in ER US carotids CBC with differential Basic metabolic panel UA CK and troponin daily, repeat 6 and 12 hr after initial draw Chest x-ray	
		Treatments: HOB elevated 30 degrees Oxygen 2 L via NC	Dr. Allison

Nursing Report

You are the day shift nurse, have just received report, and are making rounds on your patients.

You are assigned four patients. Part of your morning rounds includes a shift, head-to-toe assessment.

Your four patients include:

- Donna Turner, age 73, AA, admitted during the night with syncopal episode. Monitor NSR, no syncope, VS stable for workup today, CT scan and carotid Doppler scheduled for 9 AM.
- Bill Brown, age 67, AA, admitted 3 days ago, with angina, uncontrolled HTN. Monitor NSR, no chest pain, BP stable for discharge today.
- Marie Sanchez, age 54, admitted for chemo for liver cancer. Requires cardiac monitoring during therapy. Treatment schedule for 2 PM today. PCA morphine controlling pain. VS stable.
- Louis Bock, age 75, scheduled for cardioversion at 10 AM for uncontrolled afib. Monitor: afib 115. VS stable, no chest pain.

Prior to starting morning rounds, consider who should be assessed first?

How would you prioritize your patient assignment?

Answer:

Report on Mrs. Turner

Donna Turner, a 73-year-old African American female, admitted from the ER during the night with the diagnosis of syncopal attack. Past history of HTN, CAD, DJD. Admitted to Telemetry for monitoring and workup. CT head negative, monitor—NSR, labs WNL. INT left hand with routine NSS flush. Meds: Lisinopril, Cardizem, HCTZ daily, Motrin prn pain. Scheduled for diagnostic tests in AM. VS BP150/85, negative orthostatic drop, pulse, 87 regular, respirations 20, temperature, 97.6°F, pulse ox 96% on 2 LO_2 via nasal cannula.

Student Simulation Prep Assignment

1. Identify items and their purpose in the care of a patient with syncope.

Item	Purpose
INT	
O_2 cannula	
Monitor	

2. Identify team members and their specific roles in the care of a patient with syncope.

Team Member	Role
Primary nurse	
Physician	

3. Relevant Data Exercise

Fill in the columns below.

Relevant Data from Report	Relevant Data from Other Sources	Data Missing	Sources for Missing Data	Data Requiring Follow-up

4. Initial Focused Assessment

After reviewing the client background and nursing report, you are ready to assess your client's current status. Under each category, identify how you would target your assessment for a complete exam on a hospitalized patient.

History

Are there any questions you need to ask the patient or family to obtain additional relevant data?

Physical Exam

- General appearance:
- Integumentary:
- HEENT:
- Respiratory:
- CV:
- Breasts:
- Abdominal:
- Neuro:
- Musculoskeletal:
- Reproductive:
- Additional:
- Developmental:

What are the nursing implications considering the developmental stage of your patient?

Answer:

5. *Diagnostic tests*

What diagnostic test results relevant to the patient's current problem are needed to plan care?

Complete the table using Van Leeuwen et al, *Davis's Comprehensive Handbook of Laboratory and Diagnostic Testing with Nursing Implications* 4e, or other diagnostic test reference.

Diagnostic Test	Significance to This Patient's Problem
CT scan	
CBC with differential	
BMP -Glucose -Lytes -BUN -Creatinine	
UA	
ECG	
Ultrasound carotids	
Chest x-ray	
CK and troponin	

6. *Treatment*

Identify drugs that are used to treat a patient with syncope.

Complete the table using Deglin et al, *Davis's Drug Guide for Nurses* 12e, or other drug reference.

Medication	Dose, Route, Frequency	Indications	Side Effect	Nursing Implications
Lisinopril	10 mg daily			
Cardizem	30 mg daily			
Hydrochloro-thiazide (HCTZ)	25 mg daily			

Medication	Dose, Route, Frequency	Indications	Side Effect	Nursing Implications
Tylenol	650 mg q 4–6 hr prn for pain			

7. Nursing Problems/Diagnoses

Identify three priority nursing problems/diagnoses.

Assessment Data	Priority Problem	Intervention	Expected Patient outcome	Which Interventions Could Be Delegated to Unlicensed Personnel
1.				
2.				
3.				
4.				

Continued

Assessment Data	Priority Problem	Intervention	Expected Patient outcome	Which Interventions Could Be Delegated to Unlicensed Personnel
5.				

References

Deglin, J. H., &Vallerand, A. H. (2007).*Davis's drug guide for nurses* (10th ed.). Philadelphia: F. A. Davis.

Dillon, P. (2007). *Nursing health assessment: A critical thinking and case studies approach* (2nd ed.). Philadelphia: F. A. Davis.

Erikson, E. H. (1950). *Childhood and society*. New York: Norton.

Lagerquist, S. (2006). *Davis's NCLEX-RN success*. Philadelphia: F. A. Davis.

Van Leeuwen, A. M., Poelhuis-Leth, D. J., & Bladh, M. L. (2011). *Davis's comprehensive handbook of laboratory and diagnostic tests with nursing implications* (4rd ed.). Philadelphia: F. A. Davis.

Fundamental Skills 2

2-1 Patient Safety/What's Wrong with This Picture?

FUNDAMENTALS

STANDARD FORMS

These templates are included in the Appendix; copy before each use.

LEARNING OUTCOMES

Cognitive

The student will be able to:

1. Identify the national patient safety goals.
2. Define the principles of medical asepsis.
3. Describe the principles of body mechanics.
4. Identify fall risk factors.

Psychomotor

The student will be able to:

1. Safely administer medical/nursing interventions.
2. Properly identify the patient.
3. Perform a fall risk assessment.
4. Utilize proper body mechanics.
5. Apply principles of medical asepsis.

Affective

The student will be able to:

1. Reflect upon performance.
2. Identify strengths and areas that need improvement.
3. Develop confidence in caring for patients.
4. Identify feelings related to caring for patients.

Communication

The student will be able to:

1. Communicate effectively with the patient.
2. Practice Transparent Thinking (thinking out loud) to facilitate group problem solving.
3. Use Directed Communication (directing a message to specific individual) when delegating tasks.
4. Employ Closed-Loop Communication (acknowledgment of receipt of the message and status) to acknowledge communications from others.

Safety

The student will be able to:

Administer and maintain specific protecting interventions with attention to safety of the patient and healthcare professional.

1. Demonstrate a safe environment with attention to hazards to healthcare providers, visitors, and the client. Includes body mechanics, tripping hazards, and equipment issues.
2. Demonstrate attention to national patient safety goals. Includes patient identification standards, effective communication among healthcare providers, and safe medication administration.
3. Demonstrate attention to standard precautions. Includes hand washing, infection control measures, and use of personal protective equipment (PPE) as needed.

Leadership and Management/Delegation

The student will be able to:

1. Identify tasks that can be legally, ethically, and safely delegated to the UAP or LPN.
2. Identify and prioritize patient's needs.

OVERVIEW OF PROBLEM

2010 JCAHO National Patient Safety Goals:

- Improve accuracy of patient identification
- Improve the effectiveness of communication among caregivers
- Improve the safety of using medications
- Reduce the risk of healthcare associated infections
- Accurately and completely reconcile medications across the continuum of care
- Reduce the risk of patient harm resulting from falls

REVIEW QUESTIONS

1. Describe the six components of the Infection Chain.
   Answer:

2. Identify nursing measures that can break the infection chain.
   Answer:

3. Describe at least three principles of body mechanics.
   Answer:

4. Identify at least five risk factors for falls.
   Answer:

5. Identify three ways to identify your patient.
   Answer:

6. Identify six rights for medication administrations.
   Answer:

Related Evidence-Based Practice Guidelines

The Joint Commission National Patient Safety Goals Hospital Program. Retrieved from http://www.jointcommission.org/GeneralPublic/NPSG10_npsgs.htm

SBAR technique for communication: A situational briefing model. The Institute for Healthcare Improvement. Retrieved December 19, 2008, from http://www.ihi.org/IHI/Topics/PatientSafety/SafetyGeneral/Tools/SBARTechniqueforCommunicationASituationalBriefingModel.htm

Topics to Review Prior to the Simulation

- Medical asepsis
- Principles of body mechanics
- IV therapy
- Math calculations
- Fall risk assessment

SIMULATION

Client Background

Biographical Data

- Age: 83
- Gender: female
- Height: 5 ft 3 in
- Weight: 145 lb

Cultural Considerations

- Language: Russian
- Ethnicity: Russian
- Nationality: Russian
- Culture: language barrier

Demographic

- Marital status: widowed
- Educational level: not available
- Religion: Jewish
- Occupation: retired

Current Health Status

- Syncope and change in mental status

History

- Psychosocial history: Lives alone
  - Social support: Family nearby
- Past health history
  - Medical: HTN, CAD, CHF
  - Surgical: Negative
- Family History: + CV disease

Admission Sheet

Name:	Elena Paranosky
Age:	83
Gender:	Female
Marital Status:	Widowed
Educational Level:	High school
Religion:	Jewish
Ethnicity:	Russian
Nationality:	Russian
Language:	Russian
Occupation:	Retired

Hospital
Provider's Orders

Patient's Name: **Elena Paranosky**
Allergies: **Penicillin**

Diagnosis: Syncope and change in mental status.

Date	Time	Order	Signature
7/11/08	2 PM	Vital signs: q 4 hr with neuro check BP supine, sitting, standing	
		Diet: No added salt (NAS), 2,000 cal ADA	
		Activity: Bed rest	
		IV Therapy: 1,000 mL 5% dextrose/0.45% NSS q 12 hr	
		Medications: Toprol XL 50 mg po daily Lisinopril 10 mg po daily Lasix 20 mg po daily MVI 1 tab po daily Colace 100 mg po daily Lovenox 40 mg sq daily	
		Diagnostic studies: Lab frequency daily: Serum electrolytes Glucose BUN Creatinine CBC CK UA Carotid US–once Chest x-ray ECG CT head	
		Treatments: Oxygen 2 L via nasal cannula	
		Telemetry	Dr. I. Benoffsky

Nursing Report

Mrs. Paransoky is an 83-year-old patient of Dr. Benoffsky. She was admitted last night with the diagnosis of syncope and change in mental status. She has a history of HTN, CAD, and CHF. She lives alone; her daughter found her at home on the floor, a little confused and unsure as to what had happened. There was no apparent injury. She called 911. The patient is Russian and speaks very little English. Her daughter said she would be in early this morning.

Neurological: She slept most of the night; she is awake, alert, oriented to person, but confused to time and place, but reorients easily. PERRLA 3 mm, GCS 14.

Cardiac: Telemetry—monitor NSR, BP 140/80.

Resp: Lungs clear anterior, posterior decreased with few bibasilar crackles, pulse ox 93% on 2 L via nasal cannula.

MS: Moves all extremities, but generalized weakness.

VS: q 4 hr with neuro check, BP supine, sitting, and standing.

Accu checks with coverage ac and hs.

She has an IV #22 left hand 5 % dextrose/0.45 % NSS q 12 hr.

She is on bed rest, no added salt diet. She is scheduled for lab work and carotid US.

Student Simulator Prep Assignments

1. Identify items and their purpose in the care of a patient with syncope and altered mental status.

Item	Purpose
IV pump	
Oxygen and tubing	
Cardiac monitor	

2. Identify team members and their specific roles in a patient with syncope and altered mental status.

Team Member	Role
Primary nurse	
Secondary nurse	

3. Relevant Data Exercise: Fill in the columns below.

Relevant Data from Report	Relevant Data from Other Sources	Data Missing	Sources of Missing Data	Data Requiring follow-up

4. Initial Focused Assessment

After reviewing the patient background and nursing report, you are ready to assess your patient's current status. Under each category, identify how you would target your assessment, and what you would expect to find for the patient.

History

Are there any questions you need to ask the patient or family to obtain relevant data?

Physical Exam

- General appearance:
- Integumentary:
- HEENT:
- Respiratory:
- CV:
- Breasts:
- Abdominal:

- Neurological:
- Musculoskeletal:
- Reproductive:
- Developmental

What are the nursing implications considering the developmental stage of your patient?

Answer:

5. Diagnostic Tests

What diagnostic tests relevant to the patient's current problem are needed to plan care?

Complete the table using Van Leeuwen et al, *Davis's Comprehensive Handbook of Laboratory and Diagnostic Testing with Nursing Implications* 4e, or other diagnostic test reference.

Diagnostic Test	Significance to this Patient's Problem
CBC	
Electrolytes	
BUN and creatinine	
Glucose	
CK	
UA	
Carotid US	
ECG	
Chest x-ray	
CT of head	

6. Treatment

Identify drugs that are used to treat a patient with syncope and altered mental status.

Complete the table using Deglin et al, *Davis's Drug Guide for Nurses* 12e, or other drug reference.

Medication	Dose, Route, Frequency	Indication	Side Effect	Nursing Implications
Toprol XL	50 mg po daily			
Lisinipril	10 mg po daily			
Lasix	40 mg po daily			
MVI	1 tab po			

Continued

Medication	Dose, Route, Frequency	Indication	Side Effect	Nursing Implications
Lovenox	40 mg sq			
Colace	100 mg po			

7. Nursing Problems/Diagnoses

Identify three nursing problems/diagnoses.

Assessment Data	Priority Problem	Intervention	Expected Patient Outcome	Which Intervention Could Be Delegated to Unlicensed Personnel?
1.				
2.				
3.				

References

Deglin, J. H., & Vallerand, A. H. (2009). *Davis's drug guide for nurses* (11th ed.). Philadelphia: F. A. Davis.

Dillon, P. (2007). *Nursing health assessment: A critical thinking and case studies approach* (2nd ed.). Philadelphia: F. A. Davis.

Erikson, E. H. (1950). *Childhood and society*. New York: Norton.

The Joint Commission National Patient Safety Goals Hospital Program. Retrieved from http://www.jointcommission.org/GeneralPublic/NPSG10_npsgs.htm

Lagerquist, S. L. (2006). *Davis's NCLEX-RN success* (2nd ed.). Philadelphia: F. A. Davis.

Van Leeuwen, A. M., Poelhuis-Leth, D. J., & Bladh, M. L. (2011). *Davis's comprehensive handbook of laboratory and diagnostic tests with nursing implications.* (4th ed.). Philadelphia: F. A. Davis.

Wilkinson, J. (2007). *Fundamentals of nursing.* Philadelphia: F. A. Davis.

2-2 Admission and Care of a Client with Unstable Angina: Basic Assessment/Decision Making

FUNDAMENTALS

STANDARD FORMS

These templates are included in the Appendix; copy before each use.

LEARNING OUTCOMES

Cognitive

The student will be able to:

1. Analyze the information from the client's chart and patient's subjective and objective data.
2. Correlate signs and symptoms of headache to the pharmacodynamics of nitroglycerin.
3. Identify factors in a patient's current condition that increase risk for headache.
4. Identify the appropriate interventions for the patient with headache.
5. Differentiate roles of team members in response to a client with angina.

Psychomotor

The student will be able to:

1. Perform appropriate assessment for a patient with angina and a complaint of headache.
2. Correctly assess vital signs, including pulse ox, and document them appropriately.
3. Properly administer oral medication for headache relief.
4. Work collaboratively as part of the healthcare team.

Affective

The student will be able to:

1. Reflect on ability to apply beginning assessment skills.
2. Share factors that worked well during the simulation of care of a patient with a common reaction to a medication.
3. Share factors that needed improvement during the simulation of care of a patient with a history of chest pain taking nitroglycerin.
4. Develop self-confidence in ability to think critically using multiple assessment sources to problem solve.

Communication

The student will be able to:

1. Communicate effectively with healthcare team members in care of a patient with angina and headache.
2. Accurately and succinctly document assessments, interventions, and evaluations on appropriate forms.
3. Use SBAR when communicating with team members in the care of a patient with headache.
4. Practice Transparent Thinking (thinking out loud) to facilitate group problem solving.
5. Use Directed Communication (directing a message to specific individual) when delegating tasks.
6. Employ Closed-Loop Communication (acknowledgment of receipt of the message and status) to acknowledge communications from others.

Safety

The student will be able to:

Administer and maintain specific protecting interventions with attention to safety of the client and healthcare professional.

1. Demonstrate a safe environment with attention to hazards to healthcare providers, visitors, and the client. Includes body mechanics, tripping hazards, and equipment issues.
2. Demonstrate attention to national patient safety goals. Includes patient identification standards, effective communication among healthcare providers, and safe medication administration.
3. Demonstrate attention to standard precautions. Includes hand washing, infection control measures, and use of personal protective equipment (PPE) as needed.

Leadership and Management/Delegation

The student will be able to:

1. Identify tasks that can be legally, ethically, and safely delegated to unlicensed assistive personnel.
2. Identify and prioritize patient's needs.

Pharmacology

The student will be able to:

1. Use references to find needed drug information.
2. Identify key side effects of selected medications.

OVERVIEW OF THE PROBLEM

Definition of Angina Pectoris

Transient paroxysmal episodes of substernal or precordial pain. Two types:

- Stable: Follows an event, same severity
- Unstable: At rest or minimal exertion, recent onset, increasing severity (e.g., Prinzmetal's variant, at rest, caused by coronary spasms)

Pathophysiology

- Insufficient blood flow through coronary arteries
- Oxygen demand exceeds supply
- Temporary myocardial ischemia

Risk Factors

- Cardiovascular:
  - Atherosclerosis
  - Thromboangiitis obliterans
  - Aortic regurgitation
  - Hypertension
- Hormonal:
  - Diabetes mellitus
- Blood Disorders:
  - Anemia
  - Polycythemia vera
- Lifestyle Choices:
  - Smoking
  - Obesity
  - Cocaine use
  - Inactivity

Assessment

Subjective

- Pain—typical
  - Type: squeezing, pressing, burning
  - Location: retrosternal, substernal, left of sternum, radiates to left arm
  - Duration: short, usually 3–5 min, <30 min
- Cause: emotional stress, overeating, physical exertion, exposure to cold; may occur at rest
- Relief: rest, nitroglycerin

Note: Atypical complaints by women include jaw and upper back pain and persistent gastric upset.

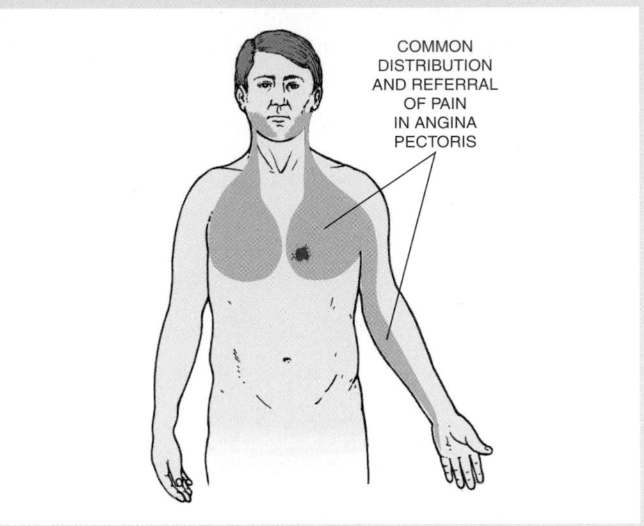

- Dyspnea
- Palpitations
- Dizziness; faintness
- Epigastric distress; indigestion; belching

Objective

- Tachycardia
- Pallor
- Diaphoresis
- EGG changes during attack

Diagnostic Tests

If ordered:

- Thallium stress test
- Cardiac catheterization
- Interventional stents

Treatment

- Oxygen
- Aspirin
- Nitroglycerine
- Morphine
- Heparin
- Fibrinolytic therapy

(AHA, ACLS protocol for Acute Coronary Syndrome, 2005)

Nursing Management

Goal: Provide relief from pain.

- Rest until pain subsides
- Nitroglycerin or amyl nitrite, beta adrenergic blockers, as ordered
- Identify precipitating factors: Large meals heavy exercise, stimulants (coffee, smoking), sex when fatigued, cold air
- Vital signs: Hypotension
- Assist with ambulation; dizziness, flushing occurs with nitroglycerin

Goal: Provide emotional support.

- Encourage verbalization of feelings, fears
- Reassurance; positive self-concept
- Acceptance of limitations

Goal: Health teaching

- Pain: Alleviation, differentiation of angina from myocardial infarction, precipitating factors
- Medication: Frequency, expected effects (headache, flushing); carry fresh nitroglycerin; loses potency after 6 mo ("stings" under tongue when potent); may use nitroglycerin paste—instruct how to apply
- Diet: Restricted calories if weight loss indicated; restricted fat, cholesterol, gas-producing foods; small, frequent meals
- Exercise: Regular, graded, to promote coronary circulation
- Prepare for coronary bypass surgery, if necessary
- Behavior modification to assist with lifestyle changes (e.g., stress reduction, stop smoking)

Evaluation/Outcome Criteria

- Relief from pain
- Fewer attacks
- No myocardial infarction
- Alters lifestyle; complies with limitations
- No smoking

REVIEW QUESTIONS

1. When admitting a patient to your unit, what is the priority initial nursing action?
   Answer:

2. What sources can you use to gather information about your patient?
   Answer:

3. What is the primary source?
   Answer:

4. What are the six rights of medication administration?
   Answer:

5. What additional items should be checked every time you administer a medication?
   Answer:

Related Evidence-Based Practice Guidelines

Diagnosis and treatment of chest pain and acute coronary syndrome *(ACS).* Institute for Clinical Systems Improvement Private Nonprofit Organization. 2004 Nov (revised 2008 Oct). 69 pages. NGC:006889

Differential diagnosis of chest pain. Finnish Medical Society Duodecim Professional Association. 2001 May 4 (revised 2008 May 16). Various pages. NGC: 006592

The Joint Commission National Patient Safety Goals Hospital Program. Retrieved from http://www.jointcommission.org/GeneralPublic/NPSG10_npsgs.htm

National Clinical Guideline Centre for Acute and Chronic Conditions. Chest pain of recent onset: assessment and diagnosis of recent onset chest pain or discomfort of suspected cardiac origin. London (UK): National Institute for Health and Clinical Excellence (NICE); 2010 Mar. 52 p. (Clinical guideline; no. 95). Retrieved from: http://www.guideline.gov/content.aspx?id=16392&search=angina

SBAR technique for communication: A situational briefing model. The Institute for Healthcare. Retrieved December 19, 2008, from http://www.ihi.org/IHI/Topics/PatientSafety/SafetyGeneral/Tools/SBARTechniqueforCommunicationASituationalBriefingModel.htm

Topics to Review Prior to the Simulation

- Vital sign assessment
- Medication administration
- History and interview techniques
- Cardiac and respiratory assessment
- Basic care for a patient experiencing a cardiac problem

The facilitator may wish to instruct students to prepare for the simulation by:

- Reviewing procedures for assessment of vital signs, medication administration, and completing the initial client physical assessment
- Developing drug cards for medications ordered for the client
- Coming prepared for a clinical day, bringing whatever equipment and resources are normally required

SIMULATION

Client Background

Biographical Data

- Age: 52
- Gender: male
- Height: 72 in
- Weight: 285 lb

Cultural Considerations

- Language: English
- Ethnicity: Irish/Scottish
- Nationality: American
- Culture: no significant cultural considerations identified.

Demographic

- Marital status: divorced
- Educational level: college
- Religion: undeclared
- Occupation: salesman

Current Health Status

Newly admitted patient just arrives from the ER to your unit. You are assigned to admit him.

History

- Psychosocial history
  - Social support: Lives alone, children in area, has two brothers and a sister also in the area, visits them frequently
- Past health history
  - Medical: Hx of hypertension and unstable angina
    - Medications at home are Toprol 50 mg po daily, aspirin 81 mg daily, and nitroglycerin 0.3 mg sublingual prn chest pain
  - Surgical: None
- Family history:
  - Father died of MI at age 62
  - Mother living in nursing home, has diagnosis of Alzheimer's disease
  - Brother (age 61) and sister (age 58) both have hypertension. Other brother (age 55) has unstable angina and had an MI 2 years ago

Admission Sheet

Name:	William Smith
Age:	52
Gender:	Male
Marital Status:	Divorced
Educational Level:	College
Religion:	Undeclared
Ethnicity:	Irish/Scottish
Nationality:	American
Language:	English
Occupation:	Salesman

Hospital
Provider's Orders

Patient's Name: William Smith
Allergies: NKDA or Food Allergies

Diagnosis: Chest Pain Unstable Angina, R/O MI

Date	Time	Order	Signature
9/25/2007	1430	Vital signs: q 4 hr	
		Diet: Cardiac soft	
		Activity: BRP	
		IV therapy: Heparin lock for venous access Flush per protocol	

Continued

Diagnosis: Chest Pain Unstable Angina, R/O MI—cont'd

Date	Time	Order	Signature
		Medications: Zantac/Rantidine tab, 150 mg, po, q 12 hr Toprol XL/metropolol tab, 50 mg po, once Aspirin 81 mg po, once daily Lovenox/enoxaparin inj 40 mg, sc, bid daily Nitroglycerin tab, 0.3 mg, sl, prn chest pain Tylenol 650 mg po q 4 hr prn Diagnostic studies; Chest x-ray, AP and lateral CBC with differential and BMP (serum electrolytes, glucose) BUN, creatinine daily Cardiac enzymes (troponin and CK) tonight at 8 PM and daily × 2	
		UA PT/INR ECG daily × 2 days Cardiac monitor	
		Treatments: O_2 via nasal cannula 4 L/min	Dr. C. J. Redstone

Nursing Report

Mr. Smith is a 52-year-old, obese male who came unaccompanied to the emergency room today with chest pain and shortness of breath via ambulance. He has a history of hypertension and angina. He has smoked one pack per day for the past 30 years. Mr. Smith reports he has had an aching feeling in the middle of his chest off and on for the past 3 days. He had been at a family wedding when he experienced a sensation of heavy pressure in his chest. He was admitted from the ER to your unit for observation and further testing to rule out a myocardial infarction. The emergency room nurse reports that a Heplock was inserted in the ER. His blood pressure ranged from 188/96 upon admission to 134/78 taken immediately before he was transferred to your unit. An ECG was taken during the attack that showed some ischemia. He has received three doses of nitroglycerin 0.3 mg sublingually in the hour prior to transfer and now reports that the pressure in his chest is gone.

Student Simulator Prep Assignments

1. Identify items and their purpose in the care of a patient with chest pain.

Item	Purpose
Stethoscope	
Watch	
Sphygmomanometer	
Thermometer	
Medication Administration Record	

2. Identify team members and specific roles in the care of a patient admitted with chest pain.

Team member	Role
Physician	
Nurse	
Laboratory personnel	
X-ray, ECG technicians	
Respiratory therapy	

3. Relevant Data Exercise

Relevant Data from Report	Relevant Data from Other Sources	Data Missing	Sources for Missing Data	Data Requiring Follow-up

4. Initial Focused Assessment

After reviewing the patient background and nursing report, you are ready to assess your patient's current status. Under each category, identify how you would target your assessment, and what you would expect to find for the patient with chest pain/unstable angina.

History

Are there any questions you need to ask the patient or family to obtain additional relevant data?

Physical Exam

- General appearance:
- Integumentary:
- HEENT:
- Respiratory:
- CV:
- Breasts:
- Abdominal:
- Neurological:
- Musculoskeletal:
- Reproductive:
- Additional:
- Renal:
- Developmental:

What are the nursing implications considering the developmental stage of your patient?

Answer:

5. *Diagnostic Tests*

What diagnostic test results relevant to the patient's current problem are needed to plan care?

Complete the table using Van Leeuwen et al, *Davis's Comprehensive Handbook of Laboratory and Diagnostic Testing with Nursing Implications* 4e, or other diagnostic test reference.

Diagnostic Test **Blood Studies**	**Significance to This Patient's Problem**
CBC with differential BMP: Serum electrolytes, glucose, BUN, creatinine	
UA	
ECG	
Chest x-ray	
Pulse oximetry	
PT/INR	
Occult blood in urine and feces	
Cardiac enzymes (troponin and CK)	

6. *Treatment*

Identify drugs that are used to treat a patient with, chest pain, unstable angina, and hypertension.

Complete the table using Deglin et al, *Davis's Drug Guide for Nurses* 12e, or other drug reference.

Medication	**Dose, Route, Frequency**	**Indications**	**Side Effect**	**Nursing Implications**
Toprol XL/ metroplol tab	50 mg, po once daily			

Medication	Dose, Route, Frequency	Indications	Side Effect	Nursing Implications
Lovenox/ Enoxaparin inj	40 mg, sc, bid			
Aspirin	81 mg po daily			

Continued

Medication	Dose, Route, Frequency	Indications	Side Effect	Nursing Implications
Nitroglycerin tab	0.3 mg, sl, prn chest pain May give up to three times 5 min apart. If no relief, call physician			

7. Nursing Problems/Diagnoses

Identify three priority nursing problems/diagnoses.

Assessment Data	Priority Problem	Intervention	Expected Patient Outcome	Which Interventions Could Be Delegated to Unlicensed Personnel?
1.				

Assessment Data	Priority Problem	Intervention	Expected Patient Outcome	Which Interventions Could Be Delegated to Unlicensed Personnel?
2.				
3.				

Continued

Assessment Data	Priority Problem	Intervention	Expected Patient Outcome	Which Interventions Could Be Delegated to Unlicensed Personnel?

References

American Heart Association (2005). *Advanced cardiovascular life support provider manual.* Dallas: American Heart Association.

Deglin, J. H., & Vallerand, A. H. (2009). *Davis's drug guide for nurses* (11th ed.). Philadelphia: F. A. Davis.

Dillon, P. (2007). *Nursing health assessment: A critical thinking and case studies approach* (2nd ed.). Philadelphia: F. A. Davis.

Doenges, M. E., Moorhouse, M. F., & Murr, A. C. (2006). *Nursing care plans: Guidelines for individualizing patient care across the life span* (7th ed.). Philadelphia: F. A. Davis.

Erikson, E. H. (1950). *Childhood and society*. New York: Norton.

Joint Commission on Accreditation of Healthcare Organizations. (2008). *Joint commission disease-specific care certification National Public Safety Goals* (prepublication version). Retrieved April 8, 2009, from http://www.jointcommission.org/NR/rdonlyres/74937937-7B39-447A-AA6F-AFD8BAEE1410/0/DSC_NPSG.pdf

Lagerquist, S. L. (2006). *Davis's NCLEX-RN success* (2nd ed.). Philadelphia: F. A. Davis.

Newfield, S. A., Hinz, M. D., Tilley, D. S., Sridaromont, K. L., & Maramba, P. J. (2007). *Cox's clinical applications of nursing diagnosis* (5th ed.). Philadelphia: F. A. Davis.

Taber's cyclopedic medical dictionary (20th ed.). (2005). Philadelphia: F. A. Davis.

Van Leeuwen, A. M., Poelhuis-Leth, D. J., & Bladh, M. L. (2011). *Davis's comprehensive handbook of laboratory and diagnostic tests with nursing implications.* (4th ed.). Philadelphia: F.A. Davis.

Wilkinson, J. M., & Van Leuven, K. (2007). *Fundamentals of nursing theory, concepts, & application.* Philadelphia: F. A. Davis.

2-3 Care of the Patient with a Colostomy

FUNDAMENTALS

STANDARD FORMS

These templates are included in the Appendix; copy before each use.

LEARNING OUTCOMES

Cognitive

The student will be able to:

1. Describe signs and symptoms of a healthy stoma.
2. Correlate signs and symptoms of infection to the physiology of wound healing.
3. Identify factors in a patient's history that increase the risk of colon cancer.
4. Identify factors in a patient's current condition that increase the risk of complications with the colostomy.
5. Identify the appropriate interventions for a patient with a colostomy.
6. Differentiate the roles of team members in response to a patient with a colostomy.

Psychomotor

The student will be able to:

1. Perform an appropriate assessment for a patient with a colostomy.
2. Initiate appropriate interventions including stoma assessment, cleansing the stoma, applying the appliance, and teaching self-care management for a patient with a colostomy.
3. Work collaboratively as part of the healthcare team in the care of a patient with a colostomy.

Affective

The student will be able to:

1. Reflect upon performance in the care of a patient with a colostomy.
2. Express personal feelings in delivering care to a patient with a colostomy.
3. Discuss feelings related to working as a member of a team in the care of a patient with a colostomy.
4. Identify factors that worked well during the simulation of care of a patient with a colostomy.
5. Identify factors that needed improvement during the simulation of care of a patient with a colostomy.
6. Develop self-confidence in the care of a patient with a colostomy.

Communication

The student will be able to:

1. Communicate effectively with healthcare team members in the care of a patient with a colostomy.
2. Communicate effectively with the patient and family in the care of a patient with a colostomy.
3. Use SBAR when communicating with team members in the care of a patient with a colostomy.
4. Practice Transparent Thinking (thinking out loud) to facilitate group problem solving.
5. Use Directed Communication (directing a message to specific individual) when delegating tasks.
6. Employ Closed-Loop Communication (acknowledgment of receipt of the message and status) to acknowledge communications from others.

Safety

The student will be able to:

Administer and maintain specific protecting interventions with attention to safety of the client and healthcare professional.

1. Demonstrate a safe environment with attention to hazards to healthcare providers, visitors, and the client. Includes body mechanics, tripping hazards, and equipment issues.
2. Demonstrate attention to national patient safety goals. Includes patient identification standards, effective communication among healthcare providers, and safe medication administration.
3. Demonstrate attention to standard precautions. Includes hand washing, infection control measures, and use of personal protective equipment (PPE) as needed.

Leadership and Management/Delegation

The student will be able to:

1. Identify tasks that can be legally, ethically, and safely delegated to unlicensed assistive personnel (UAP) or licensed practical nurse (LPN) in the care of a patient with a colostomy.
2. Identify and prioritize patient's needs in the care of a colostomy.

Teaching and Learning

The student will be able to:

1. Demonstrate to the patient how to change the colostomy appliance.
2. Describe the signs and symptoms of a functional colostomy to the patient.
3. Include the family in the teaching session with the patient's consent.
4. Evaluate the teaching session and assess the patient's knowledge.

OVERVIEW OF THE PROBLEM

Definition

Colostomies and their care.

Fecal diversion procedures create stomas, which may be temporary or permanent.

Types of stomas include:

- Temporary: The fecal stream is rerouted to allow the GI tract to heal or provide an outlet in obstruction.
- Permanent: The intestine cannot be reconnected, often performed for cancer of the colon and/or rectum.
- Continent ileostomy: A pouch is created inside the wall of the intestine. The pouch serves as a reservoir similar to the rectum. The pouch is emptied on a regular basis with a small tube.
- Ileoanal anstamosis: The large intestine is removed and the small intestine is inserted into the rectum and attached just above the anus.

Pathophysiology

Stomas are performed because of disease or trauma.

- An ileostomy may be performed for unresponsive or complicated ulcerative colitis or suspected carcinoma.
- A colostomy may be performed for colon or rectal cancer or to relieve an obstruction.

Risk Factors

Risk factors vary according to the disease process resulting in the need for a stoma. Risk factors for colonrectal cancer include:

- Male
- Middle aged
- Personal or family history of polyps or cancer
- Ulcerative colitis
- High-fat low-fiber diet
- Gardner's syndrome (autosomal dominant disease, familial adenomatous polyposis)

Assessment

Subjective

- Assess client response to stoma and stoma care

Objective

- Observe appearance of stoma—should be pink, moist
- Monitor for signs of bowel obstruction
- Check skin around stoma for signs of breakdown

Diagnostic Tests

Not applicable

Treatment

- Administer medications and IV fluids as ordered
- Irrigate if ordered

Nursing Management

Goal: Maintain fluid balance.

- Monitor I & O
- Administer IV fluids

Goal: Prevent other postoperative complications.

- Monitor for signs of intestinal obstruction
- Use aseptic technique
- Observe stoma appearance

Goal: Initiate ostomy care.

- Prevent skin breakdown
- Change appliance appropriately
- Use deodorizing drops

Goal: Promote psychological comfort.

- Support patient and family
- Assess grieving process

Goal: Initiate Health teaching.

- Self-care management
- Diet adjustments
- Signs of complications
- Community referral and follow-up care

Evaluation/Outcome Criteria

- Demonstrates self-care for independent living
- Makes dietary adjustments
- Ostomy functions well
- Adjusts to alterations in bowel elimination patterns

REVIEW QUESTIONS

1. What are the key nursing interventions for the care of a patient with a colostomy?
   Answer:

2. What are the complications of a colostomy?
   Answer:

3. What electrolyte imbalances or conditions would you observe in a patient who has had a colostomy?
   Answer:

4. What does a normal stoma look like?
   Answer:

5. What are the parts of a colostomy appliance?
   Answer:

Related Evidence-Based Practice Guidelines

American Society of Colon and Rectal Surgeons: Medical Specialty Society. (2004) Practice parameters for colon cancer. Retrieved from http://www.fascrs.org/files/pp_0804.pdf

National Guideline Clearinghouse. Registered Nurses' Association of Ontario (RNAO). Ostomy care and management. Toronto (ON): Registered Nurses' Association of Ontario (RNAO); 2009 Aug. 115 p. [101 references] Retrieved from: http://www.guideline.gov/content.aspx?id=15613&search=colostomy

National Patient Safety Goals. Retrieved from http://www.jointcommission.org/PatientSafety/NationalPatientSafetyGoals/10_hap_npsgs.htm

SBAR Technique for Communication: *A situational briefing model.* The Institute for Healthcare. Retrieved December 19, 2008, from http://www.ihi.org/IHI/Topics/PatientSafety/SafetyGeneral/Tools/SBARTechniqueforCommunicationASituationalBriefingModel.htm

Topics to Review Prior to the Simulation

- Medical/surgical nursing
- Ostomy care
- Skin and abdominal assessment
- Colon cancer
- Nutrition
- Fluid balance

SIMULATION

Client Background

Mrs. Jones had been experiencing bloody stools for over a month. She had also been complaining of increasing weakness and stomach cramps.

Biographical Data

- Age: 42
- Gender: female
- Height: 5 ft 5 in
- Weight: 140 lb

Cultural Considerations:

- Language: English as a second language, primary dialect Mandarin
- Ethnicity: Asian
- Nationality: Canadian citizen for 20 yr
- Culture: Chinese

Demographic

- Marital status: married
- Educational level: grade 12
- Religion: Catholic
- Occupation: care aide

Current health status

- Diagnosis of colon cancer and a colostomy

History

- Psychosocial history
  - Married, 4 children

Family support

- Past health history
  - Tubal ligation: 4 years ago
  - Appendectomy: 18 years ago

Admission Sheet

Name:	Mrs. Jones
Age:	42
Gender:	Female
Marital Status:	Married
Educational Level:	Grade 12 graduate
Religion:	Catholic
Ethnicity:	Asian
Nationality:	Canadian citizen–immigrated to Canada 20 years ago
Language:	English as a second language. First language Mandarin
Occupation:	Care aide

Continued

Hospital Provider's Orders		Patient's Name: Mrs. Jones Allergies: NKDA	
Diagnosis: Colon cancer–colostomy			
Date	**Time**	**Order**	**Signature**
		Vital signs: Routine	
		Diet: Full liquid diet, advance as tolerated to house diet	
		Activity: Activity as tolerated	
		IV therapy: NSS 1,000 cc at 75 cc/hr	
		Medications: Morphine 2 mg q 2 hr IV prn for pain	
		Diagnostic studies: Frequency: daily at 6 AM BMP (basic metabolic panel), CBC	
		Treatments: SCDs (sequential compression devices) until patient ambulating down hallway three times daily Incentive spirometry q 1 hr	Dr. Robinson

Nursing Report

You arrive on the unit at 0700 and have been assigned Mrs. Jones. She will require colostomy care teaching and her appliance needs to be changed. She has requested morphine 2 mg IV twice in the last 12 hr. Her husband and children are present in the room. She met with the enterostomal therapist yesterday and feels well enough to begin independent care of her colostomy.

Student Simulation Prep Assignments

1. Identify items and their purpose in the care of a patient with a colostomy.

Item	Purpose
Stethoscope	
Colostomy equipment	
Clean gloves	

2. Identify team members and their specific roles in the care of a patient with a colostomy.

Team Member	Role
Primary nurse	
WOCN or enterostomal nurse	
Family members	
Physician/surgeon	

3. *Relevant Data Exercise:* Fill in the columns below.

Relevant Data from Report	Relevant Data from Other Sources	Data Missing	Sources for Missing Data	Data Requiring Follow-up

4. *Initial Focused Assessment*

After reviewing the client background and nursing report, you are ready to assess your client's current status. Under each category, identify how you would target your assessment and what you would expect to find for the patient with a colostomy.

History

Are there any questions you need to ask the patient or family to obtain additional relevant data?

Physical Exam

- General appearance:
- Integumentary:
- HEENT:
- Respiratory:
- CV:
- Breasts:
- Abdominal:
- Neurological:
- Musculoskeletal:
- Reproductive:
- Additional:
- Developmental:

What are the nursing implications considering the developmental stage of your patient?

Answer:

5. Diagnostic Tests

What diagnostic test results relevant to the patient's current problem are needed to plan care?

Complete the table using Van Leeuwen et al, *Davis's Comprehensive Handbook of Laboratory and Diagnostic Testing with Nursing Implications* 4e, or other diagnostic test reference.

Diagnostic Test	Significance to this Patient's Problem
Stool examination	
Sigmoidoscopy	
Colonoscopy	
CT scan	
HGB	
WBC	
Electrolytes	

6. *Treatment*

Identify drugs that are used to treat a patient with a colostomy.

Complete the table using Deglin et al, *Davis's Drug Guide for Nurses* 12e, or other drug reference.

Medication	Dose, Route, Frequency	Indications	Side Effect	Nursing Implications
Morphine	2 mg IV q 2 hr prn			

7. Nursing Problems/Diagnoses

Identify three priority nursing problems/diagnoses.

Assessment Data	Priority Problem	Intervention	Expected Patient Outcome	Which Interventions Could Be Delegated to Unlicensed Personnel?
1.				
2.				
3.				

References

Deglin, J. H., & Vallerand, A. H. (2009). *Davis's drug guide for nurses* (11th ed.). Philadelphia: F. A. Davis.

Dillon, P. (2007). *Nursing health assessment: A critical thinking and case studies approach* (2nd ed.). Philadelphia: F. A. Davis.

Erikson, E. H. (1950). *Childhood and society*. New York: Norton.

Grodner, M., Long., S., & Wackingshaw, B. (2007). *Foundations and clinical applications of nutrition: A nursing approach* (4th ed.). St. Louis: Mosby.

Hausman, K. A. (2005). *Clinical companion for medical-surgical nursing: Critical thinking for collaborative care* (5th ed.). St. Louis: Saunders.

Lagerquist, S. L. (2006). *Davis's NCLEX-RN success.* (2nd ed.). Philadelphia: F. A. Davis.

Potter, P. (2007). *Basic nursing: Essentials for practice* (6th ed.). St. Louis: Mosby.

Rothrock, J. C. (2006). *Alexander's care of the patient in surgery* (13th ed.). St. Louis: Mosby.

Swearingen, P. L. (2007). *All-in-one care planning resource: Medical-surgical, pediatric, maternity, & psychiatric nursing care plans* (2nd ed.). St. Louis: Mosby.

Van Leeuwen, A. M., Poelhuis-Leth, D. J., & Bladh, M. L. (2010). *Davis's comprehensive handbook of laboratory and diagnostic tests with nursing implications* (4th ed.). Philadelphia: F.A. Davis.

Wilkinson, J. (2007). *Fundamentals of nursing.* Philadelphia: F. A. Davis.

2-4 Postoperative Assessment Following Laparoscopic Cholecystectomy

FUNDAMENTALS

STANDARD FORMS

These templates are included in the Appendix; copy before each use.

LEARNING OUTCOMES

Cognitive

The student will be able to:

1. Describe signs and symptoms of infection related to surgical wound.
2. Correlate signs and symptoms of anxiety to the pathophysiology of pain.
3. Identify the appropriate interventions for the patient with pain and anxiety.

Psychomotor

The student will be able to:

1. Perform appropriate assessment for a postoperative laproscopic cholecystectomy patient.
2. Initiate appropriate interventions: Sterile dressing change for a patient with postoperative laproscopic cholecystectomy.
3. Initiate appropriate interventions: Accurate measurement of blood pressure.

Affective

The student will be able to:

1. Identify personal feelings in delivering care to a patient with anxiety.
2. Identify factors that worked well during the simulation of care of a patient with anxiety and pain following surgery.
3. Identify factors that needed improvement during the simulation of care of a postoperative laproscopic cholecystectomy patient.

Communication

The student will be able to:

1. Communicate effectively with the patient and family in the care of a patient following laparoscopic cholecystectomy.
2. Use SBAR when communicating with team members in the care of a postoperative patient.
3. Practice Transparent Thinking (thinking out loud) to facilitate group problem solving.
4. Use Directed Communication (directing a message to specific individual) when delegating tasks.
5. Employ Closed-Loop Communication (acknowledgment of receipt of the message and status) to acknowledge communications from others.

Safety

The student will be able to:

Administer and maintain specific protecting interventions with attention to safety of the client and healthcare professional.

1. Demonstrate a safe environment with attention to hazards to healthcare providers, visitors, and the client. Includes body mechanics, tripping hazards, and equipment issues.
2. Demonstrate attention to national patient safety goals. Includes patient identification standards, effective communication among healthcare providers, and safe medication administration.
3. Demonstrate attention to standard precautions. Includes hand washing, infection control measures, and use of personal protective equipment (PPE) as needed.

Leadership and Management/Delegation

The student will be able to:

- Identify and prioritize the patient's needs regarding pain, anxiety, and postoperative interventions.

OVERVIEW OF THE PROBLEM

Definition

Cholelithiasis is the formation of stones in the gallbladder. This is one of the most common disorders of the biliary system. When stones become lodged in the neck of the cystic duct inflammation of the gallbladder occurs, which is called cholecystitis. The two disorders are often seen in the same patient.

Pathophysiology

Gallstones form when cholesterol, bile salts, and calcium precipitate from bile. This can result from metabolic or hematological disorders or biliary stasis.

Cholecystitis can be caused by bacterial infection with *Escherichia coli* (most common), *Salmonella,* and streptococci. Inflammation occurs in the mucous lining and may spread to the entire wall; the organ becomes edematous and may be filled with pus or bile.

Risk Factors

- Age: Older than 40 yr
- Female: More common in women than men
- Pregnancy: More common in women who have had more than one pregnancy
  - Use of birth control pills or hormone replacement
  - Postmenopausal women taking estrogen have higher risk than women on birth control pills
- Ethnicity: Whites have higher risk than African Americans or Asians; American Indians high risk, with Navajo and Pima the highest
- Obesity
- Sedentary lifestyle
- Family history
- High-fat, low-fiber diet
- Rapid weight loss
- Fasting
- Adhesions
- Neoplasms
- Narcotics
- History of Crohn's disease
- Cirrhosis of the liver
- Certain lipid-lowering drugs (e.g., clofibrate)

Assessment

Cholelithiasis may present as mild or severe, acute, or chronic. Some patients have no symptoms. Movement of the stones is related to the severity of symptoms. Pain occurs when a stone moves and blockage occurs. Severe pain is termed "biliary colic" and is associated with spasms that occur as the duct attempts to move the stone. Patients often present with tachycardia and diaphoresis. These episodes last up to an hour and are very debilitating.

Chronic cholecystitis symptoms:

- Fat intolerance
- Dyspepsia
- Heartburn
- Flatulence

Acute cholecystitis symptoms/findings:

Subjective

- Pain: severe colic radiating to the back, under the scapula, and to the right shoulder.
  - Right upper quadrant pain: positive Murphy's sign.
  - Spasms last until stone dislodged or relieved by medication or sometimes vomiting.
- GI
  - Indigestion
  - Anorexia
  - Nausea
  - Vomiting
  - Feeling of fullness
  - Intolerance of fatty foods

Objective

- Diarrhea
- Leukocytosis
- Fever, increased pulse, chills, jaundice
- Abdominal rigidity
- Belching, vomiting, clay-colored stools
- Dark amber urine

Diagnostic Tests

- Elevated: WBC, alkaline phosphatase, serum amylase, lipase, AST, SGOT,
- Ultrasound
- Choliangiography
- CT scan
- Endoscopic retrograde choliangiopancreatography

Treatment

- Pain control
- Antibiotics
- Solvents or medications to dissolve stones
- Lithotripsy
- Surgery

Nursing Mangement

Goal: Promote comfort

- Medications for pain, antibiotics, antispasmodics, (avoid morphine), electrolytes
- NG to low suction, T tube postoperatively, promote drainage
- Fat-free diet
- Oral dissolution therapy

Goal: Health teaching

- Signs, symptoms, and complications of disease
- Dietary restrictions: Fat free, NPO for surgery, postoperatively advance as tolerated
- Desired and side effects of medications
  - Prepare for surgery if conservative management not effective. (Teach cough, turn, deep breath, incentive spirometer, increasing activity as tolerated, and pain management)

Goal: Prevent post operative complication

- NG tube to low suction
- Position to promote T-tube drainage (if open incision)
- Keep dressing dry and intact
- Clamp tube as ordered
- Observe for abdominal distention
- IV fluids with vitamins
- Cough, turn, deep breath, incentive spirometer
- Early ambulation
- Monitor for jaundice
- Monitor for signs of hemorrhage, infection, respiratory complications

Goal postoperative health teaching

- Fat free diet for 6 weeks
- Teach signs of complications

Evaluation/Outcome Criteria

- Patient remains afebrile
- Dressing clean, dry, intact, wound healing without signs of infection
- Pain management with oral or nonpharmacological treatment
- Ambulation and ADLs performed independently
- Tolerating diet, urine and bowel function returned to baseline
- Patient able to discuss discharge instructions and follow-up care
- Possible weight reduction

REVIEW QUESTIONS

1. What nonpharmacological interventions can be used to treat anxiety and pain?
   Answer:

2. When assessing a postoperative wound, what signs might indicate infection?
   Answer:

3. What does the nurse monitor/assess in patients with pain?
   Answer:

4. What assessments following surgery are used to identify early signs of excessive bleeding?
   Answer:

5. Before applying antiembolism stockings, what test should the nurse perform and why?
   Answer:

Related Evidence-Based Practice Guidelines

Registered Nurses Association of Toronto. (2002) Assessment and management of pain. Toronto, Canada.

The Joint Commission National Patient Safety Goals Hospital Program. Retrieved from http://www.jointcommission.org/GeneralPublic/NPSG10_npsgs.htm

SBAR technique for communication: A situational briefing model. The Institute for Healthcare Improvement. Retrieved December 19, 2008, from http://www.ihi.org/IHI/Topics/PatientSafety/SafetyGeneral/Tools/SBARTechniqueforCommunicationASituationalBriefingModel.htm

Topics to Review Prior to the Simulation

- Care of the postoperative patient: pain, wound care, and aseptic dressing change
- Assessment of pain
- Fluid balance, I&O
- Medication administration, five rights: Oral
- Therapeutic communication

SIMULATION

Client Background

Biographical data

- Age: 41
- Gender: female
- Height: 5 ft 5 in
- Weight: 165 lb

Cultural considerations:

- Language: English
- Ethnicity: Irish
- Nationality: American
- Culture: American

Demographic

- Marital status: married
- Educational level: high school diploma
- Occupation: homemaker

Current health status

- Diagnosed by ultrasound with cholelithiasis and cholecystitis and underwent subsequent laparoscopic cholecystectomy

History

- Psychosocial history
  - Social support
    - Married with three children, aged: 16, 13, 9 yr
    - Mother lives nearby
- Past health history
  - Medical: gravida 3, para 3, ab 0
  - Surgical: Tonsillectomy as a child
- Family history
  - Mother has hypertension
  - Father died of cancer at 63 yr

Admission Sheet

Name:	Susan Haggerty
Age:	41
Gender:	Female
Marital Status:	Married
Educational Level:	High school diploma
Religion:	Methodist
Ethnicity:	Irish
Nationality:	American
Language:	English
Occupation:	Homemaker

Hospital
Provider's Orders

Patient's Name: Susan Haggerty
Allergies: NKDA

Diagnosis: Postop Cholecystectomy

Date	Time	Order	Signature
4/28/2008	4:30 PM	Vital signs: q 15 min × 4; q 30 min × 4; q 1 hr × 4; q 4 hr if stable	
		Diet: Clear liquids, progress as tolerated	
		Activity: Elevate head of bed, ambulate as tolerated.	

Diagnosis: Postop Cholecystectomy—cont'd

Date	Time	Order	Signature
		IV therapy: Potassium 20 mEq in D5 ½ NSS 1 L at 100 mL/hr, convert to saline lock when tolerating fluids.	
		Medications: Cefazolin 1 g IVPB q 8 hr × 2 doses If patient has a history of anaphylaxis with penicillin or known allergy to cefazolin, give: clindamycin 600 mg IVPB q 8 hr × 2 doses. Morphine 2 mg IV q 2 hr prn mild pain Percocet 2 capsules po q 4 hr prn pain when tolerating fluids Metoclopramide 10 mg IV q 6 hr prn nausea	
		Diagnostic studies: AM Labs: AST, ALT, CBC, BMP	
		Treatments: Straight cath ×1 if patient has not voided 6 hr post procedure Change dressing as needed Knee-high elastic stockings	Dr. Smith

Nursing Report

Mrs. Haggerty, 41 years old, presented to the emergency room this morning with complaints of severe right upper quadrant pain and 3 days of nausea and vomiting. She has no medical history. Ultrasound revealed cholelithiasis and cholecystitis. She underwent uncomplicated laparoscopic cholecystectomy. She received morphine 2 mg IV for pain rated 8/10, 30 min ago. She has not voided since surgery; she is tearful and anxious. Her husband is in the waiting room and was with her in the recovery room, she has three children at home. Her vital signs prior to transfer were blood pressure 137/76, pulse 88, respirations 20.

Student Simulator Prep Assignments

1. Identify items and their purpose in the care of a patient with post laparoscopic cholecystectomy.

Item	Purpose
Sphygmomanometer	
Stethoscope	
Antiembolism stockings	

2. Identify team members and their specific roles in the care of a patient with laparoscopic cholecystectomy.

Team Member	Role
Nurse	
Surgeon	

3. Relevant Data Exercise: Fill in the columns below.

Relevant Data from Report	Relevant Data from Other Sources	Data Missing	Sources for Missing Data	Data Requiring Follow-up

4. Initial Focused Assessment

After reviewing the client background and nursing report, you are ready to assess your client's current status. Under each category, identify how you would target your assessment and what you would expect to find for the patient with laparoscopic cholecystectomy.

History

Are there any questions you need to ask the patient or family to obtain additional relevant data?

Physical Exam

- General appearance:
- Integumentary:
- HEENT:
- Respiratory:
- CV:
- Breasts:
- Abdominal:
- Neurological:
- Musculoskeletal:
- Reproductive:
- Additional:
- Developmental:

What are the nursing implications considering the developmental stage of your patient?

Answer:

5. Diagnostic Tests

What diagnostic test results relevant to the patient's current problem are needed to plan care?

Complete the table using Van Leeuwen et al, *Davis's Comprehensive Handbook of Laboratory and Diagnositc Testing with Nursing Implications* 4e, or other diagnostic test reference.

Diagnostic Test	Significance to this Patient's Problem
Aspartate aminotransferase (AST)	
Alanine aminotransferase (ALT).	
WBC: Leukocytes	
CBC: Hemoglobin/Hematocrit	
BMP: Electrolytes	

6. Treatment

Identify drugs that are used to treat a patient with postlaparoscopic cholecystectomy.

Complete the table using Deglin et al, *Davis's Drug Guide for Nurses* 12e, or other drug reference.

Medication	Dose, Route, Frequency	Indications	Side Effect	Nursing Implications
Cefazolin	1 g IVPB q 8 hr × 2 doses			
Clindamycin	600 mg IVPB q 8 hr × 2 doses			

Continued

Medication	Dose, Route, Frequency	Indications	Side Effect	Nursing Implications
Metoclopramide	10 mg IV q 6 hr			
Morphine	4 mg IV prn q 2 hr			

Medication	Dose, Route, Frequency	Indications	Side Effect	Nursing Implications
Percocet	2 capsules po q 4 hr prn pain			
Potassium chloride	20 mEq in 1,000 cc D5-1/2S			

Continued

7. Nursing Problems/Diagnoses

Identify three priority nursing problems/diagnoses.

Assessment Data	Priority Problem	Intervention	Expected Patient Outcome	Which Interventions Could Be Delegated to Unlicensed Personnel?
1.				
2.				

Assessment Data	Priority Problem	Intervention	Expected Patient Outcome	Which Interventions Could Be Delegated to Unlicensed Personnel?
3.				

References

Deglin, J. H., & Vallerand, A.H. (2009). *Davis's drug guide for nurses* (11th ed.). Philadelphia: F. A. Davis.

Dillon, P. (2007). *Nursing health assessment: A critical thinking and case studies approach* (2nd ed.). Philadelphia: F. A. Davis.

Erikson, E. H. (1950). *Childhood and society*. New York: Norton.

Kozier, B., Erb, G., Berman, A., & Snyder, A. (2004). *Fundamental of nursing: Concepts, process, and practice* (7th ed). Upper Saddle River, NJ: Pearson Prentice Hall.

Lagerquist, S. L. (2006). *Davis's NCLEX-RN success.* (2nd ed.). Philadelphia: F. A. Davis.

Lewis, S. L., Heitkemper, M. M, Dirksen, S. R, Obrien, P. G., Bucher, L. B. (2007). *Medical-surgical nursing: Assessment and management of clinical problems* (7th ed.). St. Louis: Mosby.

Registered Nurses Association of Toronto. (2002). *Assessment and management of pain.* Toronto, Canada.

Van Leeuwen, A. M., Poelhuis-Leth, D. J., & Bladh, M. L. (2011). *Davis's comprehensive handbook of laboratory and diagnostic tests with nursing implications.* (4th ed.). Philadelphia: F. A. Davis.

Wilkinson, J. (2007). *Fundamentals of nursing.* Philadelphia: F. A. Davis.

2-5 Abdominal Pain

ADULT/FUNDAMENTALS

STANDARD FORMS

These templates are included in the Appendix; copy before each use.

LEARNING OUTCOMES

Cognitive

The student will be able to:

1. Identify pertinent history questions relevant to a patient with abdominal pain.
2. Identify appropriate physical assessment techniques for a patient with abdominal pain.
3. Analyzes assessment data to make appropriate clinical decisions.
4. Identify appropriate nursing interventions for a patient with abdominal pain.

Psychomotor

The student will be able to:

1. Perform appropriate symptom analysis for a patient with abdominal pain.
2. Perform appropriate physical assessment for a patient with abdominal pain.
3. Implement appropriate interventions for a patient with abdominal pain.

Affective

The student will be able to:

1. Reflect upon performance in performing an assessment on a patient with abdominal pain.
2. Identify factors that worked well during the simulation of care of a patient with abdominal pain.
3. Identify factors that needed improvement during the simulation of care of a patient with abdominal pain.
4. Develop self-confidence in assessing a patient with abdominal pain.

Communication

The student will be able to:

1. Communicate effectively with the patient with abdominal pain.
2. Accurately and succinctly document assessment findings.
3. Practice Transparent Thinking (thinking out loud) to facilitate group problem solving.
4. Use Directed Communication (directing a message to specific individual) when delegating tasks.
5. Employ Closed-Loop Communication (acknowledgment of receipt of the message and status) to acknowledge communications from others.

Safety

The student will be able to:

Administer and maintain specific protecting interventions with attention to safety of the client and healthcare professional

1. Demonstrate a safe environment with attention to hazards to healthcare providers, visitors, and the client. Includes body mechanics, tripping hazards, and equipment issues.
2. Demonstrate attention to national patient safety goals. Includes patient identification standards, effective communication among healthcare providers, and safe medication administration.
3. Demonstrate attention to standard precautions. Includes hand washing, infection control measures, and use of personal protective equipment (PPE) as needed.

OVERVIEW OF THE PROBLEM

Pain Assessment

Symptom Analysis

P = precipitating/palliative/provocative factors

- What were you doing before the pain started?
- Did anything make it better/worse?

Q = quality/quantity

- What does it feel like?
- To what degree has the pain affected your ability to perform your usual daily activities?

R = region/radiation/related symptoms

- Can you point to where it hurts?
- Do you feel the pain anywhere else?
- Do you have any other symptoms?

S = severity

- Use a scale
- On a scale of 0-10 with 10 being the worst, how bad is the pain?

T = timing

- When did it start?

- How long did it last?
- How often does it occur?

Physical Findings Related to Pain

General Appearance
- Abnormal posturing, splinting, guarding

Facial Expression
- Grimacing, frowning, crying

Gross Abnormalities
- Weight loss, muscle atrophy, deformities
- Change in vital signs

Integumentary
- Pallor, diaphoresis

HEENT
- Pained facial expression
- Clenched teeth
- Abnormal sounds, moans, and groans
- Dilated pupils

Respiratory
- Increased respiratory rate
- Atelectasis r/t limited inspiratory effort d/t pain

Cardiovascular
- Increased heart rate and blood pressure

Gastrointestinal
- Hypoactive bowel sounds

Genitourinary
- Decreased urinary output

Musculoskeletal
- Limited mobility
- Muscle tensing and spasms
- Muscle weakness and fatigue

Neurological
- Altered affect, depression
- Sensory, motor abnormalities
- Memory deficits

Immune system
- Infection

Other Regions
- Dependent on site of pain

Abdominal Assessment

Subjective

- Perform a detailed history as related to the abdomen if indicated
- Common abdominal complaints:
  - Pain, changes in weight, bowel pattern changes, indigestion, nausea and vomitting

Objective

Inspection
- Size, shape, symmetry
- Movements, respirations, pulsations, peristalsis
- Condition of skin

Auscultate
- Bowel sounds
- Vascular sounds

Percuss
- Abdomen
- Organs
- Tenderness

Palpation
- Light: surface characteristics, tenderness
- Deep: organs, masses

REVIEW QUESTIONS

1. What is the rationale for performing auscultation of the abdomen prior to palpation?
   Answer:

2. When inspecting the abdomen, you note that the abdomen is distended.
   What may account for symmetrical distention of the abdomen?
   What may account for asymmetrical distention of the abdomen?
   Answer:

3. During the abdominal assessment, your patient tells you he has pain in the left lower quadrant, in which quadrant should you begin palpation?
   Answer:

4. Your patient has referred pain. How would you define referred pain?
   Answer:

5. **a.** What does light abdominal palpation reveal?
   b. What does deep palpation reveal?
   Answer:

Related Evidence-Based Practice Guidelines

The Joint Commission National Patient Safety Goals Hospital Program. Retrieved from http://www.jointcommission.org/GeneralPublic/NPSG10_npsgs.htm

SBAR technique for communication: A situational briefing model. The Institute for Healthcare Improvement. Retrieved December 19, 2008, from http://www.ihi.org/IHI/Topics/PatientSafety/SafetyGeneral/Tools/SBARTechniqueforCommunicationASituationalBriefingModel.htm

Topics to Review Prior to the Simulation

- Health assessment (abdominal)
- Adult Medical-Surgical
- Fundamentals/postop care

SIMULATION

Client Background

Biographical data

- Age: 69
- Gender: male
- Height: 6 feet
- Weight: 225 lb

Cultural Considerations:

- Language: Spanish, little English
- Ethnicity: Hispanic
- Nationality: Mexican
- Culture: language barrier

Demographic

- Marital status: married
- Educational level: high school
- Religion: Catholic
- Occupation: retired construction worker

Current Health Status

- Patient admitted for right inguinal hernia repair

History

- Psychosocial history
  - Social support: family, lives with wife
- Past health history
  - Medical: type 2 diabetes, HTN, BPH
  - Surgical: none
- Family History: + for CV disease, DM

Admission Sheet

Name:	Sam Rivera
Age:	69
Gender:	Male
Marital Status:	Married
Educational Level:	High school
Religion:	Catholic
Ethnicity:	Hispanic
Nationality:	Mexican
Language:	Spanish, little English
Occupation:	Retired construction worker

Hospital
Provider's Orders

Patient's Name: Sam Rivera
Allergies: NKDA

Diagnosis: Right inguinal hernia repair

Date	Time	Order	Signature
3/10/09	6 PM	Admit to Medical–Surgical Unit Dx postop right inguinal herniorraphy	
		Vital signs: q 4 hr	
		Diet: NPO until awake clear, liquid to 2,000 cal ADA as tolerated	
		Activity: OOB with assistance	
		IV therapy: 1,000 mL NSS over 8 hr	
		Medications: Percocet 1 tab po q 4 hr prn pain Diovan 160 mg po daily Lisinipril 5 mg po daily Metformin 500 mg po bid	

Diagnosis: Right inguinal hernia repair—cont'd

Date	Time	Order	Signature
		Diagnostic studies: AccuCheck qid	
		Treatments: O_2 L/nasal cannula Incentive spirometry q 1 hr while awake	Dr. Dombroski

Nursing Report

Mr. Rivers, aged 69 years, patient of Dr. Dombrowski, had laporoscopic right inguinal heriniorrhaphy under general anesthesia. Patient has history of HTN, type 2 DM, BPH. Patient vital signs stable: BP 140/85, pulse 97 and regular, respirations 24 and shallow, pulse ox 95% on 2 L via nasal cannula, temperature 97.8°F. Pain 2/10. AccuCheck 115. Patient awake, alert, and oriented × 3, dressings dry and intact. Foley catheter drained 400 mL clear yellow urine and discontinued at 4 PM. 1,000 mL NSS over 8 hr. Patient for tentative discharge in AM.

Student Simulator Prep Assignments

1. Identify items and their purpose in the care of a patient with abdominal pain.

Item	Purpose
IV with pump	
O_2 cannula and rebreather mask	
Urinary straight catheter	
Gloves	
BP cuff, thermometer	

2. Identify team members and their specific roles in the care of a patient with abdominal pain.

Team Member	Role
Primary nurse	
Physician	

3. Relevant Data Exercise: Fill in columns below.

Relevant Data from Report	Relevant Data from Other Sources	Data Missing	Sources for Missing Data	Data Requiring Follow-up

4. Initial Focused Assessment

After reviewing the client background and nursing report, you are ready to assess your client's current status. Under each category, identify how you would target your assessment and what you would expect to find for the patient with abdominal pain.

History

Are there any questions you need to ask the patient or family to obtain additional relevant data?

Physical Exam

- General appearance:
- Integumentary:
- HEENT:
- Respiratory:
- CV:
- Breasts:
- Abdominal:
- Neuro:
- Musculoskeletal:
- Reproductive:
- Additional:
- Developmental:

What are the nursing implications considering the developmental stage of your patient?

Answer:

5. Diagnostic Tests

Not applicable

6. Treatment

Identify drugs that are used to treat a patient with abdominal pain.

Complete the table using Deglin et al, *Davis's Drug Guide for Nurses* 12e, or other drug reference.

Medication	Dose, Route, Frequency	Indications	Side Effect	Nursing Implications
Percocet	1 tab po q 4 hr prn			
Diovan	160 mg po daily			
Metformin	500 mg po bid			
Lisinopril	10 mg daily			

7. *Nursing Problems/Diagnoses*

Identify three priority nursing problems/diagnoses.

Assessment Data	Priority Problem	Intervention	Expected Patient Outcome	Which Interventions Could Be Delegated to Unlicensed Personnel?
1.				
2.				
3.				

References

Deglin, J. H., & Vallerand, A. H. (2009). *Davis's drug guide for nurses* (11th ed.). Philadelphia: F. A. Davis.

Dillon, P. (2007). *Nursing health assessment: A critical thinking case studies approach* (2nd ed.). Philadelphia: F. A. Davis.

Erikson, E. H. (1950). *Childhood and society*. New York: Norton.

Langerquist, S. L. (2006). *Davis's NCLEX-RN success* (2nd ed.). Philadelphia: F. A. Davis.

Van Leeuwen, A. M., Poelhuis-Leth, D. J., & Bladh, M. L. (2011). *Davis's comprehensive handbook of laboratory and diagnostic tests with nursing implications.* (4th ed.). Philadelphia: F. A. Davis.

Wilkinson, J. (2007). *Fundamentals of nursing*. Philadelphia: F. A. Davis.

2-6 Aspiration Pneumonia

ADULT/FUNDAMENTALS

STANDARD FORMS

These templates are included in the Appendix; copy before each use.

LEARNING OUTCOMES

Cognitive

The student will be able to:

1. Identify pertinent history question relevant a patient with aspiration pneumonia.
2. Identify risk factors for developing aspiration pneumonia.
3. Identify diagnostic tests that identify patients at high risk for aspiration.
4. Recognize the signs and symptoms of aspiration pneumonia.
5. Identify appropriate nursing interventions for a patient with aspiration pneumonia.
6. Describe appropriate interventions to prevent aspiration pneumonia.
7. Recognize the need to call a rapid response.

Psychomotor

The student will be able to:

1. Perform appropriate assessment for a patient with aspiration pneumonia.
2. Implement appropriate interventions for a patient with aspiration pneumonia (e.g,. nasal/oropharangeal suctioning).
3. Initiate a rapid response call.

Affective

The student will be able to:

1. Reflect upon performance in performing an assessment on a patient with aspiration pneumonia.
2. Identify factors that worked well during the simulation of care of a patient.
3. Identify factors that needed improvement during the simulation of care of a patient with aspiration pneumonia.
4. Develop self-confidence in caring for a patient with aspiration pneumonia.

Communication

The student will be able to:

1. Communicate effectively with the patient with aspiration pneumonia.
2. Use SBAR when communicating assessment findings.
3. Accurately and succinctly document assessment findings.
4. Practice Transparent Thinking (thinking out loud) to facilitate group problem solving.
5. Use Directed Communication (directing a message to specific individual) when delegating tasks.
6. Employ Closed-Loop Communication (acknowledgment of receipt of the message and status) to acknowledge communications from others.

Safety

The student will be able to:

Administer and maintain specific protecting interventions with attention to safety of the client and healthcare professional.

1. Demonstrate a safe environment with attention to hazards to healthcare providers, visitors, and the client. Includes body mechanics, tripping hazards, and equipment issues.
2. Demonstrate attention to national patient safety goals. Includes patient identification standards, effective communication among healthcare providers, and safe medication administration.
3. Demonstrate attention to standard precautions. Includes hand washing, infection control measures, and use of personal protective equipment (PPE) as needed.

Leadership and Management/Delegation

The student will be able to:

1. Identify and prioritize patient's needs in care of a patient with a aspiration pneumonia.
2. Delegate tasks appropriately.

OVERVIEW OF THE PROBLEM

Definition

Aspiration Pneumonia

Aspiration of fluids into the airways results in acute inflammation of lungs with exudate accumulation in alveoli and other respiratory passages that interferes with ventilation process.

Pathophysiology

Whether caused by infectious or noninfectious agent, clotting of an exudate rich in fibrogen results in lung consolidation.

Complications of aspiration pneumonia include:

- Lung abscess
- Acute respiratory distress syndrome (ARDS)
- Permanent lung damage
- Death

Risk Factors

- Poor cough mechanism
- Impaired swallowing
- Coma
- Anesthesia

Mechanisms

- Noninfectious: Aspiration of fluids (gastric secretions, foods, liquids, tube feedings) into the airways
- Bacterial aspiration: Related to poor cough mechanism due to anesthesia, coma (mixed flora of upper respiratory tract cause pneumonia)
- Silent aspiration: Aspiration of gastric contents without cough

Predisposing Conditions

- Patients who have difficulty swallowing, such as stroke patients
- Patients with neck injuries
- Patients with neurological impairments
- Patients with impaired level of consciousness
- Patients with drug or alcohol overdose

Prevention

Assess for those patients at risk:

- Assess ability to swallow
- Assess for drooling, pocketing of food, facial drooping, weak hoarse voice
- Assess swallow reflex
- Assess cough reflex
- Assess gag reflex
- Speech and swallow evaluation.

After speech and swallow evaluation, if patient is able to eat, follow recommendations from speech therapist; i.e., no liquids, add "thick-it" to liquids.

- Have patient sit upright during meals
- Have patient do a chin tuck, head slightly forward and flexed
- Observe patient while eating

Assessment

Subjective

- Pain on affected side or referred to abdomen, shoulder, flank area, related to breathing
- Anxious, irritable
- Nausea, anorexia
- History of aspiration

Objective

- "Wet" voice
- Productive cough
- Splinting affected side
- Sudden fever and chills
- Respiratory distress, tachypnea
- Nasal flaring
- Chest retraction
- Cyanosis
- Decreased breath sounds on affected side
- Increased breath sounds on unaffected side
- Rhonchi, crackles, wheezes
- Bronchial breath sounds over consolidation
- Dullness on percussion over consolidation
- Possible pleural friction rub

Diagnostic Tests

- Blood culture
- WBC, leukocytosis
- Elevated sed rate
- Chest x-ray: Reveals haziness or consolidation
- Sputum culture: Gram stain and culture, identifies specific organism
- Bronchoscopy: Obtain specimen
- Blood cultures: Identifies organism unless viral
- CBC: WBC leukocytosis
- Sedimentation rate: Elevated
- Arterial blood gases

Treatment

Administer antibiotics, mild analgesics, expectorants as ordered.

Nursing Management

Goal: Promote adequate ventilation

- Encourage coughing, deep breathing
- Incentive spirometer
- Chest PT
- Expectorants
- Suction prn
- Oxygen with humidification
- Change positions
- Hydration

Goal: Prevent infection

- Administer antibiotics as ordered
- Continue to assess for infection
- Maintain sterile technique
- Anti-inflammatories or steroids for aspirations pneumonia

Goal: Rest and comfort
- Control pain, avoid opioids

Goal: Promote nutrition/hydration
- Maintain hydration po or IV
- High carbohydrate/high protein diet

Goal: Health teaching
- Hand and respiratory hygiene
- Expected and side effects of medications
- Importance of taking antibiotics as prescribed
- Need for rest, ambulation as tolerated, fluids and nutrition
- Immunizations to avoid future infections

Evaluation/Outcome Criteria

- Adheres to medication regimen
- Improved pulmonary function and gas exchange
- Maintains acid base balance
- Increased energy level
- Decreased sputum production
- Stable vital signs
- Clear breath sounds
- Negative cultures
- Increased comfort level

REVIEW QUESTIONS

1. What would you expect the arterial blood gases to reveal in a patient that has aspirated?
   Answer:

2. Differentiate a silent aspiration from aspiration pneumonia.
   Answer:

3. What nursing intervention could be implemented to decrease risk for aspiration?
   Answer:

4. What signs and symptoms would indicate hypoxemia?
   Answer:

5. What assessment findings would you expect in a patient with aspiration pneumonia?
   Answer:

Related Evidence-Based Practice Guidelines

Retrieved from http://www.guideline.gov/search/search.aspx?term=aspiration+pneumonia

The Joint Commission National Patient Safety Goals Hospital Program. Retrieved from http://www.jointcommission.org/GeneraÔlPublic/NPSG10_npsgs.htm

SBAR technique for communication: A situational briefing model. The Institute for Healthcare Improvement. Retrieved December 19, 2008, from http://www.ihi.org/IHI/Topics/PatientSafety/SafetyGeneral/Tools/SBARTechniqueforCommunicationASituationalBriefingModel.htm

Topics to Review Prior to the Simulation

- Health assessment, particularly neurological, and respiratory assessment
- Adult Medical-Surgical Nursing Care
- Stroke
- Suctioning

SIMULATION

Client Background

Biographical Data

- Age: 73
- Gender: male
- Height: 6 ft
- Weight: 225 lb

Cultural Considerations

- Language: English
- Ethnicity: African American
- Nationality: American
- Culture: no significant ciltural implications identified

Demographic

- Marital status: married
- Educational level: college
- Religion: Methodist
- Occupation: retired

Current Health Status

- Patient admitted for Right CVA

History

- Psychosocial history
  - Social support: family, lives with wife
- Past health history
  - Medical: HTN and atrial fibrillation
  - Surgical: hernia repair
- Family history: + for CV disease, DM

Admission Sheet

Name:	John Brown
Age:	73
Gender:	Male
Marital Status:	Married
Educational Level:	College
Religion:	Methodist
Ethnicity:	African American
Nationality:	American
Language:	English
Occupation:	Retired

Hospital **Patient's Name: John Brown**
Provider's Orders **Allergies: NKDA**

Diagnosis: Right CVA

Date	Time	Order	Signature
3/10/09	9 AM	Admit to Telemetry Dx right CVA	
		Vital signs: q 4 hr with neuro check and NIH stroke scale	
		Diet: NPO until swallow evaluation completed	
		Activity: OOB with assistance	
		IV Therapy: Heparin 25,0000U/500 5% D/W at 1,000 units/hr	
		Medications: Coumadin per protocol Lisinopril 10 mg po daily Toprol 25 mg po daily Colace 100 mg po daily	
		Diagnostic Studies: Daily PTT, PT	
		Speech and swallow evaluation	
		Physical therapy and occupational therapy consult	
		Treatment: O_2 L/NC	
			Dr. Schram
3/10/09	3 PM	Diet: Soft with Honey Thick-it to liquids	Dr. Schram
3/13/09	9 AM	Diet: NPO	
		Activity: Bed rest	
		IV therapy: 1,000 mL NSS q 10 hr	
		Medications: Rocephin 1 g IV daily Azithromycin 500 mg IV daily	

Continued

Diagnosis: Left CVA—cont'd

Date	Time	Order	Signature
		Diagnostic studies: Stat portable CXR ABGs CBC, BMP	
		Treatments: Oxygen with nonrebreather mask	
		Cardiac monitor	Dr. Schram

Nursing Report

Mr. Brown, 73 years old, a patient of Dr. Schram, was admitted 3 days ago with diagnosis of right CVA. Patient awake, alert, and oriented ×3, has left-sided weakness, slurred speech. His cardiac monitor reveals controlled a-fib. Patient on heparin drip 1,000 units/hr, INT #22 right hand, oxygen 2 L via nasal cannula. Vital signs: BP 130/84, T 97.8° F, HR 85 irregular, respirations 22, pulse ox 93%. You are making morning rounds. Mr. Brown is eating breakfast.

Student Simulator Prep Assignments

1. Identify items and their purpose in the care of a patient with aspiration pneumonia.

Item	Purpose
IV with pump, IV antibiotics	
O_2 cannula and rebreather mask	
Monitor	
Gloves	
BP cuff, thermometer	
Suction equipment	
Lab and ABG equipment	

2. Identify team members and their specific roles in the care of a patient with aspiration pneumonia.

Team Member	Role
Primary nurse	
Physician	
Secondary nurse	
Respiratory therapist	

3. *Relevant Data Assignment:* Fill in columns below.

Relevant Data from Report	Relevant Data from Other Sources	Data Missing	Sources for Missing Data	Data Requiring Follow-up

4. *Initial Focused Assessment*

After reviewing the client background and nursing report, you are ready to assess your patient's current status. Under each category, identify how you would target your assessment and what you would expect to find for the patient with aspiration pneumonia.

History

Are there any questions you need to ask the patient or family to obtain additional relevant data?

Physical Exam

- General appearance:
- Integumentary:
- HEENT:
- Respiratory:
- CV:
- Breasts:
- Abdominal:
- Neuro:
- Musculoskeletal:
- Reproductive:
- Additional:
- Developmental

What are the nursing implications considering the developmental stage of your patient?

Answer:

5. *Diagnostic Tests*

What diagnostic test results relevant to the patient's current problem are needed to plan care?

Complete the table using Van Leeuwen et al, *Davis's Comprehensive Handbbook of Laboratory and Diagnostic Testing with Nursing Implications* 4e, or other diagnostic test reference.

Diagnostic Test	Significance to This Patient's Problem
CXR	
CBC	
BMP • Glucose • Lytes • BUN • Creatinine1	
Sputum C&S	

6. Treatment

Identify drugs that are used to treat a patient with aspiration pneumonia.

Complete the table using Deglin et al, *Davis's Drug Guide for Nurses* 12e, or other drug reference.

Medication	Dose, Route, Frequency	Indications	Side Effect	Nursing Implications
Rocephin	1 g IV daily			
Azithromycin	500 mg IV daily			
Heparin	1,000 units/hr			
Lisinopril	10 mg daily			
Toprol	25 mg daily			
Colace	100 mg daily			

7. Nursing Problems/Diagnoses

Identify three priority nursing problems/diagnoses.

Assessment Data	Priority Problem	Intervention	Expected Patient Outcome	Which Interventions Could Be Delegated to Unlicensed Personnel?
1.				
2.				
3.				

References

Deglin, J. H., & Vallerand, A. H. (2009). *Davis's drug guide for nurses* (11th ed.). Philadelphia: F. A. Davis.

Dillon, P. (2007). *Nursing health assessment. A critical thinking case studies approach (*2nd ed.). Philadelphia: F. A. Davis.

Erikson, E. H. (1950). *Childhood and society*. New York: Norton.

Lagerquist, S. L. (2006). *Davis's NCLEX-RN success* (2nd ed.). Philadelphia: F. A. Davis.

Van Leeuwen, A. M., & Poelhuis-Leth, D. J., & Bladh, M. L. (2010). *Davis's comprehensive handbook of laboratory and diagnostic tests with nursing implications* (4th ed.). Philadelphia: F.A. Davis.

Wilkinson, J. (2007). *Fundamentals of nursing*. Philadelphia: F. A. Davis.

2-7 Perioperative Care

MEDICAL-SURGICAL

STANDARD FORMS

These templates are included in the Appendix; copy before each use.

LEARNING OUTCOMES

Cognitive

The student will be able to:

1. Analyze the information from the client's chart and the subjective and objective data.
2. Identify the appropriate interventions for the patient with small bowel obstruction (SBO).
3. Describe signs and symptoms of SBO.
4. Correlate signs and symptoms of abdominal pain, nausea, and vomiting to the pathophysiology of SBO.
5. Identify factors in a patient's history that increase the risk for SBO.
6. Identify the appropriate interventions for the patient with SBO.
7. Identify appropriate interventions for the perioperative patient.
8. Provide a rationale giving the medications ordered pre- and postoperatively.
9. Identify appropriate interventions for the postoperative patient.

Psychomotor

The student will be able to:

1. Perform appropriate assessment for a patient with a complaint of SBO.
2. Correctly assess vital signs, including pulse ox, and document them appropriately.
3. Properly administer IV medication.
4. Initiate appropriate interventions including:
   - Scene 1: Assessing IV type and infusion site, insertion of NG tube, completing preop checklist, administering IV piggyback medication.
   - Scene 2: Assessing a fresh postop patient, initiate oxygen therapy, maintain NG as ordered, document all aspects of care correctly on appropriate forms.

Affective

The student will be able to:

1. Reflect on ability to apply assessment skills.
2. Share factors that worked well during the simulation of care of a patient with SBO.
3. Share factors that needed improvement during the simulation of care of a patient with SBO.
4. Develop self-confidence in ability to think critically using multiple assessment sources to problem solve.
5. Reflect upon performance in the care of a patient with SBO.
6. Identify personal feelings in delivering care to a patient with SBO.
7. Discuss feelings related to working as a member of a team in the care of a patient with SBO.

Communication

The student will be able to:

1. Communicate effectively with healthcare team members in care of a patient with SBO.
2. Accurately and succinctly document assessments, interventions, and evaluations on appropriate forms.
3. Use SBAR when communicating with team members in the care of a patient with SBO.
4. Communicate effectively with the patient and family in the care of a patient with SBO.
5. Include patient/family education about procedures and medications.
6. Document vital signs including pain, actions taken, and effect of these actions.
7. Receive and give verbal reports from ED, lab, and OR.
8. Practice Transparent Thinking (thinking out loud) to facilitate group problem solving.
9. Use Directed Communication (directing a message to specific individual) when delegating tasks.
10. Employ Closed-Loop Communication (acknowledgment of receipt of the message and status) to acknowledge communications from others.

Safety

The student will be able to:

Administer and maintain specific protecting interventions with attention to safety of the client and healthcare professional.

1. Demonstrate a safe environment with attention to hazards to healthcare providers, visitors, and the client. Includes body mechanics, tripping hazards, and equipment issues.
2. Demonstrate attention to national patient safety goals. Includes patient identification standards, effective communication among healthcare providers, and safe medication administration.
3. Demonstrate attention to standard precautions. Includes hand washing, infection control measures, and use of personal protective equipment (PPE) as needed.

Leadership and Management/Delegation

The student will be able to:

1. Use references to find needed drug information.
2. Identify key side effects of selected medications.
3. State nursing implications of medications administered.
4. Verify that preoperative consents are signed and in chart before sedation is administered.
5. Identify and prioritize patient's needs in care of a patient with SBO.
6. Identify tasks that can be legally, ethically, and safely delegated to unlicensed assistive personnel (UAP) or licensed practical nurse (LPN) in the care of a patient with SBO.

OVERVIEW OF PROBLEM

THE PERIOPERATIVE EXPERIENCE

Preoperative Preparation

Assessment

Subjective

- Understanding of proposed surgery—site, type, extent of hospitalization
- Previous experiences with hospitalization
- Age-related factors
- Allergies—iodine, latex, adhesive tape, cleansing solutions, medications
- Medication/substance use—prescribed, OTC, smoking, alcohol, recreational drugs
- Cultural and religious background

Concerns or feelings about surgery:

- Exaggerated ideas of surgical risk (e.g., fear of colostomy when none is being considered)
- Nature of anesthesia (e.g., fears of going to sleep and not waking up, saying or revealing things of a personal nature)
- Degree of pain (e.g., may be incapacitating)
- Misunderstandings regarding prognosis
- Identification of significant others as a source of client support or care responsibilities postdischarge

Objective

- Speech patterns indicating anxiety—repetition, changing topics, avoiding talking about feelings
- Interactions with others—withdrawn or involved
- Physical signs of anxiety (e.g., increased pulse and respirations, clammy palms, restlessness)
  - Baseline physiological status: vital signs; breath sounds; peripheral circulation; weight; hydration status (hematocrit, skin turgor, urine output); degree of mobility; muscle strength

Treatment

Medical and Nursing Management

Goal: Reduce preoperative and intraoperative anxiety and prevent postoperative complications.

- Preoperative teaching:
  - Provide information about hospital nursing routines and preoperative procedures to reduce fear of unknown
  - Explain purpose of diagnostic procedures to enhance ability to cooperate and tolerate procedure
  - Inform about what will occur and what will be expected in the postoperative period:
    - Will return to room, postanesthesia care unit, or intensive care unit
    - Special equipment—monitors, tubes, suction equipment
    - Pain control methods

Goal: Provide latex-free environment.

- Management of latex allergy if present. Three forms:
  - Immediate reaction—most serious, life-threatening—flushing, diaphoresis, pruritus, nausea, vomiting, cramping, hypotension, dyspnea;
  - Delayed response—most common, discomfort—localized symptoms 18 to 24 hr after contact;
  - Contact dermatitis—exposure to latex through skin, mucous membranes, inhalation, internal tissue, and intravascular; sources include gloves, anesthesia masks, tourniquets, EGG electrodes, adhesive tape, warming blankets, elastic bandages, tubes/catheters, irrigation syringes.

Goal: Instruct in exercises to reduce complications.

- Diaphragmatic breathing—refers to flattening of diaphragm during inspiration, which results in enlargement of upper abdomen; during expiration the abdominal muscles are contracted, along with the diaphragm. The client should be in a flat, semi-Fowler's, or side position, with knees flexed and hands on the mid abdomen.
  - Have the client take a deep breath through nose and mouth, letting the abdomen rise. Hold breath 3 to 5 sec.
  - Have client exhale through nose and mouth, squeezing out all air by contracting the abdominal muscles.
  - Repeat 10 to 15 times, with a short rest after each 5 to prevent hyperventilation.
  - Inform client that this exercise will be repeated 5 to 10 times every hour postoperatively.
    - Coughing—helps clear chest of secretions and, although uncomfortable, will not harm incision site.
    - Have client lean forward slightly from a sitting position, and place client's hands over incisional site; this acts as a splint during coughing.
    - Have client inhale and exhale slowly several times.
    - Have client inhale deeply, hold breath 3 sec, and cough sharply three times while exhaling—client's mouth should be slightly open.
    - Tell client to inhale again and to cough deeply once or twice. If unable to cough deeply, client should "huff" to stimulate cough.

- Turning and leg exercises—helps prevent circulatory stasis, which may lead to thrombus formation, and postoperative flatus or "gas pains," as well as respiratory problems.
  - Tell client to turn on one side with uppermost leg flexed; use side rails to facilitate the movement.
  - In a supine position, have client do five repetitions every hour of: ankle pumps, quad sets, gluteal tightenings, and straight-leg raises.
  - Apply intermittent pulsatile compression device or sequential compression device (SCD) to promote venous return.

Goal: Reduce the number of bacteria on the skin to eliminate incision contamination. Skin preparation:

- Prepare area of skin wider and longer than proposed incision in case a larger incision is necessary.
  - Gently scrub with an antimicrobial agent.
  - Note possibility of allergy to iodine.
  - Hexachlorophene should be left on the skin for 5–10 min.
  - If benzalkonium Cl (Zephiran) solution is ordered, do not soap skin before use; soap reduces effectiveness of benzalkonium by causing it to precipitate.
  - Hair should remain unless it interferes with surgical procedure.
  - Note any nicks, cuts, or irritations—potential infection sites.
  - Depilatory creams or clipping of hair is preferred to shaving with a razor; nick may result in cancellation of surgery.
  - Skin prep may be done in surgery.

Goal: Reduce the risk of vomiting and aspiration during anesthesia; prevent contamination of abdominal operative sites by fecal material.

Gastrointestinal Tract Preparation

- No food or fluid at least 6–8 hr before surgery.
- Remove food and water from bedside.
- Place NPO signs on bed or door.
- Inform kitchen and oncoming nursing staff that client is NPO for surgery.
- Give IV infusions up to time of surgery if dehydrated or malnourished.
- Enemas: Two or three may be given the evening before surgery with intestinal, colon, or pelvic surgeries; 3 days of cleansing with large-intestine procedures.
- Possible antibiotic therapy to reduce colonic flora with large-bowel surgery.
- Gastric or intestinal intubation may be inserted the evening before major abdominal surgery. Types of tubes:
  - Levin: Single lumen; sufficient to remove fluids and gas from stomach; suction may damage mucosa.
  - Salem sump: Large lumen; prevents tissue-wall adherence.
  - Miller-Abbott: Long single or double lumen; required to remove the contents of jejunum or ileum.
- Pressures: low setting with Levin and intestinal tubes; high setting with Salem sump; excessive pressures will result in injury to mucosal lining of intestine or stomach.

Goal: Promote rest and facilitate reduction of apprehension.

- Medications as ordered: On evening before surgery may give sleep medication.
- Quiet environment: Eliminate noises, distractions.
- Position: Reduce muscle tension.
- Back rub.

Goal: Protect from injury; ensure final preparation for surgery. Day of surgery:

- Operative permit signed and on chart; physician responsible for obtaining informed consent. Possible blood products consent.
- Shower or bathe.
- Dress: Hospital pajamas.
- Remove: Hair pins (cover hair); nail polish, to facilitate observation of peripheral circula tion; jewelry (or tape wedding bands securely); pierced earrings; contact lenses; dentures (store and give mouth care); give valuable personal items to family; chart disposition of items.
- Proper identification: Check band for secureness and legibility; surgical site (limb) may be marked to prevent error.
- Vital signs: Baseline data.
- Void, to prevent distention and possible injury to bladder.
- Give preoperative medication to ensure smooth induction and maintenance of anesthesia—antianxiety (e.g., midazolam, diazepam, lorazepam); narcotics (e.g., meperidine, morphine, fentanyl); anticholinergics (e.g., atropine, glycopyrrolate).
- Administered 45–75 min before anesthetic induction.
- Side rails up (client will begin to feel drowsy and lightheaded).
- Expect complaint of dry mouth if anticholinergics given.
- Observe for side effects—narcotics may cause nausea and vomiting, hypotension, arrhythmias, and/or respiratory depression.
- Quiet environment until transported to operating room.
- Anticipate antibiotics to start "on call" to OR.
- Note completeness of chart:
  - Surgical checklist completed.
  - Vital signs recorded.
  - Routine laboratory reports present.
  - Preoperative medications given.
  - Significant client observations.
- Assist client's family in finding proper waiting room.
  - Inform family members that the surgeon will contact them after the procedure is over.
  - Explain length of time client is expected to be in recovery room.

- Prepare family for any special equipment or devices that may be needed to care for client postoperatively (e.g., oxygen, monitoring equipment, ventilator, blood transfusions).

Intestinal Obstruction

Definition

Blockage of intestinal contents through the small or large intestines.

Pathophysiology

Causes

Mechanical: Physical impediments to passage of intestinal contents. E. g., adhesions, hernias, neoplasms, inflammatory bowel disease, foreign bodies, fecal impaction, congenital or radiation strictures, intussusception, or volvulus.

Paralytic: Passage open, but perastalsis ceases. E.g., Postoperative abdominal surgery, hypokalemia, MI, pneumonia, spinal injuries, peritonitis, vascular insufficiency.

Assessment

Subjective

- Proximal loop obstruction: Upper abdominal sharp, cramping, intermittent pain
- Distal loop obstruction: Poorly localized, cramping pain

Objective

Bowel sounds:

- Early: High pitched, increased
- Late: Decreased to absent
  - Obstipation: No passage of gas or stool
  - Abdominal distention
  - Vomiting
- Proximal loop: Profuse nonfecal vomiting
- Distal loop: Less frequent fecal type vomiting
  - Decreased urinary output
  - Vital signs
- Temperature: Elevated
- Pulse: Tachycardia
- Blood pressure: Hypotension
  - Shock if untreated
- Dehydration: Hemoconcentration, hypovolemia

Diagnostic Tests

- Leukocytosis
- Sodium decreased <138
- Potassium <3.5
- Bicarbonate increased >26 mEq/L
- BUN elevated >18mg/dL
- PH
  - If obstruction at gastric outlet, pH elevated, metabolic alkalosis
  - If obstruction distal duodenal or proximal jejunal, pH decreased, metabolic acidosis

Treatment

- Maintain fluid balance with IV therapy
- NPO
- Gastric decompression
- Analgesics
- Antiemetics
- Monitor labs for electrolyte imbalance
- I&O
- Position semi-Fowler's

REVIEW QUESTIONS

1. When admitting a client to your unit, what is your initial action?
   Answer:

2. What sources can you use to gather information about your client?
   Answer:

3. The primary source is_________?
   Answer:

4. When you do an abdominal assessment, in what order do you palpate, auscultate, inspect, and percuss?
   Answer:

5. When you are completing the preoperative checklist, name at least three things you need to check.
   Answer:

Related Evidenced-Based Practice Guidelines

National Guideline Clearinghouse. Retrieved from http://www.guideline.gov

Practice parameters for the prevention of venous thromboembolism. American Society of Colon and Rectal Surgeons - Medical Specialty Society. 2000 Aug (revised 2006 Oct). 7 pages. NGC:005610

Prevention of venous thromboembolism: Evidence-based clinical practice *guidelines* (8th ed.). American College of Chest Physicians: Medical Specialty Society. 2001 Jan (revised 2008 Jun). 73 pages. NGC:006665

Postoperative management in adults. A practical guide to postoperative care for clinical staff.

Scottish Intercollegiate Guidelines Network (SIGN). Edinburgh (Scotland): Scottish Intercollegiate Guidelines Network (SIGN); 2004 Aug. 56 p. (SIGN publication; no. 77). [132 references]

The Joint Commission National Patient Safety Goals Hospital Program. Retrieved from http://www.jointcommission.org/GeneralPublic/NPSG10_npsgs.htm

Scottish Intercollegiate Guidelines Network (SIGN). Postoperative management in adults. A practical guide to postoperative care for clinical staff. Edinburgh (Scotland): Scottish Intercollegiate Guidelines Network (SIGN); 2004 Aug. 56 p. (SIGN publication; no. 77). [132 references]

SBAR Technique for Communication: A situational briefing model published by The Institute for Healthcare Improvement was downloaded on December 19, 2008, from http://www.ihi.org/IHI/Topics/PatientSafety/SafetyGeneral/Tools/SBARTechniqueforCommunicationASituationalBriefingModel.htm

Topics to Review Prior to the Simulation

- Perioperative care
- Small bowel obstruction

SIMULATION

Client Background

Mr. Kelly, a 62-year-old obese, white male, PMH of HTN and S/P Rt inguinal hernia repair 2 months ago with an incidental appendectomy. He has a 2-wk history of constipation, 2-day history of severe abdominal pain, nausea and vomiting, episodes of explosive diarrhea. In the ER, an IV of 1,000 mL NS at 100 cc/hr started with a 21-gauge angiocath in the R forearm, blood work drawn (CBC, Chem-7- K+ 2.3, Na 130), given K rider 40 mEq KCl in ER, flat plate of abdomen shows diffuse air, distention. CT scan of abdomen reveals small bowel obstruction. Surgery scheduled.

Biographical Data

- Age: 62
- Gender: male
- Height: 70 in
- Weight: 250 lb

Cultural Considerations

- No significant cultural considerations identified

Demographic

- Marital status: married
- Educational level: college
- Religion: undeclared
- Occupation: teacher

Current Health Status

- Right inguinal hernia repair with incidental appendectomy two months ago. Constipation for 2 weeks, severe abdominal pain for 2 days, with nausea, vomiting and explosive diarrhea. Small bowel obstruction.

History

- Psychosocial History
  - Social support: married, one son age 26
- Past health history: HTN, S/P Rt inguinal hernia repair, obesity
- Family history: Unknown

Admission Sheet

Name:	Michael Kelly
Age:	62
Marital Status:	Married
Educational Level:	College
Religion:	Undeclared
Ethnicity:	Irish
Nationality:	United States Citzen
Language:	English
Occupation:	Teacher

Hospital Provider's Orders		Patient's Name: Michael Kelly Allergies: Sulfonamides. No food allergies	
Diagnosis: Abdominal pain, small bowel obstruction			
Date	**Time**	**Order**	**Signature**
9/25/2008	1430	Vital signs: q 4 hr	
		Diet: NPO	
		Activity: Bed rest IV therapy: D5/NS q 20 mEq KCl at 125 cc/hr	
		Medications: Morphine 6 mg IV push Flagyl 500 IVPB Levoquin 500 mg IVPB Administer first dose when called to OR	
		Insert Salem Sump 14-gauge and attach to low continuous suction Irrigate with 30 mL NSS prn	
		I&O	
		Diagnostic studies: Abdominal flat plate, CT scan of abdomen (done in ED) CXR (done in ED)	
		CBC with differential, serum electrolytes, glucose, BUN, creatinine (done in ED) Repeat K+ 1 hr following K+ rider. Routine UA stat preop Coag studies, PT, PTT, type and screen ECG stat preop	
		Continuous cardiac monitor	
		Medical consult for medical clearance preop	
		Treatments: O_2 via nasal cannula 4 L/min	Dr. C. J. Redstone

Nursing Report

Phone rings—report from ER nurse:

Mr. Kelly, a 62-year-old, obese, white male, PMH of HTN and S/P Rt inguinal hernia repair 2 months ago with an incidental appendectomy. He has a 2-wk history of constipation, 2-day history of severe abdominal pain, nausea and vomiting, episodes of explosive diarrhea. In the ER, an IV of 1,000 mL NS at 100 cc/hr started with a 21-gauge angiocath in the R forearm, you have 700 mL in the bag remaining, blood work drawn (CBC, Chem-7- K+ 2.3, Na 130), given K rider 40 mEq KCL in ER, flat plate of abdomen shows diffuse air, distention. CT scan of abdomen showed small bowel obstruction. Mr. Kelly is to be admitted unaccompanied to your surgical floor for preop prep and observation. His family has been notified and are on their way to the hospital.

Student Simulation Prep Assignments

1. Identify items and their purpose in the care of a patient with small bowel obstruction.

Item	Purpose
Stethoscope	
Watch	
Sphygmomanometer	
Thermometer	
Suction device (wall or portable)	
Correct IVs and IV pole	
Nasal cannula with O_2 source	
PCA Pump	
Tape, gauze, etc.	

2. Identify team members and their specific roles the care of a perioperative patient with SBO.

Team Member	Role
Physician	
Nurse	
Laboratory personnel	
X-ray, ECG technicians	
Respiratory therapy	

3. Relevant Data Exercise

Relevant Data from Report	Relevant Data from Other Sources	Data Missing	Sources for Missing Data	Data Requiring Follow-Up

4. Initial Focused Assessment

After reviewing the client background and nursing report, you are ready to assess your client's current status. Under each category, identify how you would target your assessment, and what you would expect to find for the patient with a small bowel obstruction?

History

Are there any questions you need to ask the patient or family to obtain additional relevant data?

Physical Exam

- General appearance:
- Integumentary:
- HEENT:
- Respiratory:
- CV:
- Breasts:
- Abdominal:
- Musculoskeletal:
- Neuro:
- Reproductive:
- Additional:
- Developmental

What are the nursing implications considering the developmental stage of your patient?

Answer:

5. Diagnostic Tests

What diagnostic test results relevant to the patient's current problem are needed to plan care?

Complete the table using Van Leeuwen et al, *Davis's Comprehensive Handbook of Laboratory and Diagnostic Testing with Nursing Implications* 4e, or other diagnostic test reference.

Diagnostic Test	Significance to This Patient's Problem
ECG	
CBC	
Coag studies, PT, PTT	
Type and screen	
Complete metabolic panel	
Routine UA	
CXR	
CT scan of abdomen	
Flat plate of abdomen	

6. Treatment

Identify drugs that are used to treat a perioperative patient with a SBO.

Complete the table using Deglin et al, *Davis's Drug Guide for Nurses* 12e, or other drug reference.

Medication	Dose, Route, Frequency	Indications	Side Effect	Nursing Implications
Morphine	6 mg IV push PCA 1 mg q 6 min, lockout at 30 mg in 4 hrs; basal rate of 2 mg/hr			
Flagyl	500 mg IVPB			

Continued

Medication	Dose, Route, Frequency	Indications	Side Effect	Nursing Implications
Levoquin	500 mg IVPB			

7. Nursing Problems/Diagnoses

Identify three priority nursing problems/diagnoses.

Assessment Data	Priority Problem	Intervention	Expected Patient Outcome	Which Interventions Could Be Delegated to Unlicensed Personnel?
1.				
2.				
3.				

References

Deglin, J. H., & Vallerand, A. H. (2009). *Davis's drug guide for nurses* (11th ed.). Philadelphia: F. A. Davis.

Dillon, P. (2007). *Nursing health assessment: A critical thinking and case studies approach* (2nd ed.). Philadelphia: F. A. Davis.

Doenges, M. E., Moorhouse, M. F., & Murr, A. C. (2006). *Nursing care plans: Guidelines for individualizing client care across the life span* (7th ed.). Philadelphia: F. A. Davis.

Erikson, E. H. (1950). *Childhood and society*. New York: Norton.

Rhoads, J., & Meeker, B. J., (2008). *Davis's clinical nursing skills.* Philadelphia: F. A. Davis.

Schnell, Z. B., Van Leeuwen, A. M., & Kranpitz, T. R. (2003). *Davis's comprehensive handbook of laboratory and diagnostic tests with nursing implications.* Philadelphia: F. A. Davis.

Taber's cyclopedic medical dictionary (18th ed.) (1997). Philadelphia: F. A. Davis.

Van Leeuwen, A. M., Poelhuis-Leth, D. J., & Bladh, M. L. (2011). *Davis's comprehensive handbook of laboratory and diagnostic tests with nursing implications.* (4th ed.). Philadelphia: F.A. Davis.

Wilkinson, J. M., & Van Leuven, K. (2007). *Fundamentals of nursing theory, concepts & application* (Vol. 1). Philadelphia: F. A. Davis.

Maternal/Newborn Nursing 3

3-1 Postpartum Hemorrhage

MATERNITY, POSTPARTUM

STANDARD FORMS

These templates are included in the Appendix; copy before each use.

LEARNING OUTCOMES

Cognitive

The student will be able to:

1. Identify factors in a patient's past obsterical history that increase risk for postpartum hemorrhage (PPH).
2. Identify factors in a patient's recent labor and delivery history that increase risk for PPH.
3. Correctly interpret the signs and symptoms of PPH.
4. Correlate signs and symptoms to the pathophysiology of PPH.
5. Identify the appropriate nursing interventions for the patient with PPH.
6. Differentiate the roles of team members in response to an obstetrical emergency.

Psychomotor

The student will be able to:

1. Perform appropriate assessment for a patient with PPH.
2. Initiate appropriate interventions for a patient with PPH.
3. Correctly set up or administer medications as ordered.
4. Work collaboratively as part of the healthcare team in the care of a patient with PPH.

Affective

The student will be able to:

1. Reflect thoughtfully upon performance of self and others in a simulated obstetrical emergency situation.
2. Identify personal feelings in a simulated obstetrical emergency situation.
3. Discuss feelings related to working as a member of a team.
4. Identify factors that worked well during the scenario.
5. Identify factors that needed improvement during the scenario.
6. Develop self-confidence in the care of a patient during a simulated obstetrical emergency.

Communication

The student will be able to:

1. Communicate effectively with healthcare team members in a simulated obstetrical emergency.
2. Communicate effectively with the patient and family in a simulated obstetrical emergency.
3. Practice Transparent Thinking (thinking out loud) to facilitate group problem solving.
4. Use Directed Communication (directing a message to specific individual) when delegating tasks.
5. Employ Closed-Loop Communication (acknowledgment of receipt of the message and status) to acknowledge communications from others.

Safety

The student will be able to:

Administer and maintain specific protecting interventions with attention to safety of the client and healthcare professional.

1. Demonstrate a safe environment with attention to hazards to healthcare providers, visitors, and the client. Includes body mechanics, tripping hazards, and equipment issues.
2. Demonstrate attention to national patient safety goals. Includes patient identification standards, effective communication among healthcare providers, and safe medication administration.
3. Demonstrate attention to standard precautions. Includes hand washing, infection control measures, and use of personal protective equipment (PPE) as needed.

Leadership and Management/Delegation

The student will be able to:

1. Identify tasks that can be legally, ethically, and safely delegated to unlicensed assistive personnel (UAP) in a simulated obstetrical emergency situation.
2. Identify and prioritize patient's needs in care of a patient with a simulated obstetrical emergency

Pharmacology

The student will be able to:

1. Identify medications used in the treatment of postpartum hemorrhage.
2. Safely administer medications in a simulated experience.

OVERVIEW OF THE PROBLEM

Definition

Postpartum hemorrhage (PPH): Loss of 500 mL of blood or more during the first 24 hr postpartum in vaginal birth; 1,000 mL in cesarean birth.

Pathophysiology

Excessive loss of blood secondary to trauma, decreased uterine contractility; results in hypovolemia.

Risk Factors

- Uterine atony
  - Uterine overdistention (multipregnancy, polyhydramnios, fetal macrosomia)
  - Multiparity
  - Prolonged or precipitous labor
  - Anesthesia
  - Fibroids
  - Oxytocin induction of labor
  - Magnesium sulfate
  - Overmassage of uterus in postpartum
  - Distended bladder
- Lacerations: cervix, vagina, perineum
- Retained placental fragments: usually delayed postpartum hemorrhage
- Hematoma: deep pelvic, vaginal, or episiotomy site

Assessment

Subjective

- Occurring late with signs of shock-anxiety, apprehension

Objective

- Uterus: Boggy, flaccid; excessive vaginal bleeding.
  - Late signs of shock: Air hunger; anxiety/apprehension, tachycardia, tachypnea, hypotension.
  - Estimated blood loss during labor and birth and in early postpartum period.
- Pain: Vulvar, vaginal, perineal.
  - Perineum: Distended due to edema; discoloration due to hematoma. May complain of rectal pressure.
  - Lacerations: Bright red vaginal bleeding with firm fundus.

Diagnostic Tests

CBC, hemoglobin, hematocrit, clotting time, platelet count.

Treatment

Medical Management

- Order oxytocics:
  - IV oxytocin infusion
  - IV or oral ergot preparations ergotrate maleate (Ergonovine); methylergonovine (Methergine); carboprost tromethamine (Hemabate), misoprostol (Cytotec)
- Order diagnostic tests
- Type and crossmatch for blood replacement
- Surgical
  - Repair of lacerations
  - Evacuation, ligation of hematoma
  - Curettage: Retained placental fragments

Nursing Management

Goal: Minimize blood loss.

- Notify physician promptly of abnormal assessment findings.
- Send blood work stat, as directed to determine blood loss and etiology.
- Fundal massage.
- Empty urinary bladder.
- Administer uterotonic medications as ordered. For ergot products and carboplast, monitor blood pressure.
- Start and monitor supplemental oxygen.

Goal: Stabilize status.

- Establish or maintain IV line.
- Administer medications as ordered to control bleeding, combat shock.
- Prepare for surgery, if indicated.

Goal: Prevent infection.

- Strict aseptic technique.

Goal: Continual monitoring: vital signs, bleeding (pad count or weigh pads, examine clots and tissue), fundal status, oxygenation, vasoconstriction, level of consciousness, urinary output.

Goal: Prevent or detect sequelae.

- Sheehan's syndrome (rare syndrome of hypopituitarism from decreased blood flow to pituitary gland in severe postpartum hemorrhage).
- Disseminated intravascular coagulation: Diffuse or widespread coagulation characterized by excessive clotting and bleeding (50% caused by obstetrical complications).

Goal: Health teaching.

- After episode reinforce perineal care, hand washing, iron supplements of other medications as ordered, adequate fluid and nutrition, monitor energy level, signs of infection or other complications.

Evaluation/Outcome Criteria

- Maternal vital signs are stable
- Bleeding is diminished or absent
- Normal diagnostic test results
- No complications (e.g., infection, thrombophlebitis, DIC)

REVIEW QUESTIONS

1. Define early PPH.
   Answer:

2. Is there a standard definition of PPH?
   Answer:

3. If not, how does that affect the ability to intervene appropriately?
   Answer:

4. Describe three potential causes of early PPH. Fill in the chart below.
   Answer:

Type	Assessment Data	Precipitating Factors	Treatment

5. List at least two potential consequences or sequelae of PPH.
Answer:

Related Evidence-Based Practice Guidelines

American College of Obstetricians and Gynecologists (ACOG). (2006, October). Postpartum hemorrhage. (ACOG Practice Bulletin No. 76). Washington, DC: Author.

Compendium of postpartum care (2nd ed) (2006). Association of Women's Health, Obstetric, and Neonatal Nurses

The Joint Commission National Patient Safety Goals Hospital Program. Retrieved from http://www.jointcommission.org/generalpublic/npsg/10_npsgs.htm

SBAR technique for communication: A situational briefing model. The Institute for Health Care. Retrieved December 19, 2008, from http://www.ihi.org/IHI/Topics/PatientSafety/SafetyGeneral/Tools/SBARTechniqueforCommunication ASituationalBriefingModel.htm

Topics to Review Prior to the Simulation

- Postpartum assessment and nursing care
- Obstetrical risk factors for developing postpartum hemorrhage
- Nursing interventions for a patient with postpartum hemorrhage
- Pharmacological (oxytocic agents) and other medical interventions for a patient with PPH

SIMULATION

Client Background

Melissa Hanson is a 31-year-old G5T3P1A0L4 who delivered a 9 lb 10 oz female via forceps at 8 AM for a prolonged second stage over a mediolateral episiotomy after a 20 hr labor augmented with Pitocin. She had epidural anesthesia. Her estimated blood loss (EBL) was 500 cc. Baseline vitals signs included BP ranging from 120/80 to 128/92, P 70, RR 12.

Biographical Data

- Age: 31
- Gender: female
- Height: 5 ft 6 in
- Weight: 120 lb

Cultural Considerations

- Language: English
- Ethnicity: Norwegian/German
- Nationality: American
- Culture: no significant cultural considerations identified

Demographic

- Marital status: married
- Educational level: high school graduate, technical school
- Religion: Lutheran
- Occupation: medical technician

Current Health Status

- Post forceps delivery

History

- Psychosocial history
  - Social support: husband, five children
- Past health history
  - Medical: not significant
  - Surgical: tonsillectomy
- Family History: not significant

Admission Sheet

Name:	Melissa Hanson
Age:	31
Gender:	Female
Marital Status:	Married
Educational Level:	High school graduate, technical school
Religion:	Lutheran
Ethnicity:	Norwegian/German
Nationality:	United States citizen
Language:	English
Occupation:	Medical technician

Hospital Provider's Orders		Patient's Name: Melissa Hanson Allergies: Aspirin	
Diagnosis: Vaginal delivery, forceps			
Date	**Time**	**Order**	**Signature**
		Admit to mother/baby unit	
		Vital signs: q ½ hr, then q 4 hr × 24, then q 8 hr	
		Diet: Regular	
		Activity: ad lib as tolerated, may shower when stable and ambulatory	
		IV therapy: Lactated Ringer's solution (LR) at 125 mL/hr, DC when vital signs are stable, vaginal bleeding normal, and tolerating po fluids well Add oxytocin 10 units to IV immediately after delivery of placenta	
		Medications: Dermoplast spray to hemorrhoids, episiotomy prn if requested, as often as 6 × per hr Tucks pads at bedside prn for hemorrhoids, may be applied to rectum as often as 6 × per hr Bisacodyl (Dulcolax) suppository 10 mg or Fleet Enema daily prn for constipation, if requested Colace tab 1 po at bedtime prn for constipation, if requested Magnesium hydroxide/aluminum hydroxide/simethicone (Maalox) 30 mL po, if requested, as often as 1 × per hr for indigestion Prenatal vitamin 1 po daily as dietary supplement Ibuprofen (Motrin) 800 mg po q 8 hr prn for cramping pain Acetaminophen (Tylenol) 325 mg 1–2 tab po q 3 hr prn for mild to moderate pain Oxycodone/acetaminophen (Percocet) 5/325 mg 1–2 tab po q 4 hr for severe pain Zolpidem (Ambien) 5 mg po at bedtime prn for sleep, if requested	
		RhoGam if RH negative and eligible	
		Rubella immunization per protocol if eligible	
		Diagnostic studies: CBC 24 hr postpartum	
		Treatments: Ice to perineum × 12 hr postpartum	
		Sitz bath q 4 hr after 12 hr for perineal discomfort	Dr. Ellis

Nursing Report

Report on admission to mother/baby unit: Ms. Hanson is being admitted to mother/baby 2 hr after delivery. She has an IV of 1,000 mL LR with 20 units of Pitocin at 125 mL/hr to be discontinued when finished if stable and tolerating po fluids. Her vital signs 30 min ago were T 99, BP 130/90, P 80, slightly weaker, RR 14, and deep, skin cool and pale, urinary output—has not voided since delivery. She is alert, oriented, and mildly anxious. Her husband is in the nursery. Pericare completed and peripads changed at 9 AM.

Student Simulation Prep Assignments

1. Identify items and their purpose in the care of a patient with PPH.

Item	Purpose
Airway and suction equipment	
Blood pressure cuff	
Blood products	
Chux pads/peripads	
Foley catheter	
Gloves	
IV equipment and solutions	
Medications	
Oxygen equipment	
Pulse oximeter	
Specimen tubes	
Stethoscope	

2. Identify team members and their specific roles in the care of a patient with PPH.

Team member	Role
Physician	
Anesthesiologist or nurse anesthetist	
Primary nurse	
Respiratory therapist	
UAP	

3. Relevant Data Exercise: Fill in the columns below.

Relevant Data from Background and Report	Relevant Data from Other Sources	Data Missing	Sources for Missing Data	Data Requiring Follow-up

Relevant Data from Background and Report	Relevant Data from Other Sources	Data Missing	Sources for Missing Data	Data Requiring Follow-up

4. *Initial Focused Assessment*

After reviewing the client background and nursing report, you are ready to assess your client's current status. Under each category, identify how you would target your assessment and what you would expect to find for the patient with PPH.

History

Are there any questions you need to ask the patient or family to obtain additional relevant data?

Physical Exam

- General appearance:
- Integumentary:
- HEENT:
- Respiratory:
- CV:
- Breasts:
- Abdominal:
- Neuro:
- Musculoskeletal:
- Reproductive:
- Additional:
- Developmental

What are the nursing implications considering the developmental stage of your patient?

Answer:

5. *Diagnostic Tests*

What diagnostic test results relevant to the patient's current problem are needed to plan care?

Complete the table using Van leeuwen et al, *Davis's Comprehensive Handbook of Laboratory and Diagnostic Testing with Nursing Implications* 4e, or other diagnostic test reference.

Diagnostic Test	Significance to This Patient's Problem
Hgb	
Hct	

6. *Treatment*

Identify drugs that are used to treat a patient with PPH.

Complete the table using Deglin et al, *Davis's Drug Guide for Nurses* 12e, or other drug reference.

Medication	Dose, Route, Frequency	Indications (reason ordered for this client)	Side Effects	Nursing Implications
Pitocin (oxytocin)	IM: 10–20 units (1–2 mL) after delivery of the placenta			

Continued

Medication	Dose, Route, Frequency	Indications (reason ordered for this client)	Side Effects	Nursing Implications
	Intravenous infusion (drip method): If the patient has an intravenous infusion of LR or NSS running, 10–40 units of oxytocin may be added to the bag, depending on the amount of solution remaining (maximum 40 units to 1,000 mL). Adjust the infusion rate to sustain uterine contraction and control uterine atony (125–200 mU/min)			
Methergine (methylergonovine)	po 200–400 mcg (0.4–0.6 mg) q 6–12 hr for 2–7 days IM, IV (rarely given IV, emergencies only, 200 mcg (0.2 mg) q 2–4 hr for up to 5 doses			

Medication	Dose, Route, Frequency	Indications (reason ordered for this client)	Side Effects	Nursing Implications
Cytotec (misoprostol)	0.8 mg rectally × 1			
Hemabate (carboprost tromethamine)	IM or intramyometrially 250 mcg (0.25 mg) of Hemabate sterile solution (1 mL). Can be repeated at intervals of 15–90 min per physician order The total dose should not exceed 2 mg (8 doses)			

7. Nursing Problems/Diagnoses

Identify three priority nursing problems/diagnoses for a patient with PPH.

Assessment Data	Priority Problem	Intervention	Expected Patient Outcome	Which Interventions Could be Delegated to Unlicensed Personnel?
1.				
2.				
3.				

Assessment Data	Priority Problem	Intervention	Expected Patient Outcome	Which Interventions Could be Delegated to Unlicensed Personnel?

References

American College of Obstetricians and Gynecologists (ACOG). (2006, October). *Postpartum hemorrhage.* (ACOG Practice Bulletin No. 76). Washington, DC: ACOG.

Benedetti, T. (2002). Obstetric hemorrhage. In S. Gabbe, J. Niebyl, & J. Simpson (Eds.). *Obstetrics: Normal and problem pregnancies* (4th ed.). New York: Churchill Livingstone.

Briggs, G.G., & Wan, S. R. (2006). Drug therapy during labor: Postpartum hemmorhage. *American Journal of Health-System Pharmacy*. *63*(12), 1131–1139. Retrieved June 16, 2008, from http://www.medscape.com/viewarticle/535774_6

Buckland, S. S., & Homer, C. S. (2007) Estimating blood loss after birth: Using simulated clinical examples. *Women Birth*, *20*(2), 85–88.

Cesario, S.K., Beck, C, Creehan, P., Watts, N. & Santa-Donata, A. *Compendium of postpartum care* (2nd ed.). (2006). Washington DC: Association of Women's Health, Obstetric, and Neonatal Nurses. & Johnson and Johnson Consumer Companies.

Deglin, J. H., & Vallerand, A. H. (2009). *Davis's drug guide for nurses* (11th ed.). Philadelphia: F. A. Davis.

Dillon, P. (2007). *Nursing health assessment: A critical thinking and case studies approach* (2nd ed.). Philadelphia: F. A. Davis.

Erikson, E. H. (1950). *Childhood and society*. New York: Norton.

Glover, P. (2003). Blood loss at delivery: How accurate is your estimation? *Australian journal of midwifery*, *16*(2), 21–24.

Lagerquist, S. L. (2006). *Davis's NCLEX-RN for success.* Philadelphia: F. A. Davis.

Lowdermilk, D. L., & Perry, S. H. (2007). *Maternity and women's health care* (9th ed.). St. Louis: Mosby.

Magann, E. F., Evans, S., Hutchinson, M., Collins, R., Howard, B., & Morrison, J. (2005). Postpartum hemorrhage after vaginal birth: An analysis of risk factors. *Southern Medical journal*, *98*(4), 419–422.

Van Leeuwen, A. M. & Poelhuis-Leth, D.J., & Bladh, M.L. (2011). *Davis's comprehensive handbook of laboratory and diagnostic tests with nursing implications* (4th ed.). Philadelphia: F. A. Davis.

3-2 Immediate Newborn Assessment

MATERNAL/CHILD

STANDARD FORMS

These templates are included in the Appendix; copy before each use.

LEARNING OUTCOMES

Cognitive

The student will be able to:

1. Determine essential assessments for the newborn with no respiratory effort upon delivery and correctly perform assessments specific to the client's priority needs in a coordinated and timely manner based on data and setting resources:
   - Interpret mother-of-baby labor history (including admit lab results) for significant factors that will influence the newborn's physiological status.
   - Perform a safety check of supplies and equipment in anticipation of newborn delivery.
   - Rapid assessment of newborn breathing, circulation, color, and tone.
2. Analyze assessment data and identify the appropriate interventions for the newborn that will address priority actions specific to client's physiological status and setting resources.
3. Engage in purposeful, efficient information sharing and plan of care implementation and evaluation when necessary.

Psychomotor

The student will be able to:

1. Demonstrate timely and efficient integration of newborn nursing interventions specific to health patterns to promote oxygenation, hydration, and skin integrity.
   - Dry, stimulate, and correctly position the newborn.
   - Administer oxygen: appropriate O_2 delivery device, rate, and flow.
   - Assign APGAR score.
   - Manage newborn thermoregulation needs.
   - Administer newborn medications when newborn is stable (AquaMEPHYTON and erythromycin eye ointment).
2. Guide and support newborn's family through the experience with communication and learning strategies specific to learning readiness, culture, age, and education level. Provides family with explanation for the following:
   - Oxygen delivery
   - Thermoregulation needs of newborn
   - Medications
3. Document and evaluate care to support continuity of care and patient outcomes.

Affective

The student will be able to:

1. Critique personal actions using a nursing framework in adapting a plan of care specific to the changing client story and setting resources.
2. Reflect upon performance in the care of a newborn with no respiratory effort
3. Discuss feelings related to working as a member of a team in the care of a newborn with no respiratory effort.
4. Identify factors that worked well during the simulation.
5. Identify factors that needed improvement during the simulation.

Communication

The student will be able to:

1. Communicate effectively with healthcare team members utilizing the SBAR reporting format.
   - Dialogue with peers, faculty, and/or charge nurse regarding client condition.
2. Communicate effectively with the newborn's family in the care of a newborn immediately following delivery.
3. Practice Transparent Thinking (thinking out loud) to facilitate group problem solving
4. Use Directed Communication (directing a message to specific individual) when delegating tasks.
5. Employ Closed loop Communication (acknowledgment of receipt of the message and status) to acknowledge communications from others.

Safety

The student will be able to:

Administer and maintain specific protecting interventions with attention to safety of the client and healthcare professional.

1. Demonstrate a safe environment with attention to hazards to employees, visitors and the client. Includes body mechanics, tripping hazards, equipment issues.
2. Demonstrate attention to national patient safety goals. Includes patient identification standards (placing newborn identification bands), and effective communication among healthcare providers, and safe medication administration.
3. Demonstrate attention to standard precautions. Includes hand washing, infection control measures, and use of PPE as needed.

Leadership and Management/Delegation

The student will be able to:

1. Identify tasks that can be legally, ethically, and safely delegated to unlicensed assistive personnel (UAP) or licensed practical nurse (LPN) in the care of a newborn immediately following delivery..
2. Identify and prioritize patient's needs in care of in the care of a newborn immediately following delivery.

OVERVIEW OF THE PROBLEM

Nursing Management of the Neonate Immediately after Birth

Effective nursing management of the newborn immediately following birth is dependent on a skilled nursing assessment. The nurse not only examines the neonate, but collects data from maternal history, including labor and delivery events, that impact neonatal health status.

Assessment

Objective

- Airway—mucus in nasopharynx, oropharynx
- APGAR score
- Number of cord vessels
- Passage of meconium stool, urine
- General physical appearance/status
  - Signs of respiratory distress
  - Skin condition
  - Cry
  - Signs of birth injury
  - General survey—body symmetry, anomalies
  - Gestational age factors
- Identify high-risk infant

Diagnostic Tests

- Blood type and RH
- Coombs test
- Cord blood gases
- Blood sugar

Nursing Management

- Ensure patent airway
- Maintain body temperature
- Identify infant
- Prevent eye infection
- Facilitate prompt identification and treatment of potential complications

Evaluation/Outcome Criteria

Successful transition to extrauterine life:

- Assessment findings within normal limits
- Responsive in bonding process with parent

REVIEW QUESTIONS

1. Review the maternal labor history and maternal admit labs. What information would indicate this newborn is at risk for respiratory depression upon birth?
   Answer:

2. What are the initial priorities in immediate care of the newborn?
   Answer:

3. Immediately after birth, the newborn is dried. Wet linen is removed and the baby is wrapped in warm blankets or placed under a radiant warmer. What is the rationale for this?
   Answer:

4. Why is it important to prevent hypothermia in the immediate newborn period? What metabolic and physiological demands does hypothermia impose?
   Answer:

5. What are the normal vital sign parameters in a term newborn?
   Answer:

6. List five signs of respiratory distress in the newborn.
   Answer:

7. What physiological assessments are conducted when evaluating the APGAR score on a newborn?
   Answer:

8. What does an APGAR score of 0–3 indicate?
   Answer:

Related Evidence-Based Practice Guidelines

American Academy of Pediatrics. Summary of Major Changes to the 2005 AAP/AHA Emergency Cardiovascular Care Guidelines for Neonatal Resuscitation. Retrieved July 2007, from www.C2005.org

National Guideline Clearing House. Neonatal resuscitation: 2005 International Consensus Conference on Cardiopulmonary Resuscitation and Emergency Cardiovascular Care Science with Treatment Recommendations. Retrieved July 2007, from www.guideline.gov

The Joint Commission National Patient Safety Goals Hospital Program. Retrieved from http://www.jointcommission.org/GeneralPublic/NPSG/10

SBAR technique for communication: A situational briefing model. The Institute for Health Care Improvement. Retrieved December 19, 2008, from http://www.ihi.org/IHI/Topics/PatientSafety/SafetyGeneral/Tools/SBARTechniqueforCommunicationASituationalBriefingModel.htm

Topics to Review Prior to the Simulation

- Normal newborn physiological transition
- Newborn assessment and care
- CPR for healthcare workers
- Pharmacology and medication administration (all routes).

SIMULATION

Client Background

Baby Boy Duyck was just born to Kristi and Joe Duyck at 39 5/7 weeks gestation. Kristi is a 28-year-old administrative secretary at a local court house. She is a G3P3 (with this birth). She had an uneventful pregnancy. She began prenatal care at 12 weeks' gestation. During the pregnancy, she took prenatal vitamins and rarely a Tylenol for lower back pain. Her CBC and metabolic profile lab results on admission were within normal limits. Kristi was admitted 4 hr ago for labor. Upon admission, her SVE (sterile vaginal exam) was 3 cm/70% effaced/−2 station. Kristi managed her pain during labor with nonpharmacological means, including deep breathing, jacuzzi, birth ball, and massage. Joe was present and supportive throughout the labor. Kristi's water broke spontaneously 20 min prior to birth and the fluid was clear. Another SVE was performed after the water broke and documented as 6–7 cm/100% effaced/0 station. Kristi then asked for pain medication (rated her pain as 10/10 in the pubic region) and was given Stadol (butorphanol) 2 mg IV which reduced her pain to 3/10. Within 5 min of receiving the Stadol, she reported that she needed to push. FHTs were 110, minimal long-term variability (LTV) with early decelerations. Uterine contractions were every 2 min, 60-sec duration, and palpated firm. SVE revealed the following: Complete/100% effaced/+1 station. Dr. Bragdon was called to attend the delivery.

Admission Sheet (Mother)

Name:	Kristi Duyck
Age:	28
Gender:	Female
Marital Status:	Married
Educational Level:	Associate degree in business
Religion:	Catholic
Ethnicity:	Polish heritage
Nationality:	American
Language:	English
Occupation:	Administrative assistant

Hospital
Provider's Orders

Patient's Name: Baby Duyck
Allergies: NKDA

Diagnosis: Term newborn

Date	Time	Order	Signature
		Routine newborn care	
		Physician's Order Record and Nursing Protocol	
		Admission: Follow protocols for blood glucose, state metabolic screening, substance abuse, and hearing screening	

Diagnosis: Term newborn—cont'd

Date	Time	Order	Signature
		24% sucrose via pacifier prn painful procedures	
		Call office or exchange for low-risk infant	
		Call attending physician immediately for the following: Sick infant, Infant less than 35 5/7 weeks gestation or less than 2,000 g (and admit to nursery), Infant at increased risk of sepsis, Infant's mother received intrapartum antibiotics, Infant's mother received group B streptococcus (GBS) prophylaxis less than 4 hr before delivery,	
		Resuscitation: Follow Neonatal Resuscitation Program guidelines for resuscitation	
		If infant required positive-pressure ventilation (PPV) for depressed respiratory effort or has a 5 min APGAR of less than 7: Obtain cord arterial and venous blood gases	
		Obtain a capillary blood glucose per unit protocol	
		Medications: Weight: ___ g AquaMEPHYTON 1 mg IM by 1 hr of age Erythromycin ophthalmic ointment 0.5% to both eyes by 1 hr of age Zinc oxide 10% prn diaper rash	
		Diet: Breast-feeding and supplementation per protocol	
		Respiratory: If infant is cyanotic, administer oxygen to keep oxygen saturation 92–98% If oxygen is administered longer than 15 min, notify physician.	Dr Bragdon

Nursing Report

Begin simulation with SBAR report. Tell the students the time is 2147 and they are attending the birth of a baby. The primary nurse's role is "baby nurse" (this nurse has responsibility of performing rapid newborn assessment, beginning resuscitation efforts, coordinating care, and assigning APGAR score).

Situation: Baby Boy Duyck is going to be born soon. Mother is complete and is having a hard time breathing to prevent pushing while we are waiting for the doctor to get here.

Background: Mrs. Duyck is a 28-year-old G3P2. Her water broke 20 min ago and the fluid was clear. After her water broke, her pain was 10/10 and her cervix was 7 cm/100% effaced/0 station, and she was requesting pain medication. She was medicated with Stadol 2 mg IV 15 min ago.

Assessment: FHTs are 110 with minimal long-term variability. Early decelerations are present. The amniotic fluid is clear. Mrs. Duyck's pain level is now 3/10. She is c/o of the urge to bear down. Contractions are every 2 min, palpate firm, 60-sec duration.

Recommendation: I already set up the newborn equipment (suction and oxygen), the medications and the chart are in the room. Anticipate a depressed baby because of the Stadol and prepare to give oxygen and perhaps Narcan.

Student Simulation Prep Assignments

1. Identify items and their purpose in an immediate newborn assessment.

Item	Purpose
Resuscitation bag and mask	
Oxygen source	
Suction catheter and suction source	
Radiant warmer	
Stethoscope	
Medications and supplies	

2. Identify team members and specific roles necessary to provide care for a newborn immediately after delivery.

Team Members	Role
Nurse	
Charge nurse	
Staff nurses	
Physician	

3. *Relevant Data Exercise:* Fill in the columns below.

Relevant Data from Background and Report	Relevant Data from Other Sources	Data Missing	Sources for Missing Data	Data Requiring Follow-up

4. Initial Focused Assessment

After reviewing the client background and nursing report, you are ready to assess your client's current status. Under each category, identify how you would target your assessment, and what you would expect to find for the newborn immediately following delivery.

History

Term gestation, uncomplicated pregnancy, lab values do not indicate infection or anemic condition, clear amniotic fluid. Anticipate normal newborn with the exception of the mother receiving Stadol 2 mg so close to delivery.

Are there any questions you need to ask the patient or family to obtain additional relevant data?

Physical Exam

- General appearance:
- Integumentary:
- HEENT:
- Respiratory:
- CV:
- Breasts.
- Abdominal:
- Musculoskeletal:
- Neuro:
- Reproductive:
- Renal:
- Genitourinary:

What are the nursing implications considering the developmental stage of your patient?

Answer:

5. Diagnostic Tests

What maternal diagnostic test results need review to anticipate the condition of the newborn?

Complete the table using Van Leeuwen et al, *Davis's Comprehensive Handbook of Laboratory and Diagnostic Testing with Nursing Implications* 4e, or other diagnostic test reference.

Maternal Lab Values

Diagnostic Test	Maternal Admit Labs	Significance to This Patient's Problem
CBC		
Electrolytes		

6. Treatment

Identify drugs that are used during the immediate newborn period.

Complete the table using Deglin et al, *Davis's Drug Guide for Nurses* 12e, or other drug reference.

Medication	Dose, Route, Frequency	Indications	Side Effect	Nursing Implications
Narcan (naloxone)	0.01 mg/kg IM or SQ As needed for neonatal respiratory depression following maternal narcotic administration			

Continued

Medication	Dose, Route, Frequency	Indications	Side Effect	Nursing Implications
AquaMEPHYTON (phytonadione)	0.5–10 mg IM within 1 hr of birth			
Erythromycin eye ointment	0.5% both eyes within hr of birth			

7. Nursing Problems/Diagnoses

Identify three priority nursing problems/diagnoses. Complete for each problem identified.

Assessment Data	Priority Problem	Intervention	Expected Patient Outcome	Which Interventions Could be Delegated to Unlicensed Personnel?
1.				
2				
3.				

References

American Academy of Pediatrics. Summary of Major Changes to the 2005 AAP/AHA. *Emergency cardiovascular care guidelines for neonatal resuscitation.* Retrieved July 2007, from www.C2005.org

Deglin, J. H., Vallerand, A. H. (2009). *Davis's drug guide for nurses* (11th ed.). Philadelphia: F. A. Davis.

Dillon, P. (2007). *Nursing health assessment: A critical thinking and case studies approach* (2nd ed.). Philadelphia: F. A. Davis.

Erikson, E. H. (1950). *Childhood and society*. New York: Norton.

Lagerquist, S. (2006). *NCLEX-RN for success.* Philadelphia: F. A. Davis.

National Guideline Clearing House. *Neonatal resuscitation: 2005 International Consensus Conference on Cardiopulmonary Resuscitation and Emergency Cardiovascular Care Science with Treatment Recommendations.* Retrieved July 2007, from www.guideline.gov

Olds, S., London, M., Ladewig, P., & Davidson, M. (2007). *Maternal-newborn nursing and women's health care* (7th ed.). Redwood City, CA: Addison-Wesley.

Van Leeuwen, A. M., Poelhuis-Leth, D. J., & Bladh, M. L. (2011). *Davis's comprehensive handbook of laboratory and diagnostic tests with nursing implications* (4th ed.). Philadelphia: F. A. Davis.

3-3 Dystocia

MATERNITY NURSING

STANDARD FORMS

These templates are included in the Appendix; copy before each use.

LEARNING OUTCOMES

Cognitive

The student will be able to:

1. Describe signs of normal labor progress.
2. Recognize signs and symptoms of dystocia.
3. Identify factors in a patient's history that increase risk for dystocia.
4. Identify the appropriate interventions for the patient with dystocia.
5. Identify risks to the patient and fetus associated with dystocia and its treatment.
6. Differentiate the roles of team members in response to a patient with dystocia.

Psychomotor

The student will be able to:

1. Perform an appropriate assessment for a patient with dystocia.
2. Initiate appropriate interventions for a patient with dystocia.
3. Work collaboratively as part of the healthcare team in the care of a patient with dystocia.

Affective

The student will be able to:

1. Reflect upon performance in the care of a patient with dystocia.
2. Identify personal feelings in delivering care to a patient with dystocia.
3. Discuss feelings related to working as a member of a team in the care of a patient with dystocia.
4. Identify factors that worked well during the simulation of care of a patient with dystocia.
5. Identify factors that needed improvement during the simulation of care of a patient with dystocia.
6. Develop self-confidence in the care of a patient with dystocia.

Communication

The student will be able to:

1. Communicate effectively with healthcare team members in care of a patient with dystocia.
2. Communicate effectively with the patient and family in the care of a patient with dystocia.
3. Use SBAR when communication with team members in the care of a patient with dystocia
4. Practice Transparent Thinking (thinking out loud) to facilitate group problem solving.
5. Use Directed Communication (directing a message to specific individual) when delegating tasks.
6. Employ Closed-Loop Communication (acknowledgment of receipt of the message and status) to acknowledge communications from others.

Safety

The student will be able to:

Administer and maintain specific protecting interventions with attention to safety of the client and healthcare professional.

1. Demonstrate a safe environment with attention to hazards to healthcare providers, visitors, and the client. Includes body mechanics, tripping hazards, and equipment issues.
2. Demonstrate attention to national patient safety goals. Includes patient identification standards, effective communication among healthcare providers, and safe medication administration.
3. Demonstrate attention to standard precautions. Includes hand washing, infection control measures, and use of personal protective equipment (PPE) as needed.

Leadership and Management/Delegation

The student will be able to:

1. Identify tasks that can be legally, ethically, and safely delegated to unlicensed assistive personnel (UAP) or licensed practical nurse (LPN) in the care of a patient with dystocia.
2. Identify and prioritize patient's needs in care of dystocia.

OVERVIEW OF THE PROBLEM

Definition

Dystocia refers to difficult or dysfunctional labor.

Pathophysiology

Interference with the normal processes and patterns of labor that may result in maternal or fetal jeopardy. Factors affecting the labor process are related to the six Ps: Powers, Passenger, Passageway, Position, Placenta, and Psychoemotional. In hypotonic dysfunction, contractions diminish in frequency, duration, and intensity, with lowered resting tone. Cervical effacement and dilatation are slowed.

Risk Factors

- Physiological response to anxiety/fear/pain
- Premature or excessive analgesia
- Maternal factors
  - Pelvic size and shape
  - Uterine or cervical abnormalities
  - Contraction ring
  - Hypertonic or hypotonic contraction patterns
  - PPROM, infection
  - Prolonged first- or second-stage labor
  - Maternal medical conditions
- Fetal factors
  - Macrosomia
  - Malpresentation, compound presentation (multifetal) or malposition
  - Congenital anomalies
  - Prolapsed cord
  - Postterm
- Placental
  - Placenta previa
  - Placental abruption
  - Placenta accreta
  - Inadequate placental perfusion

In hypotonic dysfunction, risk factors are most likely to include:

- Premature or excessive analgesia/anesthesia
- Cephalopelvic disproportion
- Overdistention of the uterus
- Fetal mal position or malpresentation
- Maternal fear or anxiety

Assessment

- Antepartal history
- Emotional status
- Maternal vitals signs
- FHR pattern
- Contraction pattern
- Vaginal discharge

Assessment of Hypotonic Dysfunction

- Onset: may be in latent, but most common during active phase
- Contractions
  - Decreased frequency
  - Shorter duration
  - Diminished intensity
  - Less uncomfortable
- Cervical changes slow or cease
- Signs of fetal distress may occur (rare)
- Maternal vital signs: fever may indicate infection
- Medical diagnosis: procedures: vaginal exam

Treatment

- Amniotomy
- Oxytocin augmentation
- If CPD, cesarean birth

Nursing Management

Goals:

- Minimize physical and psychological stress.
- Provide emotional support.
- Maintain continuous monitoring of maternal/fetal status and labor progress.
- Minimize effects of complicated labor on mother and fetus.

Evaluation/Outcome Criteria

- Restablishes normal labor pattern.
- Stable maternal status.
- Experiences successful birth of viable, healthy infant.
- Woman verbalizes understanding of process, rationale, procedures, and alternatives.

REVIEW QUESTIONS

1. Define hypotonic dysfunction during labor.
   Answer:

2. List five potential causes of hypotonic dysfunction in labor.
   Answer:

3. What medication might be used to treat hypotonic dysfunction in labor?
   Answer:

4. What potential causes of hypotonic dysfunction in labor must be ruled out before oxytocin is given?
   Answer:

5. List two other possible medical interventions for hypotonic dysfunction in labor.
   Answer:

6. What risks are associated with amniotomy?
Answer:

Related Evidence-Based Practice Guidelines

American College of Obstetricians and Gynecologists (ACOG). (2003, December). *Dystocia and augmentation of labor.* (ACOG Practice Bulletin No. 49). Washington, DC: ACOG.

American College of Obstetricians and Gynecologists (ACOG). (2005, December). Intrapartum fetal heart rate monitoring. (ACOG Practice Bulletin No. 70). Washington, DC: ACOG. (2009).

Fetal heart monitoring principles & practices (4th ed.). AWHONN.

Institute for Clinical Systems Improvement (ICSI). (2007, March). Management of labor. Bloomington, MN: ICSI.

Mayberry, L., Wood, S. H., Laura, B., Strange, L.B., Lily, L., Heisler, D. R, et al. (2000). Second-stage labor management: Promotion of evidence-based practice and a collaborative approach to patient care. AWHONN.

The Joint Commission National Patient Safety Goals Hospital Program. Retrieved from http://www.jointcommission.org/GeneralPublic/NPSG/10

SBAR technique for communication: A situational briefing model. The Institute for Health Care Improvement. Retrieved December 19, 2008, from http://www.ihi.org/IHI/Topics/PatientSafety/SafetyGeneral/Tools/SBARTechniqueforCommunicationASituationalBriefingModel.htm

Simpson, K. R. (2002). Cervical ripening & induction & augmentation of labor (2nd ed.). AWHONN

Topics to Review Prior to the Simulation

- Labor progress
- Abnormal labor patterns
- Intrapartum assessment and nursing care
- Risk factors for developing abnormal labor patterns
- Nursing interventions that are used for a patient with abnormal labor patterns
- Risks to the patient and fetus associated with abnormal labor patterns and their treatment
- Pharmacological and other medical interventions for a patient with abnormal labor patterns

SIMULATION

Client Background

Ming Rong, 26, met her American husband 2 yr ago when he was working in China. She is from a traditional Chinese family and married and immigrated to the United States last year. Although Ming agreed to move to the United States because of her husband's job, she misses her family. Ming's mother will be staying with them until after the birth of the baby. Both Ming and her husband, Brian, speak English and Chinese. Ming's mother speaks only Chinese. Brian is very supportive, and gets along well with Ming's mother but sometimes he seems ashamed of her traditional beliefs. Options for pain control during labor have been explained to Ming Rong, and although she has pain, she has declined pharmacological pain relief. Her past medical and family history is unremarkable.

Biographical Data

- Age: 26
- Gender: female
- Height: 5 ft 2 in
- weight: 100 lbs

Cultural Considerations

- Language: Chinese and English
- Ethnicity: Chinese
- Nationality: Chinese, recent immigrant to United States
- Culture: From a traditional Chinese family. The traditional Chinese woman may believe pain is an expected part of childbirth, and bearing that pain may be seen as a means of spiritual growth or the price paid for having a baby. These beliefs may influence whether or not she requests or accepts medication or other alternatives for pain control.
- In the post partum period, the nurse should assess for traditional postnatal practices such as *zuo yuezi,* which may involve dietary precautions, avoiding leaving the home, avoiding housework and limiting visitors; hygiene precautions (avoiding bathing and washing hair), supplementary feeding, and giving honeysuckle herb to the infant.

Demographic

- Marital status: married
- Educational level: Master's degree
- Religion: not known
- Occupation: interpreter

Current Health Status

- Active labor

History

- Psychosocial history
  - Social support: husband, mother staying until after birth of baby
- Past health history: unremarkable
  - Medical
  - Surgical
- Family history: unremarkable

Admission Sheet

Name:	Ming Rong Haus
Age:	26
Gender:	Female
Marital Status:	Married
Educational Level:	Master's degree
Religion:	Not identified
Ethnicity:	Chinese
Nationality:	Chinese, recent immigrant to United States
Language:	Chinese, English
Occupation:	Interpreter

Hospital
Provider's Orders

Patient's Name: **Ming Rong Haus**
Allergies: **Latex**

Diagnosis: **Intrauterine pregnancy**

Date	Time	Order	Signature
		Admit Inpatient to L and D	
		Vital signs: Per protocol	
		Diet: Clear liquids early labor, ice chips active labor	
		Activity: prn	
		IV therapy: LR at 125 mL/hr	
		Fetal monitoring according to standard unless otherwise ordered	
		Medications: Stadol 1 mg slow IV q 4 hr prn moderate to severe pain Epidural if desired Ampicillin 2 g IV, then 1 g IV q 4 hr until delivery	
		Diagnostic studies: Ultrasound for estimated fetal weight RPR, HIV prn	
		Treatments: Straight catheter prn for bladder distention	
		Remove epidural catheter prior to transfer to the postpartum unit unless other wise ordered by physician	Dr. Lane

Nursing Report

7 AM. Ming Rong Haus, G1, P0, 38 weeks' gestation has been in active labor for 2 hr. She is 5 cm dilated, 80% effaced, and station −3. She has made no progress in dilation or descent for the past 2 hr. Has not voided (HNV) since admission at 3 AM. Membranes ruptured 12 hr ago. The external fetal monitor shows a pattern of contractions 2–4 min apart lasting 60–90 sec, strong intensity by palpation. The fetal heart baseline is in the 140s with average variability and accelerations with contractions. T 99 at 4 AM, P 76, RR 19, BP 110/70 now. She has refused pain medication or an epidural. Her mother and husband are with her. She is positive for GBS, other labs are unremarkable. Her last dose of ampicillin was given at 4 AM. She has an IV of 1,000 cc LR at 125 cc/hr. She is allergic to latex.

Active Labor Assessment Protocol

- T q 4 hr
- BP, P, RR q 30 min (q 15 min if receiving oxytocin)
- Uterine activity q 15–30 min (q 15 min if receiving oxytocin)
- FHR q 15–30 min (q 15 min if receiving oxytocin)
- Intake and output q 4 hr
- Vaginal discharge q 30 min
- Behavior q 15 min
- Vaginal exam as needed to assess progress

Oxytocin Dosage Protocol

- Administer with infusion pump, 10 units of oxytocin in 1,000 cc isotonic electrolyte solution, via secondary IV
- Oxytocin secondary tubing is piggybacked to primary tubing at port closest to veinipuncture
- Oxytocin solution is labeled
- Begin at 2 mU/min
- Increase at 2 mU/min at 15- 30 min intervals until adequate progress and uterine activity pattern achieved

Student Simulation Prep Assignments

1. *Identify items and their purpose in the care of a patient with dystocia.*

Item	Purpose
Fetal monitor	
Catheter kit	
BP cuff	
Thermometer	
Stethoscope	

2. *Identify team members and their specific roles in the care of a patient with dystocia.*

Team Member	Role
Primary nurse	
Physician	

3. *Relevant Data Exercise:* Fill in the columns below.

Relevant Data from Report	Relevant Data from Other Sources	Data Missing	Sources for Missing Data	Data Requiring Follow-up

Continued

Relevant Data from Report	Relevant Data from Other Sources	Data Missing	Sources for Missing Data	Data Requiring Follow-up

4. Initial Focused Assessment

After reviewing the client background and nursing report, you are ready to assess your client's current status. Under each category, identify how you would target your assessment and what you would expect to find for the patient with dystocia in active labor.

History

Are there any questions you need to ask the patient or family to obtain additional relevant data?

Physical Exam

- General appearance:
- Integumentary:
- HEENT:
- Respiratory:
- CV:
- Breasts:
- Abdominal:
- Neuro:
- Musculoskeletal:
- Reproductive:
- Additional:
- Developmental

What are the nursing implications considering the developmental stage of your patient?

Answer:

5. Diagnostic Tests

What diagnostic test results relevant to the patient's current problem are needed to plan care?

Complete the table using Van Leeuwen et al, *Davis's Comprehensive Handbook of Laboratory and Diagnostic Testing with Nursing Implications* 4e, or other diagnostic test reference.

Diagnostic Test	Significance to This Patient's Problem
GBS rectovaginal or urine culture	
Urine ketones dipstick	

6. Treatment

Identify drugs that are used to treat a patient with dystocia.

Complete the table using Deglin et al, *Davis's Drug Guide for Nurses* 12e, or other drug reference.

Medication	Dose, Route, Frequency	Indications	Side Effect	Nursing Implications
Oxytocin	0.5–2.0 Mu/min, increase by 1–2 Mu/min q 15–60 min until pattern established, then decrease			
Stadol	1 mg IV q 4 hr prn			
Ampicillin	2 g IV loading dose, followed by 1 g IV q 4 hr			

7. Nursing Problems/Diagnoses

Identify three priority nursing problems/diagnoses.

Assessment Data	Priority Problem	Intervention	Expected Patient Outcome	Which Interventions Could be Delegated to Unlicensed Personnel?
1.				
2.				
3.				

References

American College of Obstetricians and Gynecologists (ACOG). (2003, December). *Dystocia and augmentation of labor.* (ACOG Practice Bulletin No. 49). Washington, DC: ACOG.

American College of Obstetricians and Gynecologists (ACOG). (2010), *Intrapartum fetal heart rate monitoring.* (ACOG Practice Bulletin No. 49). Washington,DC: ACOG.

Calister, L.C., Khalaf, I., Semenic, S., Kartchner, R., & Vehvilainen-Julkunen, K. (2003) The Pain of Childbirth: Perceptions of culturally diverse women. *Pain Manag Nurse* (4)4. Retrieved October 26, 2010 from: http://www.medscape.com/viewarticle/465812_5

Deglin, J. H., Vallerand, A. H. (2009). *Davis's drug guide for nurses* (11th ed.). Philadelphia: F. A. Davis.

Dillon, P. (2007). *Nursing health assessment: A critical thinking and case studies approach* (2nd ed.). Philadelphia: F. A. Davis.

Erikson, E. H. (1950). *Childhood and society*. New York: Norton.

Fetal heart monitoring principles & practices (4th ed.) (2009). AWHONN.

Institute for Clinical Systems Improvement (ICSI). (2007). *Management of labor.* Bloomington, MN: ICSI.

Lagerquist, S. L. (2006). *Davis's NCLEX-RN for success* (2nd ed.). Philadelphia: F. A. Davis.

Lowdermilk, D. L., & Perry, S. H. (2007). *Maternity and women's health care* (9th ed.). St. Louis, MO: Mosby.

Mayberry, L., Wood, S. H., Laura, B., Strange, L. B., Lily, L., Heisler, D. R, et al. (2000). *Second-stage labor management: Promotion of evidence-based practice and a collaborative approach to patient care*. AWHONN.

Raven, J.H., Chen, Q., Tolhurst, R.J., & Garner, P. (2007) Traditional beliefs and practices in the postpartum period in Fujian Province, China: a qualitative study. BMC Pregnancy and Childbirth. Retrieved October 26 from: http://www.biomedcentral.com/1471-2393/7/8

Simpson, K. R. (2002). *Cervical ripening & induction & augmentation of labor* (2nd ed.). AWHONN.

Van Leeuwen, A. M., Poelhuis-Leth, D. J., & Bladh, M. L. (2011). *Davis's comprehensive handbook of laboratory and diagnostic tests with nursing implications.* (4th ed.). Philadelphia: F. A. Davis.

3-4 Thermoregulation and Hypoglycemia

MATERNAL NEWBORN

STANDARD FORMS

These templates are included in the Appendix; copy before each use.

LEARNING OUTCOMES

Cognitive

The student will be able to:

1. Describe signs and symptoms of hypothermia and hypoglycemia.
2. Correlate signs and symptoms of hypothermia and hypoglycemia to the pathophysiology of possible diagnosis including but not limited to sepsis, meningitis, prematurity, infant of diabetic mother, inborn error of metabolism, and cold stress.
3. Identify factors in an infant's history that increase risk for hypothermia and hypoglycemia.
4. Identify factors in an infant's current condition that increase risk for hypoglycemia and hypothermia.
5. Identify the appropriate interventions for an infant with hypoglycemia and hypothermia.
6. Differentiate the roles of team members in response to an infant with hypoglycemia and hypothermia.

Psychomotor

The student will be able to:

1. Perform an appropriate assessment for an infant with hypoglycemia and hypothermia.
2. Initiate appropriate interventions including initial patient assessment, vital signs, focused health history, obtaining and interpreting blood glucose, initiation of oral feeding or intravenous dextrose, providing environmental warmth, and patient reassessment for a patient with hypoglycemia and hypothermia.
3. Work collaboratively as part of the healthcare team in the care of an infant with hypoglycemia and hypothermia.

Affective

The student will be able to:

1. Reflect upon performance in the care of an infant with hypoglycemia and hypothermia.
2. Identify personal feelings in delivering care to an infant with hypoglycemia and hypothermia.
3. Discuss feelings related to working as a member of a team in the care of an infant with hypoglycemia and hypothermia.
4. Identify factors that worked well during the simulation of care of an infant with hypoglycemia and hypothermia.
5. Identify factors that needed improvement during the simulation of care of an infant with hypoglycemia and hypothermia.
6. Develop improved self-confidence in the care of an infant with hypoglycemia and hypothermia.

Communication

The student will be able to:

1. Communicate effectively with healthcare team members in care of an infant with hypoglycemia and hypothermia.
2. Communicate effectively with the patient and family in the care of an infant with hypoglycemia and hypothermia.
3. Use SBAR when communication with team members in the care of an infant with hypoglycemia and hypothermia.
4. Practice Transparent Thinking (thinking out loud) to facilitate group problem solving.
5. Use Directed Communication (directing a message to specific individual) when delegating tasks.
6. Employ Closed-Loop Communication (acknowledgment of receipt of the message and status) to acknowledge communications from others.

Safety

The student will be able to:

Administer and maintain specific protecting interventions with attention to safety of the client and healthcare professional.

1. Demonstrate a safe environment with attention to hazards to healthcare providers, visitors, and the client. Includes body mechanics, tripping hazards, and equipment issues.
2. Demonstrate attention to national patient safety goals. Includes patient identification standards, effective communication among healthcare providers, and safe medication administration.
3. Demonstrate attention to standard precautions. Includes hand washing, infection control measures, and use of personal protective equipment (PPE) as needed.

Leadership and Management/Delegation

The student will be able to:

1. Orient members to the environment and identify available resources for use in the care of an infant with hypoglycemia and hypothermia.
2. Identify tasks that can/should be legally, ethically, and safely delegated to other members of the healthcare team in the care of an infant with hypoglycemia and hypothermia.
3. Identify and prioritize patient's needs in care of infant with hypoglycemia and hypothermia.

OVERVIEW OF THE PROBLEM

Definition

Care of the newly born infant is often routine and uneventful. This circumstance can sometimes lead to delayed recognition to the often subtle signs of impending illness or physical compromise. Thermoregulation and glucose metabolism are two areas in the care of the newly born that can offer early indication of potentially more severe patient compromise, requiring timely intervention.

Thermoregulation

Definition

Neonates are at risk for ineffective thermoregulation.

Pathophysiology

Acute cold stress can lead to hypoglycemia, increased oxygen need, and apnea.

Risk Factors

- Immature temperature regulation
- Decreased subcutaneous fat
- No shiver response
- Prematurity

Assessment

Term newborn rectal temperature norms range from 36.5 to 37.5°C and axillary temperatures range from 36 to 36.5°C. Preterm infants have ranges of rectal temperature norms of 36.2 to 37.2°C and axillary temperature norms of 36.5 to 37.3°C.

Subjective

Not applicable to newborns.

Objective

- T below 97.7°F, Cool to touch crying, worsening acrocyanosis
- Cremasteric response in males
- Mottling, cyanosis
- Hypoglycemia

Treatment

Dry and warm the newborn

Nursing Management

Goals: Establish and maintain thermal stability

- Interventions: Avoid chilling
- Dry, wrap, and apply hat or place in heated crib
- Monitor vital signs frequently

Evaluation/Outcome Criteria

T stabilizes within 8–10 hr of birth.

Hypoglycemia

Definition

Low serum glucose level, less than 40–45 mg/dL.

Pathophysiology

Low serum glucose can lead to altered cellular metabolism, cerebral irritability, and cardiopulmonary problems.

Risk Factors

- Loss of maternal glucose supply at birth
- Increased energy requirements of normal physiological activities (respiration, thermoregulation, muscular activity), decreased hepatic ability to convert amino acids
- More common in infants of diabetic mothers (IDM); preterm, postterm infants; SGA, LGA infants; smaller twin; infant of mother with preeclampsia, birth asphyxia; acute cold stress conditions causing infant hyperinsulinism; infectious processes; prolonged initiation of enteral nutrition; genetic disorders of protein and carbohydrate metabolism

Assessment

Objective

- Jitteriness
- Tremors
- Convulsions
- Lethargy
- Hypotonia
- Sweating
- Unstable temperature
- Tachypnea
- Apneic episodes
- Cyanosis
- High-pitched shrill cry
- Difficulty feeding

Diagnostic Tests

Serum glucose level, less than 40–45 mg/dL.

Treatment: Administer glucose

Nursing Management

Goals: Prevent complications.

- Interventions: Assess feeding reflexes, immediate enteral feeding and/or intravenous administration of D10W at 1–2 mL/kg (0.1–0.2 g/kg) with a maintenance infusion beginning at 4–6 mg/kg/min are the initial prescribed interventions to elevate and maintain the blood glucose into a normal range, do not feed by mouth if respirations above 60; administer oral or IV calcium if ordered; inform PCP immediately of signs of jaundice, hyperirritability, birth injury, increased ICP, hemorrhage

Evaluation/Outcome Criteria:

- Neonate makes successful transition to extrauterine life.
- Neonate responds to medical and nursing management.
- Neonate exhibits normal neurological and cardiopulmonary functioning.

REVIEW QUESTIONS

1. According to Neonatal Resuscitation Program (NRP) guidelines which four questions should a provider ask when attending a delivery?
   Answer:

2. What is the blood glucose value that signals hypoglycemia?
Answer:

3. What four ways can an infant lose body heat resulting in hypothermia?
Answer:

4. What is the first-line medication of choice, including recommended dose, to treat hypoglycemia in the newborn?
Answer:

5. What is the first intervention that should be done to prevent neonatal heat loss following birth?
Answer:

Related Evidence-Based Practice Guidelines

American Heart Association. Neonatal resuscitation guidelines (Part 13). Retrieved December 17, 2008, from http://circ.ahajournals.org/cgi/content/full/112/24_suppl/IV-188

Guidelines for glucose monitoring and treatment of hypoglycemia in breastfed neonates. Retrieved from http://www.guideline.gov/summary/summary.aspx?doc_id=11218&nbr=005865&string=neonatal+AND+hypoglycemia

The Joint Commission National Patient Safety Goals Hospital Program. Retrieved from http://www.jointcommission.org/GeneralPublic/NPSG/10

SBAR technique for communication: A situational briefing model. The Institute for Healthcare Improvement. Retrieved December 19, 2008, from http://www.ihi.org/IHI/Topics/PatientSafety/SafetyGeneral/Tools/SBARTechniqueforCommunicationASituationalBriefingModel.htm

Wight, N., Marinelli, K. A. (2006). Academy of Breastfeeding Medicine Protocol Committee. ABM clinical protocol #1: Guidelines for glucose monitoring and treatment of hypoglycemia in breastfed neonates. Academy of Breastfeeding Medicine, *1*(3), 178–184.

Topics to Review Prior to the Simulation

Infant assessment

- Care of infant during first week of life
- Thermoregulation
- Neonatal nutrition: Carbohydrate metabolism
- Identification of at risk infant population for hypoglycemia and hypothermia
- Neonatal Resuscitation Program (NRP) overview

SIMULATION

Client Background

Biographical Data

- Age: ~15 min
- Gender: female
- Height: 20 in
- Weight: 3.9 kg
- Head circ: 37 cm

Cultural Considerations

- Language: Parents, English and Spanish
- Ethnicity: Hispanic
- Nationality: American
- Culture: Latino

Demographic (Mother)

- Marital status: married
- Educational level: college graduate
- Religion: Catholic
- Occupation: teacher

Current Health Status

- Delivered 15 min ago, swaddled, quiet, centrally pink and breathing. This is a term girl of a 24-year-old G1P1 mother who received good prenatal care and experienced an uneventful pregnancy. Prenatal blood work indicated no abnormal findings. Maternal history is significant for delayed conception (2.5 yr) and for mild asthma and allergy to shellfish. The baby was delivered vaginally with an epidural, after a prolonged period of pushing (3 hr 15 min). A loose nuchal cord was resolved without a problem. Apgars were 7 and 8. The father/family member present at the bed side holding the baby near the warmer.

History

- Psychosocial history: NA
  - Social support: intact married couple. Both currently employed with mother on paid maternity leave for 4 wk. Stable housing and extended family support in area.
- Past health history
  - Medical: prolonged pushing and nuchal cord × 1
  - Surgical: NA
- Family history: grandparents with history of hypertension, coronary heart disease, stroke, and diabetes on maternal side.

Admission Sheet

Name:	Hernandez-Arias, Girl
Age:	15 min old
Gender:	Female
Marital Status:	Not applicable
Educational Level:	Not applicable
Religion:	Parents Catholic
Ethnicity:	Hispanic
Nationality:	Second-generation American
Language:	English/Spanish
Occupation:	Not applicable

Hospital
Provider's Orders

Patient's Name: **Hernandez-Arias, Girl**
Allergies: **NKDA**

Diagnosis:

Date	Time	Order	Signature
		Vital signs: Temperature, heart rate, and respiratory rate at birth then q 30 min until stable then q shift thereafter and prn	
		Weight q day	
		Diet: Breast-feed ad lib	
		Activity: As tolerated	
		Medications: Vitamin K 1 mg IM within 1 hr of birth Erythromycin ointment 1–2 cm to lower conjunctival sac to each eye × 1 at birth Hepatitis B vaccine prior to discharge Sucrose 24% solution give 1–2 mL to top of tongue 2 min prior to painful procedure plus pacifier dipped in sucrose solution. May repeat q 6 hr prn	Dr. Finn

Nursing Report

Hand off from new graduate nurse caring for mother of baby: "I have so much to do with mom, so I am glad for your help. I wrapped her up right after she was suctioned and let mom put her to breast. She didn't do much, just seemed sleepy. Her Apgars were 7 and 8. Her weight is 3.9 kg and I got an initial HR 136 and RR 40. Her name bands are on, but that is about it. She still needs a length and another set of vitals soon."

Student Simulation Prep Assignments

1. Identify items and their purpose in the care of a newborn patient with hypoglycemia and hypothermia.

Item	Purpose
Practice use heel stick technique and use of glucometer	
Overview of radiant warmer function	
Overview and practice using standardized communication tool such as SBAR with healthcare team members	
Review of NRP initial steps in newborn resuscitation	
Review of medications commonly given to newborns	

2. Identify team members and their specific roles in the care of a patient with hypoglycemia and hypothermia.

Team Member	Role
Medical intern/resident/neonatal nurse practictioner (NNP)	
Secondary nurse	
Father/family member	
Documenter	
Primary nurse	

3. Relevant Data Exercise: Fill in the columns below.

Relevant Data from Report	Relevant Data from Other Sources	Data Missing	Sources for Missing Data	Data Requiring Follow-up

4. Initial Focused Assessment

After reviewing the client background and nursing report, you are ready to assess your client's current status. Under each category, identify how you would target your assessment and what you would expect to find for the newborn patient with hypothermia and hypoglycemia.

History

Are there any questions you need to ask the patient or family to obtain additional relevant data?

Physical Exam

- General appearance:
- Integumentary:
- HEENT:
- Respiratory:
- CV:
- Breasts:
- Abdominal:
- Neuro:
- Musculoskeletal:
- Reproductive:
- Additional:
- Developmental infancy:

5. Diagnostic Tests

What diagnostic test results relevant to the patient's current problem are needed to plan care?

Complete the table using Van Leeuwen et al, *Davis's Comprehensive Handbook of Laboratory and Diagnostic Testing with Nursing Implications* 4e, or other diagnostic test reference.

Diagnostic Test	Significance to This Patient's Problem
Blood glucose	

6. Treatment

Identify drugs that are used to treat a patient with hypoglycemia.

Complete the table using Deglin et al, *Davis's Drug Guide for Nurses* 12e, or other drug reference.

Medication	Dose, Route, Frequency	Indications	Side Effects	Nursing Implications
D10W	2 mL/kg IV over 15 min now Follow with maintenance D10W infusion at 4–6 mg/kg/min			
Glucagon	0.3 mg/kg/dose IV (preferred), IM, SC q 4 hr as needed (max dose 1 mg/dose)			
Sucrose 24% solution	1–2 mL to tongue 2 min prior to painful procedure. May offer pacifier dipped in 24% sucrose solution. May repeat q 6 hr			

7. Nursing Problems/Diagnoses

Identify three priority nursing problems/diagnoses.

Assessment Data	Priority Problem	Intervention	Expected Patient Outcome	Which Interventions Could be Delegated to Unlicensed Personnel?
1.				
2.				
3.				

References

Blackburn, S. T., Mercia, Loper, D. (2004). Thermoregulation. In *Maternal, fetal & neonatal physiology: A clinical perspective.* St. Louis: Saunders.

Circulation 2005; 112, IV-188–IV-195; originally published online Nov 28, 2005; Part 13; Neonatal Resuscitation Guideline. American Heart Association. Retrieved December 17, 2008, from http://circ.ahajournals.org/cgi/content/full/112/24_suppl/IV-188

Deglin, J. H., Vallerand, A. H. (2009). *Davis's drug guide for nurses* (11th ed.). Philadelphia: F. A. Davis.

Dillon, P. (2007). *Nursing health assessment: A critical thinking and case studies approach* (2nd ed.). Philadelphia: F. A. Davis.

Erikson, E. H. (1950). *Childhood and society*. New York: Norton.

Institute for Healthcare Improvement. *SBAR: Technique for communication: A situational briefing model.* Retrieved December 18, 2008, from http://www.ihi.org/IHI/Topics/PatientSafety/SafetyGeneral/Tools/SBARTechniqueforCommunicationASituationalBriefingModel.htm

Lagerquist, S. (2006). *NCLEX-RN for success.* Philadelphia: F. A. Davis.

Liang, I. (2005). General care. In M. G. MacDonald, M. D. Mullett, & M. M. K. Seshia (Eds.). *Avery's neonatology: Pathophysiology & management of the newborn* (6th ed.) (pp. 353–357). Philadelphia: Lippincott Williams & Wilkins.

Ogata, E. S. (2005). Carbohydrate homeostasis. In M. G. MacDonald, M. D. Mullett, & M. M. K. Seshia (Eds.). *Avery's neonatology: Pathophysiology & management of the newborn* (6th ed.) (pp. 876–879). Philadelphia: Lippincott Williams & Wilkins.

Van Leeuwen, A. M., Poelhuis-Leth, D. J., & Bladh, M. L. (2011). *Davis's comprehensive handbook of laboratory and diagnostic tests with nursing implications.* (4th ed.). Philadelphia: F. A. Davis.

Wight, N., & Marinelli, K. A. (2005). Academy of Breastfeeding Medicine Protocol Committee. ABM clinical protocol #1: Guidelines for glucose monitoring and treatment of hypoglycemia in breastfed neonates. *Breastfeed medicine, 1*(3), 178–184.

Zenk, K. E., Sills, J. H., & Koeppel, R. M. (2003). *Neonatal medications & nutrition: A comprehensive guide* (3rd ed.). Santa Rosa, CA: NICU INK.

3-5 Postoperative Cesarean Section

MATERNAL-CHILD

STANDARD FORMS

These templates are included in the Appendix; copy before each use.

LEARNING OUTCOMES

Cognitive

The student will be able to:

1. Determine essential assessments for the postoperative obstetrical client and correctly perform assessments specific to the client's priority needs in a coordinated and timely manner based on data and setting resources:
   - Focused postoperative assessment: neurological, cardiac, respiratory, mobility
   - Vital signs including pain
   - Intake and output
   - Dressing
   - Fundus
   - Lochia
2. Analyze assessment data and identify the appropriate interventions for the postoperative obstetrical patient that will address priority actions specific to client's physiological status, age, culture, and setting resources.
3. Engage in purposeful, efficient information sharing and plan of care implementation and evaluation when necessary.

Psychomotor

The student will be able to:

1. Demonstrate timely and efficient integration of postoperative nursing interventions specific to health patterns to promote oxygenation, hydration, mobility, elimination, and skin integrity.
   - Assist client with incentive spirometer (IS) and turn, cough, and deep breathe (TCDB).
   - Monitor fluid balance: Check IV fluid type and infusion rate, monitor urine output, monitor lochia: color, amount, odor.
   - Administer medications with attention to The Joint Commission National Patient Safety goals for safe medication delivery: Pain medication.
2. Guide and support client and family through the postoperative experience with communication and learning strategies specific to learning readiness, culture, age, and education level. Provides client with explanation for the following:
   - Medications
   - TCDB and IS
   - Lochia and uterine involution
   - Potential for disturbed body image related to unexpected cesarean delivery

Affective

The student will be able to:

1. Critique personal actions using a nursing framework in adapting a plan of care specific to the changing client story and setting resources.
2. Reflect upon performance in the care of a postoperative obstetrical patient with cesarean delivery.
3. Identify personal feelings in delivering care to a postoperative obstetrical patient with cesarean delivery.
4. Discuss feelings related to working as a member of a team in the care of a postoperative patient.
5. Identify factors that worked well during the simulation.
6. Identify factors that needed improvement during the simulation.

Communication

The student will be able to:

1. Communicate effectively with healthcare team members utilizing the SBAR reporting format.
2. Dialogue with peers, physician, faculty, and/or charge nurse regarding client condition.
3. Communicate effectively with the patient in the care of a postoperative patient.
4. Practice Transparent Thinking (thinking out loud) to facilitate group problem solving.
5. Use Directed Communication (directing a message to specific individual) when delegating tasks.
6. Employ Closed-Loop Communication (acknowledgment of receipt of the message and status) to acknowledge communications from others.

Safety

The student will be able to:

Administer and maintain specific protecting interventions with attention to safety of the client and healthcare professional.

1. Demonstrate a safe environment with attention to hazards to healthcare providers, visitors, and the client. Includes body mechanics, tripping hazards, and equipment issues.
2. Demonstrate attention to national patient safety goals. Includes patient identification standards, effective communication among healthcare providers, and safe medication administration.

3. Demonstrate attention to standard precautions. Includes hand washing, infection control measures, and use of personal protective equipment (PPE) as needed.

Leadership and Management/Delegation

The student will be able to:

1. Identify tasks that can be legally, ethically, and safely delegated to unlicensed assistive personnel (UAP) or LPN in the care of a postoperative cesarean section patient.
2. Identify and prioritize patient's needs in care of a postoperative cesarean section patient.

OVERVIEW OF THE PROBLEM

Definition

Cesarean section is an incision through the abdominal wall and uterus to give birth. Indications can be fetal or maternal.

- Fetal:
  - Fetal distress
  - Fetal medical jeopardy: RH or ABO incompatibility
  - Fetal malposition or malpresentation
- Maternal
  - Uterine dysfunction; rupture
  - Placental disorders
  - Severe maternal preeclampsia, ecclampsia
  - Fetopelvic disproportion
  - Sudden maternal death
  - Failed induction

Method

Low-segment incision is the method of choice.

Assessment

Objective

- Maternal physical status: Vital signs, labor status, contractions, status of membranes, bleeding
- Fetal status: FHR pattern; amniotic fluid—color, amount; biophysical profile; gestational age, lung maturity; fetal size, presentation, position

Subjective

- Maternal emotional response
- Maternal understanding of indications for procedures and implications
- Other, as for any abdominal surgery

Diagnostic Tests

- As expected for abdominal surgery
- In addition: Type Rh, Coombs, rubella titer, GBS culture, RPR, or VDRL

Nursing Management

Preoperative

Goal: Safeguard fetal well-being:

- Monitor FHR pattern
- Notify NICU and neonatology for suspected complications

Goal: Provide health teaching:

- Explain preoperative and operative procedures and rationale
- Other, as for abdominal surgery
- Prepare for operative birth

Postoperative

- Same as for any abdominal surgery
- Same as for postpartum care

Evaluation/Outcome Criteria

- Verbalizes understanding of indication for cesarean birth
- Successful birth of viable healthy infant
- No evidence of surgical or birth complications
- No evidence of interference with newborn attachment
- Expresses satisfaction with birth experience

REVIEW QUESTIONS

1. What are the priority assessments for postoperative clients?
   Answer:

2. What are the major complications associated with postoperative obstetrical clients?
   Answer:

3. Postoperative obstetrical clients are at higher risk for fluid and electrolyte imbalances. What essential assessments are required to monitor fluids and electrolytes?
   Answer:

4. Your postoperative client's urinary output has been 60 mL/hr for the past 2 consecutive hr. Is this amount acceptable? What other assessments would be done to evaluate the client's fluid balance?
   Answer:

5. Deep vein thrombosis (DVT) is a complication associated with surgery. List interventions to prevent DVT.
Answer:

Related Evidence-Based Practice Guidelines

National Guideline Clearing House. Postoperative management in adults. A practical guide to postoperative care for clinical staff. Retrieved July 2007, from www.guideline.gov

Smith, S. (2006) *Sandra Smith's review for NCLEX-RN* (11th ed.). Los Altos, CA: National Nursing Review.

Smith, S., Duell, D., & Martin, B. (2008). Clinical nursing skills. Upper Saddle River, NJ: Pearson Education.

The Joint Commission National Patient Safety Goals Hospital Program. Retrieved from http://www.jointcommission.org/GeneralPublic/NPSG/10

SBAR technique for communication: A situational briefing model. The Institute for Healthcare Improvement retrieved December 19, 2008, from http://www.ihi.org/IHI/Topics/PatientSafety/SafetyGeneral/Tools/SBARTechniqueforCommunicationASituationalBriefingModel.htm

Topics to Review Prior to the Simulation

- Postoperative care for abdominal surgery: Assessments, anticipated interventions, and expected outcomes

Postpartum care

- Cesarean: Pathophysiology associated with abdominal surgery, potential complications, and associated obstetrical concerns
- Atelectasis: Pathophysiology and anticipated interventions
- Patient medications: Dose, route, essential assessments to be completed prior to medication delivery, patient education, and compatibility

SIMULATION

Client Background

Beth Simmons is a 24-year-old, 5 ft 4 in, 160-lb, white, English-speaking woman. She is a math teacher at a local high school. Past medical history is negative for smoking, drugs, or ETOH abuse. She denies previous surgeries or hospital admissions. Ms. Simmons is married, obstetrical history: G1P1, 40 +3/7 weeks' gestation. Blood type O+, rubella immune, Hep B negative, GBS negative, HIV negative. Ms. Simmons was admitted at 0300 today in active labor with spontaneous rupture of membranes (SROM) reported by the patient at 0230 for clear, odorless fluid. Sterile vaginal exam (SVE) at 0300 was 4 cm/80% effaced/–3 station. SROM confirmed by FERN test and positive nitrazine test. She received an epidural at 1300, SVE at that time was 5 cm/90% effaced/–3 station. The epidural provided excellent pain relief, patient rated her pain as 10/10 before the epidural and 1/10 after the epidural. At 1350, SVE was unchanged. An intrauterine pressure catheter was placed which revealed adequate uterine contractions as evidenced by 200 Montevideo units (MVUs). At 1500, SVE remained unchanged and the decision to delivery by cesarean was discussed related to failure to progress. Consent was obtained. Ms. Simmons delivered a 10 lb 2 oz boy at 1612. She returned to the obstetrical unit for recovery. The recovery phase was uneventful and she is now 8 hr postoperative.

Biographical Data

- Age: 24
- Gender: female
- Height: 5 ft 4 in
- Weight: 160 lb

Cultural Considerations

- Language: English
- Ethnicity: English/German
- Nationality: American
- Culture: no significant cultural consideration identified

Demographic

- Marital status: married
- Educational level: college
- Religion: Catholic
- Occupation: high school math teacher

Current Health Status

- Cesarean section for failure to progress

History

- Psychosocial history
  - Social support: husband
  - Negative smoking, alcohol, or drugs
- Past health history
  - Medical: no previous hospital admissions
  - Surgical: no previous surgeries
  - Ob history: grava 1 para 1
- Family history: none significant

Admission Sheet

Name:	Beth Simmons
Age:	24
Gender:	Female
Marital Status:	Married
Educational level:	College
Religion:	Catholic
Ethnicity:	English/German
Nationality:	American
Language:	English
Occupation:	Math teacher, high school level
Lab Values:	On admission

Diagnostic Test	Normal Range	Patient Values
CBC	WBC 5,000–10,000	WBC 12,000
	Neutrophils 1,935–7,942	Neutrophils 7,000
	RBC 4.5–5.3 mill	RBC 5 mL
	Hgb 13 to 18 g/100 mL	Hgb 14 g/100 mL
	Hct 37–49%	Hct 39%
	Platelet 150,000–400,000/mm^3	Platelets 250,000 mm^3
Electrolytes	Na 136–145 mEq/L	Na 138 mEq/L
	K 3.5–5.1 mEq/L	K 5.0 mEq/L
	Cl 98–107 mEq/L	Cl 100 mEq/L
	Ca 8.6–10.2 mg/dL	Ca 9.0 mg/dL

Hospital
Provider's Orders

Patient's Name: Beth Simmons
Allergies: NKDA

Diagnosis: Cesarean section

Date	Time	Order	Signature
		Admit to obstetrical unit: s/p cesarean section	
		Vital signs: q 4 hr, include pulse ox	
		Diet: Clear liquids, advance as tolerated	
		Activity: Turn/position q 2 hr	
		IV therapy: LR with 20 units Pitocin at 150 mL/hr × 1 then LR 100 mL/hr	
		Medications: Dermoplast spray to perineum prn Tucks pads (witch hazel) to perineum/hemorrhoids prn	

Continued

Diagnosis:	Cesarean section—cont'd		
Date	**Time**	**Order**	**Signature**
		Hemabate 250 mcg IM as needed for excessive bleeding; can be repeated at intervals of 15–90 min per provider's order, not to exceed 2 mg (8 doses)	
		Morphine sulfate 5 mg IV push q 2–4 hr prn for breakthrough pain	
		Tylenol 1,000 mg po q 8 hr prn mild pain	
		Toradol 10 mg IV q 6 hr × 8 doses for maintenance pain control	
		May remove Foley when U/O greater than 80 mL/hr × 6 hr	
		Incentive spirometer at bedside: TCDB (turn, cough, deep breathe) q 2 hr while awake	
		Oxygen 2–4 L prn via NC to keep O_2 sats >90%	Dr. Chorpenning

Medication Administration Record

Name:	Simmons, Beth
DOB:	06/04/85
Allergies:	NKDA
Diagnosis:	Cesarean section
Physician:	Dr. Chorpenning
Comments:	
Administration Period:	

Medication	Start	Stop	Shift 1 0600–1359	Shift 2 1400–2159	Shift 3 2200–0559
Toradol 10 mg IV q 6 hr × 8 doses	Today	After 8 doses	0600 1200	1800	2400 (first dose)
Dermoplast spray prn to perineum					
Hemabate 250 mcg IM prn excessive bleeding	Today				
Tucks pads prn to perineum or hemorrhoids	Today				
Tylenol 1,000 mg po q 8 hr prn mild pain	Today				
Morphine sulfate 5 mg IV q 2–4 hr prn severe pain	Today			(1920) 5 mg in recovery Lck (2120) 5 mg Lck (Lck = nurses initials)	

Injection Sites	Initial	Signature	Initial	Signature	Initial	Signature
I. Right deltoid area	Lck	Lckrautscheid, RN				
II. Left deltoid						
III. Right gluteal area						
IV. Left gluteal						
V. Right abdomen						
VI. Left abdomen						
VII. Right thigh						
VIII. Left thigh						

Nursing Report:

The time now is 2300, the beginning of night shift.

Situation: Beth Simmons is a G1P1 who delivered a 10 lb 2 oz boy at 1612 by cesarean for failure to progress. She is 7 hr postoperative and the primary concern is pain relief. She rates her pain as 8/10 over the incision area, she has been receiving morphine 5 mg IV for pain and this reduces her pain to a 4/10. She describes the pain as burning and the pain is made worse by turning, coughing, and deep breathing.

Background: She is O+, rubella immune, Hep B negative, GBS negative. Membranes were ruptured for 14 hr prior to delivery. She is breast-feeding; her husband is present and supportive.

Assessment: She has fine crackles in bilateral lower lobes, these clear with coughing and when she uses her incentive spirometer, heart is normal sinus rhythm, she is afebrile, her dressing is clean, dry, intact. She last received morphine 5 mg IV about 2 hr ago and this reduced her pain from a 8/10 to 4/10. She has an IV infusing, LR with 20 units Pitocin at 150 mL/hr by gravity. She is not passing gas yet. Her incentive spirometer is at the bedside and I have to encourage her to use it. Urine output is 60 mL/hr.

Recommendation: Complete your shift assessment. Double check her pain level. See how she does with Toradol versus the morphine. You might need to call for PCA orders.

Student Simulation Prep Assignments

1. Identify items and their purpose in the care of a postoperative cesarean section section patient.

Item	Purpose
BP cuff, stethoscope, thermometer	
Watch with second hand	
Goggles	
Stethoscope	
Pulse oximeter	
IV therapy supplies	
Medications	

2. Identify team members and their specific roles in the care of a postoperative cesarean section patient.

Team Member	Role
Nurse	
Charge nurse	
Certified nurses aid	
Physician	
Respiratory therapy	
Pharmacist	

3. Relevant Data Exercise: Fill in columns below.

Relevant Data from Report	Relevant Data from Other Sources	Data Missing	Sources for Missing Data	Data Requiring Follow-up

4. Initial Focused Assessment

After reviewing the client background and nursing report, you are ready to assess your client's current status. Under each category, identify how you would target your assessment, and what you would expect to find for the patient with cesarean section.

History

Are there any questions you need to ask the patient or family to obtain additional relevant data?

Physical Exam

- General appearance:
- Integumentary:
- HEENT:
- Respiratory:
- CV:
- Breasts.
- Abdominal:
- Neuro:
- Musculoskeletal:
- Reproductive:
- Additional:
- Developmental

  What are the nursing implications considering the developmental stage of your patient?

  Answer:

5. Diagnostic Tests

What diagnostic test results relevant to the patient's current problem are needed to plan care?

Complete the table using Van Leeuwen et al, *Davis's Comprehensive Handbook of Laboratory and Diagnostic Testing with Nursing Implications* 4e, or other diagnostic test reference.

Diagnostic Test	Significance to This Patient's Problem
CBC	
Electrolytes	

6. Treatment

Identify drugs that are used to treat a patient with cesarean section.

Complete the table using Deglin et al, *Davis's Drug Guide for Nurses* 12e, or other drug reference.

Medication	Dose, Route, Frequency	Indications	Side Effect	Nursing Implications
Morphine	5 mg IV push q 2-4 hr			
Tylenol	1,000 mg po q 8 hr prn			
Hemabate	250 mcg IM as needed			
Toradol	10 mg IV q 6 hr × 8 doses			
Dermoplast spray	Apply a thin layer by holding the can 6–12 in from affected area. Use 4–6 times/day			
Tucks pads	Apply one pad to affected area 4–6 times/day			

7. Nursing Problems/Diagnoses

Identify three priority nursing problems/diagnoses.

Assessment Data	Priority Problem	Intervention	Expected Patient outcome
1.			

Continued

Assessment Data	Priority Problem	Intervention	Expected Patient outcome
2.			
3.			

References

Deglin, J. H., Vallerand, A. H. (2009). *Davis's drug guide for nurses* (11th ed.). Philadelphia: F. A. Davis.

Dillon, P. (2007). *Nursing health assessment: A critical thinking and case studies approach* (2nd ed.). Philadelphia: F. A. Davis.

Drugs.com. *Anesthetics (Topical).* Retrieved August 3, 2008, from http://www.drugs.com/cons/dermoplast-topical.html#GXX02

Erikson, E. H. (1950). *Childhood and society*. New York: Norton.

Lagerquist, S. (2006). *NCLEX-RN success.* Philadelphia: F. A. Davis.

National Guideline Clearing House. *Postoperative management in adults. A practical guide to postoperative care for clinical staff.* Retrieved July 2007, from www.guideline.gov

Smith, S. (2006) *Sandra Smith's review for NCLEX-RN* (11th ed.). Los Altos, CA: National Nursing Review.

Smith, S., Duell, D., & Martin, B. (2008). *Clinical nursing skills.* Upper Saddle River, NJ: Pearson Education.

Van Leeuwen, A. M., Poelhuis-Leth, D. J., & Bladh, M. L. (2011). *Davis's comprehensive handbook of laboratory and diagnostic tests with nursing implications.* (4th ed.). Philadelphia: F. A. Davis.

3-6 Precipitous Delivery

MATERNITY NURSING

STANDARD FORMS

These templates are included in the Appendix; copy before each use.

LEARNING OUTCOMES

Cognitive

The student will be able to:

1. Describe signs and symptoms of an active labor patient.
2. Correlate signs and symptoms of an active labor patient to the pathophysiology of labor.
3. Identify factors in a patient's history that increase risk for postdelivery complications.
4. Identify factors in a patient's current condition that increase risk for a precipitous delivery.
5. Identify the appropriate interventions for the patient in active labor.
6. Differentiate the roles of team members in response to a patient in active labor and delivering.

Psychomotor

The student will be able to:

1. Perform appropriate admission assessment for a term patient presenting in active labor.
2. Prepare a patient room for delivery of a full-term infant.
3. Initiate appropriate interventions for the patient presenting in active labor.
4. Activate the appropriate healthcare team members in preparation for a precipitous full-term delivery.
5. Work collaboratively as part of the healthcare team in the care of a patient in active labor.

Affective

The student will be able to:

1. Reflect upon performance in the care of a patient in active labor.
2. Identify personal feelings in delivering care to peripartum patient.
3. Discuss feelings related to working as a member of a team in the care of the laboring patient throughout the various stages of the scenario.
4. Identify factors that worked well during the simulation of care of the active labor patient.
5. Identify factors that needed improvement during the simulation of care.
6. Develop self-confidence in the care of the active labor patient experiencing imminent delivery.

Communication

The student will be able to:

1. Communicate effectively with healthcare team members.
2. Utilize a family-patient center approach in communicating throughout the care of the patient.
3. Use SBAR when communicating with team members.
4. Will practice Transparent Thinking (thinking out loud) to facilitate group problem solving.
5. Use Directed Communication (directing a message to specific individual) when delegating tasks.
6. Employ Closed-Loop Communication (acknowledgment of receipt of the message and status) to acknowledge communications from others.

Safety

The student will be able to:

Administer and maintain specific protecting interventions with attention to safety of the client and healthcare professional.

1. Demonstrate a safe environment with attention to hazards to healthcare providers, visitors, and the client. Includes body mechanics, tripping hazards, and equipment issues.
2. Demonstrate attention to national patient safety goals. Includes patient identification standards, effective communication among healthcare providers, and safe medication administration.
3. Demonstrate attention to standard precautions. Includes hand washing, infection control measures, and use of personal protective equipment (PPE) as needed.

Leadership and Management/Delegation

The student will be able to:

1. Identify tasks that can be legally, ethically, and safely delegated to unlicensed assistive personnel (UAP) in the care of the patient in precipitous
2. Identify and prioritize patient's needs within each stage of labor.

OVERVIEW OF THE PROBLEM

Definition

Precipitous labor is labor that lasts less than 3 hr from onset of contraction to delivery.

Pathophysiology

Precipitous labor is characterized by abrupt onset of higher intensity contractions occurring in a shorter period of time unlike the gradual increase in frequency, intensity, and duration of contractions typical of most spontaneous labors.

Risk factors

It occurs at the highest rate in women ages 35–39 and lowest in women less than 20.

It is important for the labor nurse to assess for a history of rapid labors. Such a history, especially if patient lives a significant distance from the hospital, can be a valid indication for induced labor to control the time and setting of delivery.

Complications

Complications are reduced when dilatation and effacement occurs as rapidly as contractions. The risk for maternal and fetal injury increases if contractions are of higher intensity and dilatation and effacement do not keep pace. Precipitous labor may result from tetanic uterine contractions leading to maternal and fetal complications such as:

- Lacerations
- Uterine rupture
- Amniotic fluid embolism
- Postpartum hemorrhage
- Fetal hypoxia
- Intracranial hemorrhage

Assessment for Imminent birth

- Strong contractions
- Bearing down efforts
- Perineal bulging; crowning
- Mother states, "Baby is coming."

Treatment

Vaginal delivery is indicated when the maternal pelvis is adequate. Administer pharmacological agents if ordered such as tocolytics to control and slow labor progress.

Nursing Management

- Assess for history of rapid labors
- Closely monitor woman with a previous history
- Anticipate use of scheduled induction
- Do not leave patient alone
- Reassure mother to reduce anxiety and fear
- Safely delay birth—encourage panting, side-lying position

Emergency Birth

- Prevent infection
- Prevent hypoxia
- Minimize maternal and fetal trauma and complications
- Assist birth
- Facilitate drainiage of mucus and fluid, clear infant airway
- Prevent placental transfusion
- Prevent hypothermia and maintain infant's temperature
- Establish and maintain infant respirations
- Initiate CPR if infant HR less than 60
- Encourage bonding
- Maintain legal accountability as birth attendant

Evaluation/ Outcome Criteria

- Experiences normal spontaneous birth of viable infant over intact perineum
- Uncomplicated fourth stage of labor
- Expresses satisfaction in management of emergency birth

REVIEW QUESTIONS

1. Identify the difference between true and false labor for a client presenting to the triage unit.

Factor	True Labor	False Labor
Contractions		
Show		
Cervix		
Fetal movement		

2. Determine reassuring versus nonreassuring fetal heart rate patterns related to the intrapartal client.
Answer:

3. Identify appropriate components of an assessment of the client in the second stage of labor.
Answer:

4. Discuss the nursing care of the client during the second stage of labor.
Answer:

Related Evidence-Based Practice Guidelines

Review the Cochrane database. Available at Guidelines.gov

Simpson, K., & Creehan, P. (2008). AWHONN perinatal nursing (3rd ed.). Philadelphia: Lippincott Wilkinson & Williams.

Mattson, S., & Smith, J. (2004). Core curriculum for maternal newborn nursing (3rd ed.). St. Louis: Elsevier.

The Joint Commission National Patient Safety Goals Hospital Program. Retrieved from http://www.jointcommission.org/GeneralPublic/NPSG/10

SBAR technique for communication: A situational briefing model. The Institute for Healthcare Improvement. Retrieved December 19, 2008, from http://www.ihi.org/IHI/Topics/PatientSafety/SafetyGeneral/Tools/SBARTechniqueforCommunicationASituationalBriefingModel.htm

Topics to Review Prior to the Simulation

- Labor and delivery process and complications
- Intrapartal fetal assessment
- Intrapartal nursing assessment and skills, including tests for rupture of membranes
- Medication administration

SIMULATION

Client Background

Gerlinde Jean St. Baptist, a 19-year-old gravida 3 para 1 with 1 elective AB arrives to the L&D triage with her auntie at her side. She states she is having contractions "what seems like nonstop." Her auntie adds that she has been leaking fluid from her bottom for the past few hours. The nurse interviews the patient and determines she had late prenatal care with the local prenatal community clinic. Ms Jean St. Baptist presents a small prenatal care card from the clinic which indicates that she is 37 2/7 weeks' pregnant confirmed by ultrasound. She has blood type A positive, VDRL negative, as well as RPR negative. She was last seen in the clinic 2 days ago for what she states as back pain. The nurse does note that her GBS status is positive.

Biographical Data

- Age: 19
- Gender: female
- Height: 5 ft 5 in
- Weight: 150 lb

Cultural Considerations

- Language: English/Creole
- Ethnicity: Haitian American
- Nationality: Haitian
- Culture: Haitian
- The crucial period of childbearing for Haitian women is after the baby has been born. It is a time of elaborate and well-defined beliefs and practices. Such traditions not only provide Haitians with spiritual and emotional support, they also influence perceptions and choices within this population on a wide range of issues. Conversely, pregnancy, labor, and birth are seen as inevitable courses.

Haitians may believe that a uterine "cold" could be caused by exposure to cold air. Use of a sanitary pad may be seen as a way to prevent cold air entering the vagina.

Demographic

- Marital status: single
- Educational level: high school
- Religion: Catholic
- Occupation: home health aide, currently unemployed

Current Health Status

- Has been experiencing "nonstop" contractions for several hours. In addition, she has felt some fluid "leaking" from her vagina for the last few hours.

History

- Psychosocial history
  - Social support: father deceased (MVA 5 yr ago), Mother is "in and out" of her life. She currently resides out of state with her new husband. Patient has been living with her auntie for 2 yr. She states that her auntie is very supportive. "When she found out I was pregnant, she hugged me and told me that she would help me through it." Is unsure of who is the FOB. She states she expects no support from the FOB.
- Past health history
  - Medical: Patient receives all primary care through the local community health clinic. States that she remembers her mother telling her that she is allergic to penicillin, that she had it when she had her tonsils removed and developed a rash. Currently receiving care through the perinatal community health clinic: A positive, VDRL/RPR negative, Rh negative, GBS positive. NSVD 2 yr ago, male, 9 lb. She reports no medical issues.
  - Surgical: Tonsillectomy at age 4. Episiotomy with first delivery. Elective termination of pregnancy at 10 wk 4 yr ago. She reports no other surgical history.
- Family history
  - Poor historian: states that she is unaware of any relevant family history.

Admission Sheet

Name:	Gerlinde Jean St. Baptist
Age:	19
Gender:	Female
Marital Status:	Single
Educational Level:	High School
Religion:	Catholic
Ethnicity:	Haitian American
Language:	English/Creole
Occupation:	Unemployed

Hospital
Provider's Orders

Patient's Name: Gerlinde Jean St. Baptist
Allergies: Penicillin, rash

Diagnosis: Labor check

Date	Time	Order	Signature
		Vital signs:	
		2 hr labor check while in triage	
		Apply continuous External Fetal Monitor and TOCO meter. Obtain 30 min strip, if fetal heart rate is reassuring, then may monitor intermittently (30 min on and 30 min off) to allow for ambulation/ comfort activities	
		Diet: Clear liquid	
		Activity: May ambulate if reactive fetal heart tracing	
		Medications: None	
		Diagnostic studies: None	
		Perform an initial vaginal exam, reassess in 2 hr prn	
		Assess vaginal fluid using Nitrazine paper. If positive, obtain a FERN slide and send to lab for confirmation	

Diagnosis: Labor check—cont'd

Date	Time	Order	Signature
		UA STAT Draw: CBC, RPR, type and screen	
		Call healthcare provider with results	Dr Mendez

Nursing Report

ER nurse provides the L&D triage nurse the following report:

Situation: Ms. Gerlinde Jean St. Baptist, G3, T1, A1, P0, L1, presents at 37 2/7 weeks' gestation with complaints of "nonstop" contractions for several hour and now feels fluid leaking from her vagina. Her auntie is at the bed side and supportive.

Background: Late prenatal care through the local perinatal community health clinic. She was last seen in the clinic 2 days ago for what she states as back pain.

Patient presents prenatal visit information card: Blood type A positive, VDRL negative, BGS positive, RPR negative.

Assessment: Patient seems really uncomfortable. Her underpants were very wet.

Recommendations: Notify the CNM on call.

Student Simulation Prep Assignments

1. Identify items and their purpose in the care of a patient with precipitous labor.

Item	Purpose
IV catheter 18 g	
Nitrazine	
FERN slide	
Telephone	
IV equipment (tubing), IV labels	
IV pump	
Oxygen via mask and nasal cannula	
Foley	
Gloves	
3-cc and 10-cc syringes	
Specimen tubes, vacutainer, and tourniquet	
Alcohol wipes	
BP cuff, thermometer, stethoscope	
Sterile gloves	
Delivery instruments 2 Kelly clamps Mayo scissors Cord clamp	

Continued

Item	Purpose
Bulb suction	
Basin for the placenta	
Peripad	
Blue waterproof pads	
Fetal monitor	
Fetal monitor belts	
Fetal monitor paper	
Baby warmer	
Birthing bed	
Ambu bag for neonate	
Suction catheters for the neonate	
Warm baby blankets	

2. Identify team members and their specific roles in the care of a patient with precipitous labor.

Team Member	Role
Nurse midwife	
UAP	
Triage nurse	
Labor nurse	
Newborn nurse	

3. Relevant Data Exercise: Fill in the columns below.

Relevant Data from Background and Report	Relevant Data from Other Sources	Data Missing	Sources for Missing Data	Data Requiring Follow-up

4. Initial Focused Assessment

After reviewing the client background and nursing report, you are ready to assess your client's current status. Under each category, identify how you would target your assessment and what you would expect to find for the patient with a precipitous delivery of a full-term baby.

History

Are there any questions you need to ask the patient or family to obtain additional relevant data?

Physical Exam

- General appearance:
- Integumentary:

- HEENT:
- CV:
- Breasts:
- Abdominal:
- Neuro:
- Musculoskeletal:
- Reproductive:
- Additional:
- Developmental

What are the nursing implications considering the developmental stage of your patient?

Answer:

5. *Diagnostic Tests*

What diagnostic test results relevant to the patient's current problem are needed to plan care?

Complete the table using Van Leeuwen et al, *Davis's Comprehensive Handbook of Laboratory and Diagnostic Testing with Nursing Implications* 4e, or other diagnostic test reference.

Diagnostic Test	Significance to This Patient's Problem
The nitrazine test	
FERN	
U/A	
CBC	
Rapid plasma reagin (RPR)	
Type and screen, Rh	
Venereal Disease Research Laboratory test (VDRL)	
Group B streptococcus (GBS)	

6. *Treatment*

Identify drugs that are used to treat a patient with precipitous labor.

Complete the table using Deglin et al, *Davis's Drug Guide for Nurses* 12e, or other drug reference.

Medication	Dose, Route, Frequency	Indications	Side Effect	Nursing Implications
Ampicillin	2 g IVPB			

Continued

Medication	Dose, Route, Frequency	Indications	Side Effect	Nursing Implications
Nubain	20 mg IVP q 3 hr prn			
Pitocin	10 units/500 mL D5W. Start at 1–3 mU/min IV			

Medication	Dose, Route, Frequency	Indications	Side Effect	Nursing Implications

7. Nursing Problems/Diagnoses

Identify three priority nursing problems/diagnoses.

Assessment Data	Priority Problem	Intervention	Expected Patient Outcome	Which Interventions Could be Delegated to Unlicensed Personnel?
1.				

Continued

Assessment Data	Priority Problem	Intervention	Expected Patient Outcome	Which Interventions Could be Delegated to Unlicensed Personnel?
2.				

Assessment Data	Priority Problem	Intervention	Expected Patient Outcome	Which Interventions Could be Delegated to Unlicensed Personnel?
3.				

Continued

Assessment Data	Priority Problem	Intervention	Expected Patient Outcome	Which Interventions Could be Delegated to Unlicensed Personnel?

References

Andrews, M. A., Boyle, J S., Carr, T. J. (1999) *Transcultural concepts in nursing care.* (4th ed.). Philadelphia: Lippincott Williams & Wilkins.

Deglin, J. H., & Vallerand, A. H. (2009). *Davis's drug guide for nurses* (11th ed.). Philadelphia: F. A. Davis.

Dillon, P. (2007). *Nursing health assessment: A critical thinking and case studies approach* (2nd ed.). Philadelphia: F. A. Davis.

Erikson, E. H. (1950). *Childhood and society*. New York: Norton.

Hogan, M., & Glazebrook, R. (2003). *Maternal-newborn nursing reviews & rationales*. Upper Saddle River, NJ: Prentice Hall.

Lagerquist, S. (2006). *NCLEX-RN success.* Philadelphia: F. A. Davis.

Lowdermilk, D. L., & Perry, S. E. (2007). *Maternity and women's health care* (9th ed.). St. Louis: Mosby.

Mattson, S., & Smith, J (Eds.). (2004). *Core curriculum for maternal-newborn nursing* (3rd ed.). St. Louis: Elsevier Saunders.

Simpson, K., & Creehan, P. (2008). *AWHONN perinatal nursing* (3rd ed.). Philadelphia: Lippincott Wilkinson & Williams.

Van Leeuwen, A. M., Poelhuis-Leth, D. J., & Bladh, M. L. (2011). *Davis's comprehensive handbook of laboratory and diagnostic tests with nursing implications.* (4th ed.). Philadelphia: F. A. Davis.

Ward, S., & Hisley, S. (2009). *Maternal child nursing care: Optimizing outcomes for mothers, children and families*. New York: F. A. Davis.

Pediatric Nursing

4

4-1 Pediatric Asthma

EMERGENCY NURSING/ACUTE CARE/GENERAL PEDIATRICS

STANDARD FORMS

These templates are included in the Appendix; copy before each use.

LEARNING OUTCOMES

Cognitive

The student will be able to:

1. Identify the signs and symptoms of the child in respiratory distress.
2. Identify appropriate intervention for a pediatric patient with an asthma exacerbation.
3. Describe the physiological process that occurs with asthma (inflammation and constriction).
4. Calculate the dosage of medication based on weight for a pediatric asthma patient.
5. Give a concise and thorough report using SBAR format to transfer care to another nurse.

Psychomotor

The student will be able:

1. Perform an appropriate assessment for a pediatric patient with respiratory distress.
2. Initiate appropriate interventions, such as start and maintain IV, obtain stat vital signs, and administer appropriate medications.
3. Manage the care of a patient requiring nebulized medications.
4. Demonstrate and educate the patient on the proper technique for utilizing a peak flow meter.

Affective

The student will be able to:

1. Reflect upon performance in a simulated situation of care for a patient with acute respiratory distress/asthma exacerbation.
2. Identify elements that worked well during the simulation.
3. Identify areas that need improvement.
4. Reflect on overall feeling about the simulation.
5. Discuss feelings related to working as a team member.
6. Develop self-confidence in caring for a pediatric patient with respiratory distress.
7. Perform self-reflective evaluation.

Communication

The student will be able to:

1. Communicate effectively with healthcare team members in the care of a pediatric patient with acute respiratory distress.
2. Communicate effectively with the patient and family members during the care of a pediatric patient with respiratory distress.
3. Use SBAR format when communicating with healthcare team members.
4. Work collaboratively as part of the healthcare team.
5. Accurately and succinctly document assessments, interventions, and evaluations.
6. Practice Transparent Thinking (thinking out loud) to facilitate group problem solving.
7. Use Directed Communication (directing a message to specific individual) when delegating tasks.
8. Employ Closed-Loop Communication (acknowledgment of receipt of the message and status) to acknowledge communications from others.

Safety

The student will be able to:

Administer and maintain specific protecting interventions with attention to safety of the client and healthcare professional.

1. Demonstrate a safe environment with attention to hazards to healthcare providers, visitors, and the client. Includes body mechanics, tripping hazards, and equipment issues.
2. Demonstrate attention to national patient safety goals. Includes patient identification standards, effective

communication among healthcare providers, and safe medication administration.

3. Demonstrate attention to standard precautions. Includes hand washing, infection control measures, and use of personal protective equipment (PPE) as needed.

Leadership and Management/Delegation

The student will be able to:

1. Identify tasks that can be legally, ethically, and safely delegated to unlicensed assistive personnel (UAP) or LPN in the care of a patient with asthma.
2. Identify and prioritize patient's needs in the care of a patient with asthma.

OVERVIEW OF THE PROBLEM

Definition

Asthma is a reactive airway disease (RAD), a complex inflammatory process that can result in airway tissue damage, characterized by airway inflammation and hyperresponsiveness to a variety of stimuli (triggers), such as allergens, cold, dust, smoke, exercise, medications (e.g., ASA), and food additives.

Pathophysiology

The trigger initiates a release of inflammatory mediators, such as histamine, that leads to airway obstruction through smooth muscle constriction, microvascular leakage, mucous plugging, and swelling. Allergic or antigenic stimuli activate inflammatory (mast) cells signalling the immune system to release proinflammatory substances. Inflammatory cells migrate to the inflamed respiratory tract; proinflammatory mediators activate migrating cells resulting in tissue damage. Status asthmaticus is a life-threatening asthma attack that does not respond to standard treatment and is a medical emergency.

Types of Asthma

- Immunological or allergic asthma: Atopic (hypersensitivity state may have hereditary influence); immunoglobulin E usually elevated.
- Nonimmumniological or nonallergic asthma; repeated respiratory infections; usually >35 yr.
- Mixed combined immunological and nonimmunological asthma.

Risk Factors

- History of allergies, seasonal or environmental
- Recurrent respiratory infection
- Family history of asthma

Assessment

Subjective

- History of URI, allergies, family history of asthma
- Tightness of chest, dyspnea
- Anxiety, restlessness
- Cough

Objective

- Peak flowmeter levels drops
- Increased respirations
- Shortness of breath
- Expiratory wheezes, crackles
- Hyperresonnance to percussion
- Retraction
- Use of accessory muscles
- Tachycardia, tachypnea
- Dry, hacking, paroxysmal, persistent cough, especially at night
- General appearance:
  - Pallor
  - Cyanosis
  - Diaphoresis
  - Barrel chest
  - Distended neck veins
  - Orthopnea
- Thick mucous sputum
- Anxiety
- Decreased level of alertness, such as severe drowsiness or confusion

Diagnostic Tests

- Forced vital capacity (FVC), decreased
- Forced expiratory volume in 1 sec (FEV1), decreased
- Peak expiratory flow rates, decreased
- Residual volume, increased

Treatment

- Administer corticosteroids as ordered: Medrol, prednisone.
- Administer broncodilators, beta-adrenergic agonists (albuterol, metaproterenol).

Maintenance

- Steroids
- Leukotriene inhibitors/receptor antagonists
- Theophylline
- Beta agonists
- Mast cell stabilizers
- Administer antibiotics as ordered: infection is a common trigger.

Nursing Management

Goal: Promote pulmonary ventilation

- Interventions: Position to promote lung expansion (high Fowler's, leaning forward).
- Rescue: Oxygen therapy as ordered
- Respiratory assessment
- Rest

Goal: Facilitate expectoration of secretions

- Interventions: Humidification; administer fluids as ordered.

Goal: Reduce anxiety

- Interventions: Provide relief of hypoxia; remain with child, offer support; administer sedation as ordered; encourage parents to remain with child

Goal: Health teaching

- Management of disease: Review home medications; review breathing exercises; teach use of peak expiratory flowmeter.
- Facilitate child's assuming control over personal care as appropriate to developmental level

Evaluation/Outcome Criteria

- Adequate oxygenation is provided, as evidenced by pink nail beds and mucous membranes, and ease in respiratory effort.
- Anxiety is relieved.
- Child demonstrates mastery and confidence in skills necessary to manage disease.

REVIEW QUESTIONS

1. Childhood asthma attacks are often triggered by irritants. Name at least three triggers.
   Answer:

2. List three developmental milestones that should be easily accomplished by a 5-year-old child.
   Answer:

3. Children will often have atypical presentation of asthma symptoms. List at list three symptoms that could be associated with childhood asthma.
   Answer:

4. List common medication classes used to control asthma.
   Answer:

5. List three psychosocial complications of a child with asthma.
   Answer:

Related Evidence-Based Practice Guidelines

Search The National Guideline Clearing House at http://www.guideline.gov asthma

The Joint Commission National Patient Safety Goals Hospital Program. Retrieved from http://www.jointcommission.org/generalpublic/npsg/10_npsgs.htm

SBAR technique for communication: A situational briefing model. The Institute for Healthcare Improvement. Retrieved December 19, 2008, from http://www.ihi.org/IHI/Topics/PatientSafety/SafetyGeneral/Tools/SBARTechniqueforCommunicationASituationalBriefingModel.htm

Topics to Review Prior to the Simulation

- Pediatric respiratory assessment
- Medication administration, nebulizer

SIMULATION

Client Background

Anita Miller is a 5-year-old female who presents to the emergency department with her mother after becoming short of breath at a birthday party. The patient's mother states that Anita was at a party at a friend's house where there was a dog. Mother states patient was in the emergency department 1 month ago after exposure to an animal at a friend's house. Anita has had eight visits to the emergency department for asthma exacerbations in the past year and has never had to be hospitalized. Anita used albuterol as needed for symptom control and denies other medications.

Biographical Data

- Age: 5
- Gender: female
- Height: 3 ft 6 in
- Weight: 40 lb

Cultural Considerations

- Language: English
- Ethnicity: Irish
- Nationality: American
- Culture: no significant cultural considerations identified

Demographic

- Marital status: N/A
- Educational level: Attending kindergarten
- Religion: Catholic
- Occupation: N/A

Current Health Status

- Asthma

History

- Psychosocial history
  - Social support: lives with both parents, no siblings, mother with patient
- Past health history
  - Medical: eight visits to the emergency department for asthma exacerbations in the past year and has never had to be hospitalized
  - Surgical: none
- Family history: none significant

Admission Sheet (source: parent)

Name:	Anita Miller
Age:	5
Gender:	Female
Marital Status:	Single
Educational Level:	Attends kindergarten
Religion:	Catholic
Ethnicity:	Irish
Nationality:	American
Language:	English
Occupation:	N/A

Hospital
Provider's Orders

Patient's Name: Anita Miller
Allergies: NKDA

Diagnosis: Asthma

Date	Time	Order	Signature
6/20/07	8 PM		
		Admitting diagnosis: Respiratory distress/asthma exacerbation	
		Vital signs: q 4 hr	
		Diet: Regular diet	
		Activity: Bed rest	
		Diagnostic tests: Peak flow function	
		Medications: Albuterol 5 mg neb × 3 Atrovent 0.5 mg neb × 1 (power source O_2) Prednisolone 1 mg/kg po	
		Oxygen: NRB or NC to maintain saturation 95%	
		Radiology: CXR	Dr. B. Hart

Nursing Report

No report. You are the ER nurse and first to see patient.

Student Simulation Prep Assignments

1. Identify items and their purpose in the care of a pediatric patient with asthma.

Item	Purpose
O_2 NRB mask, cannula, nebulizer, bag valve mask	
Monitor	
Peak flowmeter	

2. Identify team members and their specific roles in the care of a patient with asthma.

Team Member	Role
Physician	
Primary nurse	
Secondary nurse	

3. Relevant Data Exercise: Fill in columns below.

Relevant Data from Report	Relevant Data from Other Sources	Data Missing	Sources for Missing Data	Data Requiring Follow-up

4. *Initial Focused Assessment*

After reviewing the client background and nursing report, you are ready to assess your client's current status. Under each category, identify how you would target your assessment and what you would expect to find for the pediatric patient with asthma.

History

Are there any questions you need to ask the parent or family to obtain additional relevant date?

Physical Exam

- General appearance:
- Integumentary:
- HEENT:
- Respiratory:
- CV:
- Breasts:
- Abdominal:
- Neuro:
- Musculoskeletal:
- Reproductive:
- Renal:
- Additional:
- Developmental:

What are the nursing implications considering the developmental stage of your patient?

Answer:

5. *Diagnostic Tests*

What diagnostic test results relevant to the patient's current problem are needed to plan care?

Complete the table using Van Leeuwen et al, *Davis's Comprehensive Handbook of Laboratory and Diagnostic Testing with Nursing Implications* 4e, or other diagnostic test reference.

Diagnostic Test	Significance to this Patient's Problem
Peak Flow	

6. *Treatment*

Identify drugs that are used to treat a patient with pediatric asthma.

Complete the table using Deglin et al, *Davis's Drug Guide for Nurses* 12e, or other drug reference.

Medication	Dose, Route, Frequency	Indication	Side Effect	Nursing Implications
Albuterol	5 mg nebulized			
Atrovent	0.5 mg nebulized			

Medication	Dose, Route, Frequency	Indication	Side Effect	Nursing Implications
Prednisone	1 mg/kg			

7. Nursing Problems/Diagnoses

Identify three priority nursing problems/diagnoses.
Complete for each problem identified.

Assessment Data	Priority Problem	Intervention	Expected Outcome	Which Interventions Could Be Delegated to Unlicensed Personnel?
1.				
2.				
3.				

References

American Heart Association. (2006). Heartsaver first aid with CPR and AED. Dallas: AHA.

Deglin, J. H., & Vallerand, A. H. (2009). *Davis's drug guide for nurses* (11th ed.). Philadelphia: F. A. Davis.

Dillon, P. (2007). *Nursing health assessment: A critical thinking case studies approach* (2nd ed.). Philadelphia: F. A. Davis.

Erikson, E. H. (1950). *Childhood and society*. New York: Norton.

Lagerquist, S. L. (2006). *Davis's NCLEX-RN for success* (2nd ed.). Philadelphia: F .A. Davis.

Van Leeuwen, A. M., Poelhuis-Leth, D. J., & Bladh, M. L. (2011). *Davis's comprehensive handbook of laboratory and diagnostic tests with nursing implications.* (4th ed.). Philadelphia: F. A. Davis.

Wong, D., & Hockenberry-Eaton, M. (2001). *Wong's essentials of pediatric nursing* (6th ed.). St. Louis: Mosby.

4-2 Head Injury

PEDIATRIC

STANDARD FORMS

These templates are included in the Appendix; copy before each use.

LEARNING OUTCOMES

Cognitive

The student will be able to:

1. Describe signs and symptoms of an epidural hematoma.
2. Correlate signs and symptoms of an epidural hematoma to the pathphysiology of increased intracranial pressure (IICP).
3. Differentiate between the signs and symptoms of an epidural hematoma and of a subdural hematoma.
4. Identify the appropriate interventions for the patient with an epidural hematoma.
5. Differentiate the roles of team members in response to a patient with an epidural hematoma.

Psychomotor

The student will be able to:

1. Perform neurological assessment for a patient with an epidural hematoma.
2. Initiate appropriate interventions for a patient with an epidural hematoma: Start IV, administer medications, prep for OR.
3. Work collaboratively as part of the healthcare team in the care of a patient with an epidural hematoma.

Affective

The student will be able to:

1. Reflect upon performance in the care of a patient with a epidural hematoma.
2. Identify personal feelings in delivering care to a patient with an epidural hematoma.
3. Discuss feelings related to working as a member of a team in the care of a patient with an epidural hematoma.
4. Identify factors that worked well during the simulation of care of a patient with an epidural hematoma.
5. Identify factors that needed improvement during the simulation of care of a patient with an epidural hematoma.
6. Develop self-confidence in the care of a patient with an epidural hematoma.

Communication

The student will be able to:

1. Communicate effectively with healthcare team members in the care of a patient with an epidural hematoma.
2. Communicate effectively with the patient and family in the care of a patient with an epidural hematoma.
3. Use SBAR format when communicating with team members in the care of a patient with an epidural hematoma.
4. Practice Transparent Thinking (thinking out loud) to facilitate group problem solving.
5. Use Directed Communication (directing a message to specific individual) when delegating tasks.
6. Employ Closed-Loop Communication (acknowledgment of receipt of the message and status) to acknowledge communications from others.

Safety

The student will be able to:

Administer and maintain specific protecting interventions with attention to safety of the client and healthcare professional.

1. Demonstrate a safe environment with attention to hazards to healthcare providers, visitors, and the client. Includes body mechanics, tripping hazards, and equipment issues.
2. Demonstrate attention to national patient safety goals. Includes patient identification standards, effective communication among healthcare providers, and safe medication administration.
3. Demonstrate attention to standard precautions. Includes hand washing, infection control measures, and use of personal protective equipment (PPE) as needed.

Leadership and Management/Delegation

The student will be able to:

1. Identify tasks that can be legally, ethically, and safely delegated to unlicensed personnel (UAP) or licensed practical nurse (LPN) in the care of a patient with an epidural hematoma.
2. Identify and prioritize patient's needs in care of a patient with an epidural hematoma.

Spiritual

The student will be able to:

1. Identify spiritual needs of patient and family.
2. Implement appropriate interventions to meet the spiritual needs of patient and family.

OVERVIEW OF THE PROBLEM

Definition

Four types of primary head trauma:

- Concussion: Injury results in brief loss of consciousness due to paralysis of neuronal function. Recovery usually total.
- Contusion: Injury results in bruising of brain tissue.
- Laceration: Injury results in tearing of brain tissue or blood vessel from sharp bone fragment or object, or tearing force.
- Fracture: Injury results in linear, depressed, or basilar fracture: Linear may result in epidural bleed; depressed may tear dura and result in spinal fluid leak; basilar is the worst, may result in meningitis or brain abscess, bleeding from nose or ears, CSF leak, Battle's sign (bruising over mastoid process), raccoon eyes (periorbital ecchymosis).

Secondary head trauma response to primary trauma:

- Hematomas
- Epidural (extradural) bleed between skull and dura due to tear of middle meningeal artery. Usually, but not always, injury followed by brief loss of consciousness followed by lucid period with progressive lethargy to coma. Increase irritability, headache, and vomiting may occur. A surgical emergency; untreated leads to herniation and death.
- Subdural bleed between arachnoid and dura layers usually due to tear or rupture of a vein. May be acute, subacute, or chronic. Signs and symptoms (s/s) related to (r/t) increased intracranial pressure(ICP) such as headache, change in level of consciousness:
  - Acute: s/s appear within 48 hr of injury
  - Subacute: s/s appear within 2–14 days after injury.
  - Chronic: s/s appear within weeks to months after seemingly minor injury.
- Intracerebral bleed: bleeding within the brain itself.

Pathophysiology

- Depressed neuronal activity in reticular activating system (RAS) leads to altered level of consciousness.
- Depressed neuronal activity in lower brain stem affects eyes, CNs II, III, IV, VI.
- Depression of respiratory center affects respirations and can lead to respiratory arrest.

Risk Factors

- Trauma/accidents.
- Abuse: Children with sudural hematoma with retinal hemorrhages: suspect shaken baby syndrome (SBS).

Assessment

Subjective

- History of head trauma
- LOC
- Headache
- Vision changes
- Nausea
- Dizziness
- Loss of balance

Objective

Physical findings:

- Obvious laceration or fracture.
- Drainage from ears, nose: Test for CSF (halo or ring sign: blood in center surrounded by yellow ring) or + for glucose.
- Projectile vomiting, hematemesis (vomiting three or more times by children with head injury warrants immediate medical attention).
- Vital signs associated with increased ICP:
  - BP: Assess for widening pulse pressure.
  - Pulse: Assess for bradycardia, tachycardia.
  - Respirations: Assess for change in pattern (Cheyne-Stokes, Biot's), deep and sonorous, hiccups.
- Temperature: Assess for elevation.
- Neurological exam:
  - Change in mental status (loss of consciousness in child following head trauma warrants immediate medical attention).
  - Use Glasgow Coma Scale (GCS): Generally, the lower the score, the worse the prognosis.
  - Pupils: Test reaction, speed and equality (unequal or dilated pupils in an unresponsive child is a neurological emergency).
  - Extremities: Paresis or paralysis.
  - Reflexes: Hyper/hypotonia.
  - Check Babinski, check gag, corneal reflexes.

Diagnostic Tests

- CT scan
- Lumbar puncture
- EEG
- Blood chemistries

Treatment

- Dependent on type of injury and signs and symptoms.
- Craniotomy if indicated

Nursing Management

- Goal: Sustain vital functions and minimize or prevent complications.

Interventions

- Airway: Maintain patent airway; ET if indicated; oxygen (hypoxia and hypercapnea potent cerebral vasodilator that increases ICP); avoid aggressive suctioning because it may increase ICP
- If spinal cord injury suspected, immobilize head and neck
- Position patient at 30 degrees; supine position may increase ICP
- Monitor vital signs:
  - Assess for signs of increased ICP
  - Assess for Cushing's triad (widening pulse pressure, bradycardia with full bounding pulse, and irregular respirations)
  - Cooling measures: Treat temperature elevation with Tylenol or cooling blanket; fever increases ICP

- Neurological assessment:
  - Sensory and motor function
  - Pupil assessment
  - LOC: GCS: best eye, best verbal, best motor. Report any change in GCS and level of consciousness
- Seizure precautions:
- NPO, fluid restriction, strict I&O
- Prepare patient for surgery (epidural hematoma), craniotomy
- Medications:
  - Steroids
  - Hyperosmolar diuretic (mannitol, urea)
  - Antacids or H_2 antagonists: prevent stress ulcers
  - Antibiotics: prevent infection
  - Anticonvulsants (Dilantin, phenobarbitol)
  - Analgesic/antipyretic (Tylenol—morphine contraindicated)
- Report signs of restlessness immediately
- Diet: NPO. Monitor blood chemistries
- Goal: Provide comfort and emotional support

Interventions

- Skin care, oral hygiene, wrinkle-free linens.
- Lubricate eyes.
- Perform ROM as tolerated.
- Avoid restraints.
- Encourage family communication.

Evaluation/Outcome Criteria

- Alert, oriented without residual effects.
- No signs of increased ICP.
- Regains motor and sensory function.
- Resumes self-care activities.

REVIEW QUESTIONS

1. How would you differentiate a subdural hematoma from an epidural hematoma?
Answer:

2. Name three areas that are included in a neurological examination.
Answer:

3. Name three nursing interventions that reduce/prevent increased ICP.
Answer:

4. What five areas should be assessed when checking pupillary reaction?
Answer:

5. Name three signs and symptoms associated with head injury.
Answer:

Related Evidence-Based Practice Guidelines

Search National Guideline Clearinghouse at http://www.guideline.gov, Head Injury.or epidural hematoma

SBAR technique for communication: A situational briefing model. The Institute for Healthcare Improvement. Retrieved December 19, 2008, from http://www.ihi.org/IHI/Topics/ PatientSafety/SafetyGeneral/Tools/SBARTechniqueforCommunicationASituationalBriefingModel.htm

Topics to review prior to the simulation

- Neurological assessment
- Head injury

SIMULATION

Client Background

Biographical Data

- Age: 9
- Gender: female
- Height: 5 ft
- Weight: 75 lb

Cultural Considerations

- Language: English
- Ethnicity: Irish
- Nationality: American
- Culture: no significant cultural considerations identified

Demographic

- Marital status: N/A
- Educational level: grade school
- Religion: Catholic
- Occupation: student

Current Health Status

- Fell off bike and hit head 2 hr ago.

History

- Psychosocial history
  - Social support: family
- Past health history
  - Medical: negative medical problems
  - Surgical: no surgeries
- Family History: N/A

Admission Sheet

Name:	Caitlyn Doyle
Age:	9
Gender:	Female
Marital Status:	N/A
Educational Level:	Student
Religion:	Catholic
Ethnicity:	Irish
Nationality:	American
Language:	English
Occupation:	Student

Hospital
Provider's Orders

Patient's Name: CAITLYN DOYLE
Allergies: NKDA

Diagnosis: Head Trauma

Date	Time	Order	Signature
		Vital signs: q 1 hr with neuro check	
		Diet: NPO	
		Activity: Bed rest	
		IV therapy: NSS KVO	
		Medications: Mannitol 1 g/kg over 30 min IV Dilantin 5 mg/kg in 3 divided doses/24 hr IV Tylenol 10 mg/kg suppository Ancef 25 mg/kg in 4 divided doses/24hr IV Pepcid 0.5 mg/kg IV	
		Diagnostic studies: CT scan of head C-spine x-ray CBC, BMP, Serum osmolality, T&S, PT, PTT, UA	
		Treatments: HOB elevated 30 degrees Oxygen 2 L via NC	
		Cardiac monitor	Dr. Robinson

Nursing Report

Caitlyn Doyle, 9-year-old female, brought to the emergency department by her mother. The child is awake but drowsy, crying and complaining of a headache. The child walks in with mother. The mother states her daughter fell off her bike and hit her head.

Student Simulation Prep Assignments

1. Identify items and their purpose in the care of a patient with a head injury.

Item	Purpose
IV with pump	
O_2 cannula	
Monitor	

2. Identify team members and their specific roles in the care of a patient with a head injury.

Team Member	Role
Triage nurse	
Primary nurse	
Secondary nurse	
Physician	
Pastoral care	

3. Relevant Data Exercise: Fill in columns below.

Relevant Data from Report	Relevant Data from Other Sources	Data Missing	Sources of Missing Data	Data Requiring Follow-up

4. Initial Focused Assessment

After reviewing the client background and nursing report, you are ready to assess your client's current status. Under each category, identify how you would target your assessment and what you would expect to find for the patient with a head injury

History

Are there any questions you need to ask the patient or family to obtain additional relevant data?

Physical Exam

- General appearance:
- Integumentary:
- HEENT:
- Respiratory:
- CV:
- Breasts:
- Abdominal:
- MS:

- Neuro:
- Reproductive:
- Developmental:

What are the nursing implications considering the developmental stage of your patient?

Answer:

5. Diagnostic Tests

What diagnostic test results relevant to the patient's current problem are needed to plan care?

Complete the table using Van Leeuwen et al, *Davis's Comprehensive Handbook of Laboratory and Diagnostic Testing with Nursing Implications* 4e, or other diagnostic test reference.

Diagnostic Test	Significance to This Patient's Problem
CT Scan	
CBC	
PT, PTT	
T&S	
BMP	
UA	
Serum osmolality	

6. Treatment

Identify drugs that are used to treat a patient with

What diagnostic test results relevant to the patient's current problem are needed to plan care?

Complete the table using Deglin et al, *Davis's Drug Guide for Nurses* 12e, or other drug reference.

Medication	Dose, Route, Frequency	Indications	Side Effect	Nursing Implications
Mannitol	1 g/kg			
Dilantin	5 mg/kg in 3 divided doses/24 hr			
Tylenol	10 mg/kg			

Continued

Medication	Dose, Route, Frequency	Indications	Side Effect	Nursing Implications
Ancef	25 mg/kg in 4 divided doses/24 hr			
Pepcid	0.5 mg/kg			

7. Nursing Problems/Diagnoses

Identify three priority nursing problems/diagnoses.

Assessment Data	Priority Problem	Intervention	Expected Patient Outcome	Which Interventions Could Be Delegated to Unlicensed Personnel?
1.				
2.				
3.				

References

Deglin, J. H., & Vallerand, A. H. (2009). *Davis's drug guide for nurses* (11th ed.). Philadelphia: F. A. Davis.

Dillon, P. (2007). *Nursing health assessment: A critical thinking case studies approach* (2nd ed.). Philadelphia: F. A. Davis.

Erikson, E. H. (1950). *Childhood and society*. New York: Norton.

Ignatavicius, D., & Workman, M. (2002). *Medical-surgical nursing critical thinking for collaborative care* (4th ed.). Philadelphia: Saunders.

Lagerquist, S. L. (2006). *Davis's NCLEX-RN for success.* Philadelphia: F. A. Davis.

Van Leeuwen, A. M., Poelhuis-Leth, D. J., & Bladh, M. L. (2011). *Davis's comprehensive handbook of laboratory and diagnostic tests with nursing implications.* (4th ed.). Philadelphia: F. A. Davis.

4-3 Fracture/Suspected Child Abuse

PEDIATRICS

STANDARD FORMS

These templates are included in the Appendix; copy before each use.

LEARNING OUTCOMES

Cognitive

The student will be able to:

1. Describe signs and symptoms of a femur fracture.
2. Correlate signs and symptoms of a femur fracture to the pathophysiology of neurovascular compromise.
3. Identify factors in a patient's history that increase risk for child abuse.
4. Identify factors in a patient's current condition that increase risk for neurovascular compromise.
5. Identify the appropriate interventions for the patient with a femur fracture.
6. Identify the appropriate diagnostic evaluation for the patient with an orthopedic injury and suspected child abuse.
7. Differentiate the roles of team members in response to a patient with an orthopedic injury and suspected child abuse.

Psychomotor

The student will be able to:

1. Perform appropriate assessment for a patient with a femur fracture in the setting of suspected child abuse.
2. Initiate appropriate interventions for a patient with a femur fracture:
   - Immobilization.
   - Pain management.
   - Head-to-toe assessment to rule out other traumatic injuries.
   - Maintain patient safety.
   - Facilitate additional diagnostic workup for suspected child abuse.
   - Contact appropriate Child Protective Services (CPS) for region of practice.
   - Objectively document findings.
3. Work collaboratively as part of the healthcare team in the care of a patient with a femur fracture in the setting of suspected child abuse.

Affective

The student will be able to:

1. Reflect upon performance in the care of a patient with a femur fracture in the setting of suspected child abuse.
2. Identify personal feelings in delivering care to a patient with a femur fracture in the setting of suspected child abuse.
3. Discuss feelings related to working as a member of a team in the care of a patient with a femur fracture in the setting of suspected child abuse.
4. Identify factors that worked well during the simulation of care of a patient with a femur fracture in the setting of suspected child abuse.
5. Identify factors that needed improvement during the simulation of care of a patient with femur fracture in the setting of suspected child abuse.
6. Develop self-confidence in the care of a patient with a femur fracture in the setting of suspected child abuse.

Communication

The student will be able to:

1. Communicate effectively with healthcare team members in care of a patient with a femur fracture in the setting of suspected child abuse.
2. Communicate effectively with the patient and family in the care of a patient with a femur fracture in the setting of suspected child abuse.
3. Use SBAR format when communicating with team members about the care of a patient with a femur fracture in the setting of suspected child abuse.
4. Objectively document findings on assessment of a patient with a femur fracture in the setting of suspected child abuse.
5. Practice transparent thinking (thinking out loud) to facilitate group problem solving.
6. Use directed communication (directing a message to specific individual) when delegating tasks.
7. Employ Closed-Loop Communication (acknowledgment of receipt of the message and status) to acknowledge communications from others.

Safety

The student will be able to:

Administer and maintain specific protecting interventions with attention to safety of the client and healthcare professional.

1. Demonstrate a safe environment with attention to hazards to healthcare providers, visitors, and the client. Includes body mechanics, tripping hazards, and equipment issues.
2. Demonstrate attention to national patient safety goals. Includes patient identification standards, effective

communication among healthcare providers, and safe medication administration.
3. Demonstrate attention to standard precautions. Includes hand washing, infection control measures, and use of personal protective equipment (PPE) as needed.

Leadership and Management/Delegation

The student will be able to:
1. Identify tasks that can be legally, ethically, and safely delegated to unlicensed assistive personnel (UAP) or licensed practical nurse (LPN) in the care of a patient with a femur fracture in the setting of suspected child abuse.
2. Identify and prioritize patient's needs in care of a femur fracture in the setting of suspected child abuse.

Patient Care Outcomes

The student will recognize the importance of these patient care outcomes:
1. Safe disposition of child post-discharge.
2. Accurate reporting of suspected child abuse to local child protective agency and police.
3. Developmental considerations of child who is potentially being abused.

OVERVIEW OF THE PROBLEM

Two problems discussed: Child maltreatment and extremity fractures.

Child Maltreatment

Definition

Child abuse can be physical, psychological, sexual, or neglect. For information from the CDC regarding this topic, see the following link:
- CDC Child Maltreatment Surveillance at http://www.cdc.gov/ncipc/dvp/CMP/CMP-Surveillance.htm

Documentation and Reporting of Suspected Child Maltreatment

Documentation of suspected child maltreatment must be thorough and objective. Careful documentation of the reported history and physical findings can have important legal implications. Go to the following site for a tool to use for documentation on page 18 of its guideline.
- http://www.luhs.org/depts/emsc/Child%20Abuse.Neglect% 20Guideline.doc

Mandated reporters are required by law to report suspected cases of child maltreatment to child protective agencies. State statutes define mandated reporters as well as the conditions for reporting. In most states, mandated reporters include but are not limited to physicians, nurses, prehospital providers, social workers, teachers, psychiatrists, childcare providers, and law enforcement. It is important to be knowledgeable of the child abuse laws within one's state of practice. It is not the mandated reporter's responsibility to prove the abuse, but rather to report suspicion of abuse.

Pathophysiology

- Characteristics: Victims are powerless, may blame themselves. Abusers often blame the victim, have poor impulse control, use power to threaten the victim.

Risk Factors

Abuse can be a learned response, previous history of abuse within the family.
Any child can become a victim.

Assessment

Subjective

History
- Delay in seeking medical care
- Major discrepancies in the history between different person's versions
- History and observed injuries
- History and the child's developmental capabilities
- History of multiple visits for a variety of injuries

Objective

Physical Exam
- Withdrawn, apathetic, does not cry
- Does not turn to caregivers for comfort
- Unusual fear or desire to please caregiver
- Poor hygiene, malnourished
- Presence of suspicious evidence of physical injury:
  - Multiple bruises
  - Welts
  - Abrasions, especially central injuries (buttocks, trunk)
  - Bite marks
  - Burn marks
  - Rope marks
  - Handprints
  - Fingernail marks
  - Old bruises or fractures in various stages of healing (especially in child less than 3 years)
- Caregiver behavior: exaggerated concern

Some cultural and religious health practices can be misdiagnosed as child maltreatment if healthcare providers do not remain cognizant of the family's ethnicity and cultural beliefs regarding healthcare; for example:
- Cupping: Asia, Europe, Russia, Middle East. Heated cup containing steam applied to specific points on the body. As steam cools, a vacuum is created producing circular, ecchymotic areas on the skin.
- Coining: Vietnam. Coin repeatedly rubbed lengthwise on oiled skin, which may produce lesions resembling welts.
- Burning: Southeast Asia. Small areas of skin are burned to treat various ailments.

- Moxibustion: Southeast Asia. Stick of burning wormwood, incense, or yarn is placed over an affected area of the body. May produce lesions resembling cigarette burns, usually in a pyramid pattern.
- Topical garlic: Yemenite Jews. Crushed garlic is applied to wrists, which can result in blisters or garlic burns.
- Remedies containing lead: Mexico, Southeast Asia, India.

Certain medical conditions in addition to normal skin pigmentation variations in some ethnic groups can be misdiagnosed as child maltreatment; for example:

- Mongolian spots frequently confused with bruising
- Erythema multiforme
- Idiopathic thrombocytopenic purpura
- Leukemia
- Hemophilia
- Osteogenesis imperfecta

Nursing Management

Interventions

- Provide safe environment
- Conduct interview in private; separate child and caregiver if indicated
- Treat physical injuries
- Document physical injuries
- Maintain supportive nonjudgmental approach
- Mandatory reporting
- Encourage individual and family therapy

Evaluation/Outcome Criteria

- Physical injuries have been treated
- Plan established for safety and protection against further injury
- Abuser has agreed to seek help

Extremity Fractures

Definition

Two types of extremity fractures:

- Closed: Bone fragments remain under skin surface
- Open: Bone fragments have broken through skin surface increasing infection risk

Assessment

Subjective

- Tingling
- Numbness
- Nausea
- Pain/tenderness
- History of trauma
- Muscle spasm

Objective

- Change in function
- Deformities
- Ecchymosis
- Localized edema
- Crepitation

Diagnostic Tests

- X-ray

Treatment

- Immobilization
- Cast includes joints above and below fracture

Nursing Management

Goal: Promote healing and prevent complications.

Interventions

- Appropriate diet and fluid to promote healing and prevent constipation and kidney stones
- Developmentally appropriate activities to reduce perceptual deprivation

Goal: Prevent further injury or trauma

Interventions

- Maintain proper alignment
- Maintain skin integrity
- Assess neurovascular function—the five Ps (pain, paralysis, paresthesia, pulses, pallor), temperature changes, maintain mobility, cast care

Goal: Provide care related to use of assistive devices

- Teach proper use of crutches

Goal: Provide safety measures

- Monitor for signs of complications such as thrombophlebitis, fat embolism, nerve compression, avascular necrosis, infection, delayed union/nonunion, skin breakdown, duodenal distress (with spica cast)

Goal: Health teaching

- Explain purpose of cast
- Signs and symptoms of complications
- Isometric exercises
- Safe use of crutches

Evaluation/Outcome Criteria

- No further injury or complications related to immobilization
- Bone remains in alignment and begins to heal
- Elevates limb to relieve edema
- Understands prevention of potential complications
- Begins to use affected limb
- Demonstrates correct technique for ambulation

REVIEW QUESTIONS

1. Mandated reporters are state defined and legally required to report suspected cases of child maltreatment
   a) True
   b) False
   Answer:

2. List four categories of child mistreatment
   Answer:

3. Some medical conditions can be mistaken for child maltreatment. List three:
Answer:

4. You are caring for a child with an arm fracture that has been recently casted. Upon routine assessment you notice that his fingers are swollen, capillary refill is sluggish, and he is stating that his arm feels "funny." What should your first action be?
Answer:

5. List the five Ps used to evaluate neurovascular status in a patient with an extremity fracture:
Answer:

Related Evidence-Based Practice Guidelines

Cincinnati Children's Hospital Medical Center. (2006, December). Evidence-based care guideline for femoral shaft fractures. Cincinnati: Author. Guidelines. Retrieved from http://www.guideline.gov

The Joint Commission National Patient Safety Goals Hospital Program. Retrieved from http://www.jointcommission.org/generalpublic/npsg/10_npsgs.htm

Kellogg, N. D. (2007). American Academy of Pediatrics Committee on Child Abuse and Neglect. Evaluation of suspected child physical abuse. Pediatrics, 119(6), 1232–1241.

SBAR technique for communication: A situational briefing model. The Institute for Healthcare Improvement. Retrieved December 19, 2008, from http://www.ihi.org/IHI/Topics/PatientSafety/SafetyGeneral/Tools/SBARTechniqueforCommunicationASituationalBriefingModel.htm

Topics to Review Prior to the Simulation

- Neurovascular assessment in an extremity fracture
- Identification, documentation, and reporting of suspected child abuse

SIMULATION

Client Background

Biographical Data

- Age: 3
- Gender: female
- Height: 96 cm
- Weight: 15 kg

Cultural Considerations

- Language: English/Spanish
- Ethnicity: Hispanic
- Nationality: American
- Culture: Potential language barrier

Demographic

- Marital status: N/A
- Educational level: N/A
- Religion: Catholic
- Occupation: N/A

Current Health Status

- Femur fracture

History

- Psychosocial history
  - Social support: parents: father present, mother at home with two younger siblings
- Past health history
  - Medical: none, up-to-date (UTD) on immunizations
  - Surgical: none
- Family history: none

Admission Sheet

Name:	Jessica Ramirez
Age:	3
Gender:	Female
Marital Status:	N/A
Educational Level:	N/A
Religion:	Catholic
Ethnicity:	Hispanic
Nationality:	American

Admission Sheet—cont'd

Language:	English/Spanish
Occupation:	N/A

Hospital Provider's Orders

Patient's Name: Jessica Ramirez
Allergies: NKA

Diagnosis: Right femur fracture

Date	Time	Order	Signature
		Vital signs: q 4 hr	
		Neurovascular checks to RLE q 4 hr	
		Diet: NPO	
		Activity: Bed rest	
		IV therapy: NSS 50 mL/hr	
		Medications: Morphine 1.5 mg IV q 4 hr prn severe pain (IV 0.1 mg/kg/dose) Acetaminophen 225 mg po q 6 hr prn pain (po 15 mg/kg/dose) Diazepam 3 mg IV q 2–4 hr prn muscle spasm right leg (IV 0.2 mg/kg/dose)	
		Diagnostic studies: Right femur x-ray Skeletal survey CBC, BMP, PT/PTT	
		Treatments: Splint to right leg, elevation	
		Orthopedics consult	
		Case management consult	
		Child life specialist	Dr. Daniels

Nursing Report

Jessica Ramirez, 3-year-old Hispanic female, carried into ED by father. The child is quiet and will not make eye contact with staff. Father initially states to triage nurse child tripped running and fell 2 days ago and now will not walk. When questioned later by physician, father states that child fell down stairs. Child appears clean, dressed appropriately for weather. Eyes downward, being held by father but does not seem affectionate toward him. When legs palpated while in father's arms, child winces on palpation of right femur. Will not bear weight on right leg. Swelling noted to right femur.

Student Simulation Prep Assignments

1. Identify items and their purpose in the care of a patient with a femur fracture.

Item	Purpose
IV with pump	
Orthopedic splinting supplies/pillows	

2. *Identify team members and their specific roles in the care of a patient with a femur fracture in the setting of suspected child abuse.*

Team Member	Role
Triage nurse	
ED nurse	
ED physician	
Admitting physician	
Case manager	
Child Protection Services (CPS)	

3. *Relevant Data Exercise:* Fill in columns below.

Relevant Data from Report	Relevant Data from Other Sources	Data Missing	Sources for Missing Data	Data Requiring Follow-up

4. *Initial Focused Assessment*

After reviewing the client background and nursing report, you are ready to assess your client's current status. Under each category, identify how you would target your assessment and what you would expect to find for the patient with a femur fracture in the setting of suspected child abuse.

History

Are there any questions you need to ask the patient or family to obtain additional relevant data?

Physical Exam

- General appearance:
- Integumentary:
- HEENT:
- Respiratory:
- CV:
- Breasts:
- Abdominal:
- Neuro:
- Musculoskeletal:
- Reproductive:
- Additional:
- Developmental

What are the nursing implications considering the developmental stage of your patient?

Answer:

5. Diagnostic Tests

What diagnostic test results relevant to the patient's current problem are needed to plan care?

Complete the table using Deglin et al, *Davis's Drug Guide for Nurses* 12e, or other drug reference.

Diagnostic Test	Significance to this Patient's Problem
CBC	
BMP	
PT/PTT	
Right femur x-ray	
Skeletal survey	

6. Treatment

Identify drugs that are used to treat a patient with a femur fracture.

Complete the table using Van Leeuwen et al, *Davis's Comprehensive Handbook of Laboratory and Diagnostic Testing with Nursing Implications* 4e, or other diagnostic test reference.

Medication	Dose, Route, Frequency	Indications	Side Effect	Nursing Implications
Morphine	1.5 mg IV q 4 hr prn severe pain (IV 0.1 mg/kg/dose)			
Acetaminophen	225 mg po q 6 hr prn pain (po 15 mg/kg/dose)			
Diazepam	3 mg IV q 2–4 hr prn muscle spasm right leg (IV 0.2 mg/kg/dose)			

7 Nursing Problems/Diagnoses

Identify three priority nursing problems/diagnoses.

Assessment Data	Priority Problem	Intervention	Expected Patient Outcome	Which Interventions Could Be Delegated to Unlicensed Personnel?
1.				
2.				
3.				

References

American College of Surgeons Committee on Trauma (2008). *Advanced trauma life: Support for doctors, Student course manual* (8th ed.). Chicago: ACS.

Deglin, J. H., & Vallerand, A. H. (2009). *Davis's drug guide for nurses* (11th ed.). Philadelphia: F. A. Davis.

Dillon, P. (2007). *Nursing health assessment: A critical thinking and case studies approach* (2nd ed.). Philadelphia: F. A. Davis.

Emergency Nurses Association (2004). *Emergency nursing pediatric course* (3rd ed.). Des Plaines, IL: ENA.

Erikson, E. H. (1950). *Childhood and society*. New York: Norton.

Van Leeuwen, A. M., Poelhuis-Leth, D. J., & Bladh, M. L. (2011). *Davis's comprehensive handbook of laboratory and diagnostic tests with nursing implications.* (4th ed.). Philadelphia: F. A. Davis.

Pdfs for Hip spica teaching Retrieved from
Cincinnati Childrens Hospital
http://www.cincinnatichildrens.org/health/info/orthopaedics/home/hip-spica.htm
Vanderbilt Childrens Hospital
www.vanderbiltchildrens.com/uploads/documents/ortho-hc0425.pdf
Seattle Childrens Hospital
www.seattlechildrens.org/child_health_safety/pdf/flyers/PE005.pdf
Phoenix Childrens Hospital
www.phoenixchildrens.com/emily-center/child-health-topics/handouts/Spica-Care-788.pdf

Neurovascular assessment. Retrieved from http://www.snjourney.com/ClinicalInfo/Systems/PDF/NeuroVas%20Assessment.pdf

IV therapy. Retrieved from http://www.rch.org.au/clinicalguide/cpg.cfm?doc_id=5203

4-4 Meningitis

PEDIATRICS

STANDARD FORMS

These templates are included in the Appendix; copy before each use.

LEARNING OUTCOMES

Cognitive

The student will be able to:

1. Identify pertinent history question relevant a patient with meningitis.
2. Differentiate bacterial from viral meningitis.
3. Identify risk factors for meningitis.
4. Correlate the pathophysiology associated with the signs and symptoms of meningitis.
5. Identify appropriate diagnostic studies for a patient with meningitis.
6. Describe appropriate treatment for a patient with meningitis.

Psychomotor

The student will be able to:

1. Obtain a pertinent health history from a patient with meningitis.
2. Perform appropriate assessment for a patient with meningitis.
3. Implement patient safety standards for a patient with meningitis.

Affective

The student will be able to:

1. Reflect upon performance in performing an assessment on a patient with meningitis.
2. Identify factors that worked well during the simulation of care of a patient with meningitis.
3. Identify factors that needed improvement during the simulation of care of a patient with meningitis.
4. Develop self-confidence in performing an assessment on a patient with meningitis.

Communication

The student will be able to:

1. Communicate effectively with the patient with meningitis.
2. Use SBAR format when communicating assessment findings.
3. Accurately and succinctly document assessment findings.
4. Practice Transparent Thinking (thinking out loud) to facilitate group problem solving.
5. Use Directed Communication (directing a message to specific individual) when delegating task.
6. Employ Closed-Loop Communication (acknowledgment of receipt of the message and status) to acknowledge communications from others.

Safety

The student will be able to:

Administer and maintain specific protecting interventions with attention to safety of the client and healthcare professional.

1. Demonstrate a safe environment with attention to hazards to healthcare providers, visitors, and the client. Includes body mechanics, tripping hazards, and equipment issues.
2. Demonstrate attention to national patient safety goals. Includes patient identification standards, effective communication among healthcare providers, and safe medication administration.
3. Demonstrate attention to standard precautions. Includes hand washing, infection control measures, and use of personal protective equipment (PPE) as needed.

Leadership and Management/Delegation

The student will be able to:

1. Identify and prioritize patient's needs in care of a patient with meningitis.
2. Delegate tasks appropriately.
3. Develop a teaching plan for the patient and family with meningitis.
4. Make appropriate referrals for the patient with meningitis.

OVERVIEW OF THE PROBLEM

Definition

Meningitis is an inflammation of the spinal cord or brain membranes usually caused by an infectious agent.

Pathophysiology

Infectious meningitis is a medical emergency.

Causes

- Bacterial: *Streptococcus pneumoniae* and *Neiserria meningitidis* most common bacterial causes
- Viral: Usually self-limiting, not as serious and life-threatening as bacterial meningitis
- Other: Mycobacteria, fungal, amebas, noninfectious

Prevention

- *Haemophilus influenzae* vaccine
- Menomune vaccine (for some meningococcal bacteria) for college students
- Treat close contacts prophylactically
- Isolation

Risk Factors

- Upper respiratory infection
- Otitis media
- Sinusitis
- Pneumonia
- Sickle cell anemia
- Trauma
- Surgical procedure
- Immunocompromised disorders
- Chronic debilitating illnesses

Assessment

Subjective

- History of recent URI or acute otitis media
- Headache, neck pain, nuchal rigidity, back pain r/t meningeal irritation
- Photophobia
- Nausea, vomiting
- Any rashes: Streptococcal, flat red macular/papule rash; *Neiserria,* red flat patches

Objective

- Acute onset, initial sign may be a seizure
- Chills, fever
- Changes in level of consciousness, delirium, stupor r/t increased ICP
- Opisthotonos position; head hyperextended, bulging fontanels infants d/t meningeal irritation
- Hyperactive reflexes r/t to CNS irritability
- + Kernig's sign (with knee flexed, extensions of knee causes pain in hamstrings)
- + Brudzinski's sign (when patient flexes head to chest causes hips to flex)
- Cranial nerve VIII, hearing may be affected
- Cranial nerves III, IV, VI, EOM may be affected
- Cranial nerve VII, facial muscles may be affected
- Papilledema r/t increased ICP
- Complications: Seizures, hemiparesis, SIADH, disseminated intravascular coagulopathy (DIC), death

Diagnostic Tests

- CBC
- Lumbar puncture: CSF for Gram stain, C&S provides definitive diagnosis
- CT scan if neurological deficits present

Treatment

- Antibiotics for bacterial meningitis
- Supportive care

Nursing Management

Goal: Prevent spread of infection

- Standard precautions
- Strict hand hygiene
- Respiratory isolation minimum of 24 hr after start of antibiotics
- Supervise visitors in isolation techniques
- Identify patient contacts who are at risk
- Cultures and prophylactic antibiotics: antibiotics should be started immediately and continued for 10–14 days (until CSF is negative or patient clinically improved)
- Restrain if necessary to protect IV access

Goal: Promote safety and prevent complications:

- Administer IV meds slowly in dilute form to prevent phlebitis
- Steroids (Decadron)
- Position HOB elevated 30 degrees to prevent increased intracranial pressure (IICP). If opisthotonos, side lying; prevent straining, coughing to prevent IICP
- Quiet environment, minimal stimuli, restrict visitors, avoid bright lights d/t photophobia
- Analgesics for pain (headaches)
- Antipyretics for fever
- Maintain hydration with IVs or po fluids (NPO or clear liquids initially), monitor I&O
- Maintain seizure precautions. Administer anticonvulsants if ordered (Dilantin and lorazepam may be used for seizures)
- Monitor neuro assessment (Glasgow Coma Scale), vital signs

Goal: Maintain adequate nutrition and fluid balance:

- If NPO, IV therapy
- Diet for age when tolerated
- Monitor I&O, daily weights

Evaluation/Outcome Criteria

- No spread of infection
- Safety is maintained
- Adequate fluid and nutritional intake maintained
- Child recovers with no permanent neurological damage

REVIEW QUESTIONS

1. What findings of the C&S of the CSF would indicate bacterial meningitis?
   Answer:

2. What signs and symptoms would indicate increased intracranial pressure?
   Answer:

3. Describe the mechanism resulting in the following signs and symptoms of meningitis? Nuchal rigidity, headache, photophobia, seizures, papilledema.
   Answer:

4. What nursing intervention could be implemented to decrease ICP?
   Answer:

5. Which type of meningitis (bacterial or viral) is considered life threatening?
   Answer:

Related Evidence-Based Practice Guidelines

Search The National Guideline Clearinghouse at http://www.guideline.gov meningitis

The Joint Commission National Patient Safety Goals Hospital Program. Retrieved from http://www.jointcommission.org/generalpublic/npsg/10_npsgs.htm

SBAR technique for communication: A situational briefing model. The Institute for Healthcare Improvement. Retrieved December 19, 2008, from http://www.ihi.org/IHI/Topics/PatientSafety/SafetyGeneral/Tools/SBARTechniqueforCommunicationASituationalBriefingModel.htm

Topics to Review Prior to the Simulation

- Health assessment/neuro
- Infectious disease/isolation

SIMULATION

Client Background

Biographical Data

- Age: 19
- Gender: female
- Height: 5 ft 3½ in
- Weight: 105 lb

Cultural Considerations

- Language: English
- Ethnicity: Irish
- Nationality: American
- Culture: no significant cultural considerations identified

Demographic

- Marital status: single
- Educational level: college student
- Religion: Catholic
- Occupation: student

Current Health Status

- c/o headache, back pain, nausea and vomiting

History

- Psychosocial history
  - Social support: family
- Past health history
  - Medical: negative
  - Surgical: negative
- Family history: not available

Admission Sheet

Name:	Nancy Egger
Age:	19 yr
Gender:	Female
Marital Status:	Single
Educational Level:	College student

Continued

Admission Sheet—cont'd

Religion:	Catholic
Ethnicity:	Irish
Nationality:	American
Language:	English
Occupation:	Student

Hospital Provider's Orders

Patient's Name: Nancy Egger

Allergies: NKDA

Diagnosis: R/O meningitis

Date	Time	Order	Signature
		Admit to ICU	
		Respiratory isolation	
		Vital signs: q 1 hr with neuro check	
		Diet: NPO for 24 hr then advance to clear liquids as tolerated	
		Activity: Bed rest	
		IV therapy: 1,000 mL LR q 8 hr	
		Insert Foley catheter	
		Medications: Rocephin 2 g IV daily Vancomycin 1 g IV daily Decadron 0.15 mg/kg IV q 6 hr Tylenol 650 mg po/suppository Q 4 hr prn pain or fever Dilaudid 1 mg IV push q 4 hr prn pain Compazine 5 mg IV q 6 hr prn nausea and vomiting Regular Humilin insulin coverage sliding scale <150 no coverage 150–200 2 units Regular Humilin insulin 200-250 4 units Regular Humilin insulin 250–300 6 units Regular Humilin insulin >300 call physician	
		Diagnostic studies: LP done in ER CT scan head Repeat CBC, BMP, in AM Routine UA	

Diagnosis: R/O meningitis—cont'd

Date	Time	Order	Signature
		Viral studies Preg test	
		Treatments: Oxygen 2 L via NC	
		Cardiac monitor	Dr. Robert Kelly

Triage Nursing Report

Nancy Egger, 19-year-old white female, college student presents in ED with parents with the chief complaint of headache, back pain, nausea, and vomiting. Mother states daughter is a student at the University of Pittsburgh. Had three episodes of rash and fever while at school during the fall semester. Was seen at student health services for two of the episodes, at which time she was treated symptomatically and told that it was most likely viral.

While home on semester break, developed fever and red, flat sparse rash on chest, abdomen, and legs again. Seen by PCP, labs drawn: CBC, sed rate, Epstein-Barr virus, Mono Spot, parvovirus. c/o headache, back pain, nausea, and vomiting next morning. PCP notified. Patient instructed to go directly to ED. Lab results: WBC 26,000 with increase in neutrophils, elevated sed rate, negative Epstein-Barr virus, Mono Spot, and parvovirus.

Student Simulation Prep Assignments

1. Identify items and their purpose in the care of a patient with meningitis.

Item	Purpose
IV with pump, IV antibiotics	
O_2 cannula	
Monitor	
Gloves	
BP cuff, thermometer	
Pen light	
Isolation set up	
LP equipment	

2. Identify team members and their specific roles in the care of a patient with meningitis.

Team Member	Role
Primary nurse	
Physician	
Secondary nurse	

3. Relevant Data Assignment: Fill in columns below.

Relevant Data from Report	Relevant Data from Other Sources	Data Missing	Sources for Missing Data	Data Requiring Follow-up

4. Initial Focused Assessment

After reviewing the client background and nursing report, you are ready to assess your client's current status. Under each category, identify how you would target your assessment and what you would expect to find for the patient with meningitis

History

Are there any questions you need to ask the patient or family to obtain additional relevant data?

Physical Exam

- General appearance:
- Integumentary:
- HEENT:
- Respiratory:
- CV:
- Breasts:
- Abdominal:
- MS:
- Neuro:
- Reproductive:
- Additional:
- Developmental

What are the nursing implications considering the developmental stage of your patient?

Answer:

5. Diagnostic Tests

What diagnostic test results relevant to the patient's current problem are needed to plan care?

Complete the table using Van Leeuwen et al, *Davis's Comprehensive Handbook of Laboratory and Diagnostic Testing with Nursing Implications* 4e, or other diagnostic test reference.

Diagnostic Test	Significance to this Patient's Problem
CT scan	
CBC	
BMP Glucose Electrolytes BUN Creatinine	
CSF for C&S	
UA	
Pregnancy test	

6. Treatment

Identify drugs that are used to treat a patient with meningitis.

Complete the table using Deglin et al, *Davis's Drug Guide for Nurses* 12e, or other drug reference.

Medication	Dose, Route, Frequency	Indication	Side Effect	Nursing Implications
Rocephin	2 g IV daily			
Vancomycin	1 g IV daily			
Decadron	0.15 mg/kg IV q 6 hr			

Continued

Medication	Dose, Route, Frequency	Indication	Side Effect	Nursing Implications
Tylenol	650 mg po/ suppository q 4 hr prn pain/fever			
Dilaudid	1 mg IV q 4 hr prn severe pain			
Compazine	5 mg IV q 6 hr prn nausea and vomiting			
Regular Humalin insulin	As per sliding scale			

7. Nursing Problems/Diagnoses

Identify three priority nursing problems/diagnoses.

Assessment Data	Priority Problem	Intervention	Expected Patient Outcome	Which Interventions Could Be Delegated to Unlicensed Personnel?
1.				

Assessment Data	Priority Problem	Intervention	Expected Patient Outcome	Which Interventions Could Be Delegated to Unlicensed Personnel?
2.				
3.				

References

Deglin, J. H., & Vallerand, A. H. (2009). *Davis's drug guide for nurses* (11th ed.). Philadelphia: F. A. Davis.

Dillon, P. (2007). *Nursing health assessment: A critical thinking case studies approach* (2nd ed.). Philadelphia: F. A. Davis.

Erikson, E. H. (1950). *Childhood and society*. New York: Norton.

Goroll, A., & Mulley Jr., A. (2000). *Primary care medicine* (4th ed.). Philadelphia: Lippincott Williams & Wilkins.

Lagerquist, S. L. (2006). *Davis's NCLEX-RN for success* (2nd ed.). Philadelphia: F. A. Davis.

Mattson Porth, C. (2005). *Pathophysiology concepts of altered health states* (7th ed.). Philadelphia: Lippincott Williams & Wilkins.

Van Leeuwen, A. M., Poelhuis-Leth, D. J., & Bladh, M. L. (2011). *Davis's comprehensive handbook of laboratory and diagnostic tests with nursing implications.* (4th ed.). Philadelphia: F. A. Davis.

4-5 Spleen Injury

PEDIATRICS

STANDARD FORMS

These templates are included in the Appendix; copy before each use.

LEARNING OUTCOMES

Cognitive

The student will be able to:

1. Describe signs and symptoms of blunt abdominal trauma.
2. Correlate signs and symptoms of a splenic injury to the pathophysiology of hypovolemic shock.
3. Identify factors in a patient's history that increase risk for blunt abdominal trauma.
4. Identify factors in a patient's current condition that increase risk for hypotension, bleeding.
5. Identify appropriate interventions for the patient with blunt abdominal trauma and signs of hypovolemic shock.
6. Differentiate the roles of team members in response to a patient with blunt abdominal trauma.

Psychomotor

The student will be able to:

1. Perform an appropriate assessment for a patient with blunt abdominal trauma.
2. Initiate appropriate interventions for a patient with blunt abdominal trauma and signs of hypovolemic shock.
3. Work collaboratively as part of the healthcare team in the care of a patient with blunt abdominal injury.

Affective

The student will be able to:

1. Reflect upon performance in the care of a patient with blunt abdominal trauma.
2. Identify personal feelings in delivering care to a patient with blunt abdominal trauma.
3. Discuss feelings related to working as a member of a team in the care of a patient with blunt abdominal trauma.
4. Identify factors that worked well during the simulation of care of a patient with blunt abdominal trauma and signs of hypovolemic shock.
5. Identify factors that needed improvement during the simulation of care of a patient with abdominal trauma and signs of hypovolemic shock
6. Develop self-confidence in the care of a patient with blunt abdominal trauma.

Communication

The student will be able to:

1. Communicate effectively with healthcare team members in the care of a patient with blunt abdominal trauma.
2. Communicate effectively with the patient and family in the care of a patient with blunt abdominal trauma.
3. Use SBAR format when communicating with team members about the care of a patient with blunt abdominal trauma showing signs of hypovolemic shock.
4. Practice Transparent Thinking (thinking out loud) to facilitate group problem solving.
5. Use Directed Communication (directing a message to specific individual) when delegating tasks.
6. Employ Closed-Loop Communication (acknowledgment of receipt of the message and status) to acknowledge communications from others.

Safety

The student will be able to:

Administer and maintain specific protecting interventions with attention to safety of the client and healthcare professional.

1. Demonstrate a safe environment with attention to hazards to healthcare providers, visitors, and the client. Includes body mechanics, tripping hazards, and equipment issues.
2. Demonstrate attention to national patient safety goals. Includes patient identification standards, effective communication among healthcare providers, and safe medication administration.
3. Demonstrate attention to standard precautions. Includes hand washing, infection control measures, and use of personal protective equipment (PPE) as needed.

Leadership and Management/Delegation

The student will be able to:

1. Identify tasks that can be legally, ethically, and safely delegated to unlicensed assistive personnel (UAP) or licensed practical nurse (LPN) in the care of a patient with blunt abdominal trauma.
2. Identify and prioritize patient's needs in care of blunt abdominal trauma.

Overview of the Problem

Definition

Abdominal trauma is an injury to the abdomen. It may be blunt or penetrating and may involve damage to the abdominal organs.

Pathophysiology

Intra-abdominal injuries secondary to blunt force occur with collisions between the injured person and the external environment resulting in acceleration or deceleration forces acting on the person's internal organs. Blunt force injuries to the abdomen can generally be explained by three mechanisms.

The first occurs when shear forces cause hollow, solid, visceral organs and vascular pedicles to tear, especially at relatively fixed points of attachment.

The second is when intra-abdominal contents are crushed between the anterior abdominal wall and the vertebral column or posterior thoracic cage. Solid viscera such as the spleen, liver, and kidneys are especially vulnerable.

The third is when external compression forces result in a sudden and dramatic rise in intra-abdominal pressure and culminate in rupture of a hollow viscous organ.

Risk Factors

- Occurs slightly more often in males

Assessment for Splenic Injury

Subjective

- Left upper quadrant pain
- Left shoulder pain (Kehr's sign)

Objective

- Moderate rigidity
- Hypotension, shock

Treatment

- Prehospital care:
  - ABCs with spinal immobilization
  - Institute shock measures
- Assess for other injuries based on mechanism
- In-hospital care:
  - Assess respiratory and hemodynamic status
  - Maintain airway and ventilation
  - IV therapy as ordered
  - CVP and arterial lines if indicated
  - Insert Foley catheter if indicated (low-grade lacerations are admitted to med/surg with activity restrictions and accurate I/O)
  - Prepare for angiography/embolization or splenectomy if indicated
  - Administer postsplenectomy vaccinations if indicated

Nursing Management

- Observe for rigidity
- Assess for hematuria
- Auscultate bowel sounds
- Palpate for tenderness
- Assist with diagnostic peritoneal lavage to confirm bleeding into the peritoneal cavity
- Prepare for angiography if indicated
- Postsplenic embolization care:
  - Prepare for exploratory laparotomy if indicated
  - Insert NG tube to check for upper GI bleeding— not a common practice unless patient is intubated or develops an ileus
- Monitor vitals signs and signs of shock

Current practice is nonoperative management of pediatric splenic injuries unless the patient becomes hemodynamically unstable. The next course of action after fluids and blood products is usually angiography with embolization if active extravasation is present. Splenectomy is a last resort only and rarely done.

REVIEW QUESTIONS

1. Name three goals in the treatment of shock.
   Answer:

2. Complete the following table:

Type of Shock	Causes	Signs	Priority Intervention
Hypovolemic			

Continued

Type of Shock	Causes	Signs	Priority Intervention
Distributive			
Cardiogenic			
Obstructive			

3. Describe the difference between compensated and decompensated (hypotensive) shock.
   Answer:

4. What are three primary functions of the spleen?
   Answer:

5. True or False: Abdominal organs are more exposed in younger children due to their shorter rib cages, predisposing them to easier injury.
   Answer:

Related Evidence-Based Practice Guidelines

Practice management guidelines for the evaluation of blunt abdominal trauma. Retrieved from http://www.east.org/tpg/bluntabd.pdf

Practice Management Guidelines for the Nonoperative Management of Blunt Injury to the Liver or Spleen retrieved from http://www.east.org/tpg/livspleen.pdf

IV Therapy http://www.rch.org.au/clinicalguide/cpg.cfm?doc_id=5203

The Joint Commission National Patient Safety Goals Hospital Program. Retrieved from http://www.jointcommission.org/generalpublic/npsg/10_npsgs.htm

SBAR technique for communication: A situational briefing model published by The Institute for Healthcare Improvement was downloaded on December 19, 2008, from http://www.ihi.org/IHI/Topics/PatientSafety/SafetyGeneral/Tools/tTechniqueforCommunicationASituationalBriefingModel.htm

Topics to Review Prior to the Simulation

- Anatomy and physiology of the spleen
- Types of shock (hypovolemic, cardiogenic, distributive, obstructive)

SIMULATION

Client Background

Biographical Data

- Age:14
- Gender: male
- Height: 5 ft 5 in
- Weight: 154 lb

Cultural Considerations

- Language: English
- Ethnicity: German heritage
- Nationality: American
- Culture: no significant cultural implications identified

Demographic

- Marital status: N/A
- Educational level: Freshman in high school
- Religion: Lutheran
- Occupation: student

Current Health Status

- Admitted to med/surg after sustaining a small splenic laceration while playing football

History

- Psychosocial history
  - Social support: parents present
- Past health history
  - Medical: none, up-to-date (UTD) on immunizations, PCN allergy
  - Surgical: appendectomy age 8
- Family history: noncontributory

Admission Sheet

Name:	Joshua Eck
Age:	14
Gender:	Male
Marital Status:	N/A
Educational Level:	High school freshman
Religion:	Lutheran
Ethnicity:	German
Nationality:	American
Language:	English
Occupation:	Student

Hospital
Provider's Orders

Patient's Name: Joshua Eck
Allergies: PCN

Diagnosis: Splenic laceration

Date	Time	Order	Signature
		Vital signs: q 4 hr	
		Diet: NPO	
		Activity: Bed rest	
		IV therapy: NSS at 100 mL/hr	

Continued

Diagnosis: Splenic laceration—cont'd

Date	Time	Order	Signature
		Medications: Fentanyl 70 mcg IV q 4 hr prn pain (2 mcg/kg/dose q 2-4 hr) Zofran 4 mg IV q 8 hr prn nausea/vomiting Pepcid 20 mg IV q HS	
		Diagnostic studies: H&H q 12 hr CBC q AM CT abdomen/pelvis with IV contrast	
		Type and cross for 2 units PRBC	
		Monitor Intake/Output	Dr. Shudder

Nursing Report

Joshua Eck, 14-year-old male, admitted to med/surg after sustaining a small splenic laceration while playing football. He was wearing full padding and was tackled while running with the football, landing on the ball. He presented to the ED complaining of left-sided chest and left upper quadrant abdominal pain. CT of his chest, abdomen, and pelvis showed a small splenic laceration without active bleeding. He is being admitted to med/surg for close observation and pain control. He arrived to the pediatric unit 1 hr ago with his parents. You are beginning your shift and have been assigned to care for Joshua.

Student Simulation Prep Assignments

1. Identify items and their purpose in the care of a patient with spleen injury.

Item	Purpose
IV with pump	

2. Identify team members and their specific roles in the care of a patient with a spleen injury.

Team Member	Role
Primary nurse	
Surgical resident	
Nursing assistant/technical partner	
Primary ICU nurse	

3. *Relevant Data Exercise:* Fill in the columns below.

Relevant Data from and Report	Relevant Data from Other Sources	Data Missing	Sources for Missing Data	Data Requiring Follow-up

4. *Initial Focused Assessment*

After reviewing the client background and nursing report, you are ready to assess your client's current status. Under each category, identify how you would target your assessment and what you would expect to find for the patient with a spleen laceration.

History

Are there any questions you need to ask the patient or family to obtain additional relevant data?

Physical Exam

- General appearance:
- Integumentary:
- HEENT:
- Respiratory:
- CV:
- Breasts:
- Abdominal:
- Neuro:
- Musculoskeletal:
- Reproductive:
- Developmental:

What are the nursing implications considering the developmental stage of your patient?

Answer:

5. *Diagnostic Tests*

What diagnostic test results relevant to the patient's current problem are needed to plan care?

Complete the table using Van Leeuwen et al, *Davis's Comprehensive Handbook of Laboratory and Diagnostic Testing with Nursing Implications* 4e, or other diagnostic test reference.

Diagnostic Test	Significance to This Patient's Problem
CBC	
BMP	
Lactate	
Type and cross for PRBC	
CT abdomen and pelvis with IV contrast	
Angiography with embolization	

6. Treatment

Identify drugs that are used to treat a patient with spleen injury.

Complete the table using Deglin et al, *Davis's Drug Guide for Nurses* 12e, or other drug reference.

Medication	Dose, Route, Frequency	Indications	Side Effects	Nursing Implications
Fentanyl	2 mcg/kg/dose IV q 2–4 hr			
Pepcid	20 mg IV at bedtime			
Zofran	4 mg IV q 8 hr			

7. Nursing Problems/Diagnoses

Identify three priority nursing problems/diagnoses .

Assessment Data	Priority Problem	Intervention	Expected Patient Outcome	Which Interventions Could Be Delegated to Unlicensed Personnel?
1.				
2.				
3.				

References

American College of Surgeons Committee on Trauma (2008). *Advanced trauma life support for doctors, student course manual* (8th ed.). Chicago: ACS.

Deglin, J. H., & Vallerand, A. H. (200). *Davis's drug guide for nurses* (11th ed.). Philadelphia: F. A. Davis.

Dilln, P. (2007). *Nursing health assessment: A critical thinking and case studies approach* (2nd ed.). Philadelphia: F. A. Davis.

Durning, M. (2009). *Davis's comprehensive handbook of laboratory and diagnostic tests with nursing implications* (3rd ed.). Philadelphia: F. A. Davis.

Erikson, E. H. (1950). *Childhood and society*. New York: Norton.

IV therapy. Retrieved from http://www.rch.org.au/clinicalguide/cpg.cfm?doc_id=5203

The Joint Commission National Patient Safety Goals Hospital Program. Retrieved from http://www.jointcommission.org/generalpublic/npsg/10_npsgs.htm

Lagerquist, S. L. (2006). *Davis's NCLEX-RN for success* (2nd ed.). Philadelphia: F. A. Davis.

Pediatric advanced life support provider manual (2006). American Heart Association and American Academy of Pediatrics.

Practice management guidelines for the evaluation of blunt abdominal trauma. Retrieved from http://www.east.org/tpg/bluntabd.pdf

SBAR technique for communication: A situational briefing model. The Institute for Healthcare Improvement. Retrieved December 19, 2008, from http://www.ihi.org/IHI/Topics/PatientSafety/SafetyGeneral/Tools/SBARTechniqueforCommunicationASituationalBriefingModel.htm

Van Leeuwen, A. M., Poelhuis-Leth, D. J., & Bladh, M. L. (2011). *Davis's comprehensive handbook of laboratory and diagnostic tests with nursing implications.* (4th ed.). Philadelphia: F. A. Davis.

Adult Health Nursing 5

5-1 Intestinal Obstruction

MEDICAL-SURGICAL OR FUNDAMENTALS

STANDARD FORMS

These templates are included in the Appendix; copy before each use.

LEARNING OUTCOMES

Cognitive

The student will be able to:

1. Describe signs and symptoms of an intestinal obstruction.
2. Compare observed clinical manifestations with the pathophysiology of intestinal obstruction.
3. Summarize factors in a patient's history which may predispose the person to an intestinal obstruction.
4. Determine appropriate interventions for the patient with a nasogastric tube for decompression.
5. Integrate theoretical concepts with the care of a patient with an intestinal obstruction.
6. Recognize and correct medication errors.
7. Delineate assessment parameters which would indicate optimal functioning of a nasogastric tube for decompression.

Psychomotor

The student will be able to:

1. Perform an appropriate focused assessment for a patient with an intestinal obstruction and a nasogastric tube for decompression.
2. Manage a nasogastric tube. The management should include interventions to ensure patency, trouble shoot for malfunction, and tube irrigation.
3. Manipulate suction equipment.
4. Ascertain that medical orders for treatment are appropriately implemented.
5. Demonstrate the use of standard precautions throughout the care of a patient with an intestinal obstruction.

Affective

The student will be able to:

1. Reflect upon performance in a simulated situation and care of a patient with an intestinal obstruction.
2. Express personal feelings in delivering care to a patient with an intestinal obstruction.
3. Identify elements of the simulation which promoted the patient's physical and psychological well-being.
4. Identify elements of the simulation which could have been done differently in order to promote the patient's physical and psychological well-being.
5. Consistently act in a professional manner during the simulated care of a patient with an intestinal obstruction.

Communication

The student will be able to:

1. Recognize the need to notify the prescriber with changes in the condition of a patient with an intestinal obstruction.
2. Communicate effectively with healthcare team members in the care of a patient with an intestinal obstruction, using the SBAR format.
3. Demonstrate therapeutic dialogue with the patient and family members during the care of a patient with an intestinal obstruction.
4. Accurately document the care given to a patient with an intestinal obstruction.
5. Practice Transparent Thinking (thinking out loud) to facilitate group problem solving
6. Use Directed Communication (directing a message to specific individual) when delegating tasks.
7. Employ Closed-Loop Communication (acknowledgment of receipt of the message and status) to acknowledge communications from others.
8. Work collaboratively as part of the healthcare team in the care of a patient with an intestinal obstruction.

Safety

The student will be able to:

Administer and maintain specific protecting interventions with attention to safety of the client and healthcare professional.

1. Demonstrate a safe environment with attention to hazards to healthcare providers, visitors, and the client.

Includes body mechanics, tripping hazards, and equipment issues.

2. Demonstrate attention to national patient safety goals. Includes patient identification standards, effective communication among healthcare providers, and safe medication administration.
3. Demonstrates attention to standard precautions. Includes hand washing, infection control measures, and use of personal protective equipment (PPE) as needed.

Leadership and Management/Delegation

The student will be able to:

1. Identify tasks that can be legally, ethically, and safely delegated to unlicensed assistive personnel (UAP) or licensed practical nurse (LPN) in the care of a patient with an intestinal obstruction.
2. Prioritize the care of a patient with an intestinal obstruction and nasogastric decompression.

OVERVIEW OF THE PROBLEM

Definition

Two types of intestinal obstruction:

- Mechanical: A physical blockage which interferes with the passage of intestinal contents. Mechanical obstructions are most common in the small intestine. Adhesions are the most common cause of small bowel obstruction, followed by hernias and tumors. Other causes of mechanical obstruction include inflammatory bowel disease, stool impactions, strictures, and intussusception.
- Nonmechanical (also known as paralytic ileus): There is no physical obstruction present, but peristalsis is markedly diminished, or totally absent. Nonmechanical obstruction may by due to neuromuscular or vascular disturbances. The most common cause of a nonmechanical obstruction is paralytic ileus. This usually is a result of handling the bowel during surgery. Other causes of nonmechanical obstruction include inflammatory response, abdominal trauma, hypokalemia, spinal injuries, or vascular insufficiency.

Pathophysiology

In both types of obstruction, the contents of the intestine back up above the level of the obstruction. This accumulation of intestinal contents results in distension. The distension leads to increased peristalsis in an attempt to clear the intestine of the accumulated secretions. The increased peristaltic activity causes more secretions to be formed. More distension follows, which causes edema in the bowel. The edema results in increased capillary permeability. The fluid trapped in the intestines causes a decreased amount of absorption into the vascular space. The lack of vascular fluid leads to hypovolemia and electrolyte imbalance.

Risk Factors

- Previous or recent abdominal surgery
- Previous history of bowel obstruction

Assessment

Subjective

- Determine location, duration, severity, and timing of abdominal pain. Obstructions in the small intestine most commonly cause colicky, cramping, intermittent pain, which often comes in wavelike contractions. There may be vomiting, constipation, or diarrhea. As the obstruction progresses, an unpleasant breath odor will be present. Large intestinal obstructions usually cause nagging, cramping abdominal pain.
- Question the client about the presence and frequency of flatus.
- Assess for the presence of vomiting. If present, assess the frequency, color, odor, and amount of vomitus. Large amounts of nonfecal vomitus are most common with small bowel obstructions. Less frequent, but fecal vomitus is common with large bowel obstructions.

Objective

- Inspection: Note the presence of scars and distension.
- Auscultate bowel sounds and note their location and duration. Bowel sounds are initially loud and high pitched, becoming absent as muscular atony occurs.
- Palpation: Areas of pain, tenderness, guarding.
- Accurate measurement of intake and output. (Urine output is usually decreased.)
- Vital signs: Temperature: commonly elevated. A high temperature (>100.3°F) may indicate the presence of infection. Heart rate: usually tachycardic. Amplitude may be thready due to the lack of fluid in the vascular space. Blood pressure: usually hypotension; again due to the hypovolemia. An untreated obstruction may progress to shock due to hypovolemia.

Diagnostic Tests

WBC: usually elevated. Electrolytes: sodium and potassium will be decreased. BUN and creatinine will rise if inadequate circulatory volume is contributing to renal failure. Flat plate and upright abdominal x-ray, abdominal ultrasound, or CT scans may be done to confirm the diagnosis. If the obstruction is at the gastric outlet, pH will be elevated, indicating metabolic alkalosis. If the obstruction is in distal duodenal or proximal jejunum, the pH will drop, indicating metabolic acidosis.

Treatment

- If no improvement with conservative treatment, or if condition worsens, emergency surgery may be required. The surgery may include resection of the obstructed bowel and joining the remaining healthy bowel together. If the obstruction is extensive, a partial or total colectomy may be required.

Nursing Management

Medical and nursing management will depend on the severity of the obstruction.

Goal: Maintain fluid and electrolyte status:

- Rest the bowel: NPO status, NG for decompression.
- Intravenous fluids: Usually normal saline or lactated Ringer's solution. Potassium may be added if there is adequate renal function and laboratory data reflect hypokalemia.
  - Strict intake and output and daily weights should be instituted.
  - Monitor CVP for hydration status.
- Monitor success of treatment: Laboratory data, auscultate bowel sounds, return of bowel function (flatus, stool), monitor abdominal girth for reduction of abdominal distension, intakc and output.

Goal: Relieve pain and nausea: analgesics and antiemetics as ordered. Nonpharmacological pain control: relaxation, massage, etc.

- Promote restful environment, limit visitors per client wishes. Frequent skin and mouth care. Assess pain frequently, and medicate before pain is out of control.
- If opioids are ordered for pain, monitor the patient response carefully, especially if hypovolemia is present.
- A stimulant such as neostigmine may be ordered for nonmechanical obstructions such as paralytic ileus. This is a rare treatment.

Goal: Prevent respiratory complications.

- Encourage coughing, deep breathing, incentive spirometry.
- Semi-Fowler's or position of comfort.

Evaluation/Outcome Criteria

- Fluid and electrolyte balance is maintained
- Obstruction is resolved
- Pain is managed or decreased
- Fluids tolerated by mouth
- Complications such as shock, perforation, and peritonitis are avoided

REVIEW QUESTIONS

1. Define intestinal obstruction.
   Answer:

2. What is the recommended method to assure position of a nasogastric tube?
   Answer:

3. What objective signs would be seen in a patient with a small bowel obstruction?
   Answer:

4. What is the most common complication which a patient with a small bowel obstruction might experience?
   Answer:

5. What are three collaborative goals for the treatment of a patient with a small bowel obstruction, and what are nursing interventions which may be used to reach each goal?
   Answer:

Collaborative Goal	Examples of Nursing Interventions
1.	
2.	

Continued

Collaborative Goal	Examples of Nursing Interventions
3.	

Related Evidence-Based Practice Guidelines

Insertion and management of nasogastric tubes for adults. Retrieved from http://www.joannabriggs.edu/protocols/protnasotube.php

The Joint Commission National Patient Safety Goals Hospital Program. Retrieved from http://www.jointcommission.org/generalpublic/npsg/10_npsgs.htm

Reising, D., & Neal, R. (2005). Enteral tube feeding: What you think are the best practices may not be. American Journal of Nursing, *105*(3), 415.

SBAR Technique for Communication: A situational briefing model published by The Institute for Healthcare Improvement and was downloaded on December 19, 2008, from http://www.ihi.org/IHI/Topics/PatientSafety/SafetyGeneral/Tools/SBARTechniqueforCommunicationASituationalBriefingModel.htm

Topics to Review Prior to the Simulation

- Nasogastric tube management: ensuring patency, how the tube functions, purpose of the tube, etc.
- Pathophysiology of a small bowel obstruction. What signs and symptoms would you expect to see in a patient with a small bowel obstruction?
- Focused abdominal physical assessment nursing interventions for a patient with a nasogastric tube.

The instructor may also wish to assign these articles:

Best, C. (2005). Caring for a patient with a nasogastric tube. Nursing Standard, *20*(3), 59-67.

Ellett, M. (2004). What is known about methods of correctly placing gastric tubes in adults and children? Gastroenterology Nursing, *27*(6), 253-259.

Sumar, S. (2005). Methods to check correct placement of a nasogastric tube: Beware of the pitfalls. *Age and Aging*, *34*(3), 415.

SIMULATION

Client Background

Emily Grace is a 45-year-old woman who was admitted to a medical-surgical unit with a small bowel obstruction. She has had a 4-day history of abdominal pain and vomiting, with up to 12 vomiting episodes per day. The vomitus is blood streaked at times. Her medical history includes an 8-year history of hypertension and type 2 diabetes for 12 years. Recent surgeries include an appendectomy 3 years ago.

Biographical Data:

- Age: 45
- Gender: female
- Height: 5 ft 8 in
- Weight: 180 lb

Cultural Considerations

- Language: English
- Ethnicity: Hispanic
- Nationality: American
- Culture: no significant cultural considerations identified

Demographic

- Marital status: married
- Educational level: community college
- Religion: Episcopal
- Occupation: administrative assistant

Current Health Status

- 4-day history of abdominal pain and vomiting, with up to 12 vomiting episodes per day. The vomitus is blood streaked at times.

History

- Psychosocial history
  Social support: married
- Past health history
  - Medical: 8-year history of hypertension and type 2 diabetes for 12 years.
  - Surgical: recent surgeries include an appendectomy 3 years ago
- Family History: none significant

Admission Sheet

Name:	Emily Grace
Age:	45
Gender:	Female
Marital Status:	Married
Educational Level:	Community College
Religion:	Episcopal
Ethnicity:	Hispanic
Nationality:	American
Language:	English
Occupation:	Administrative assistant

Hospital
Provider's Orders

Patient's Name: **Emily Grace**
Allergies: **Penicillin and Compazine**

Diagnosis: **Small bowel obstruction**

Date	Time	Order	Signature
		Admit to medical-surgical unit	
		Vital signs: q 4 hr	
		Diet: NPO—may have occasional ice chips	
		Activity: up as tolerated with assistance Assess for falls, and institute fall precautions	
		IV therapy: D5 0.45% NS with 20 mEq KCl/L @ 125 cc/hr	
		Medications: Ciprofloxacin 400 mg IV q 12 hr Metronidazole 1200 mg IV infused over 1 hr for 1 dose and then 500 mg IV q 6 hr Morphine sulfate 2 mg IV q 2–4 hr as needed Acetaminophen 650 mg rectally q 4 hr prn temp >100.3°F.	

Continued

Diagnosis: Small bowel obstruction—cont'd			
Date	**Time**	**Order**	**Signature**
		Promethazine hydrochloride 10 mg IV q 4–6 hr as needed for vomiting or nausea Lisinopril 20 mg per NG tube every day Regular insulin: sliding scale q 4 hr. Subcutaneous administration: BG 70–150: give 0 units BG 151–200: give 2 units BG 201–250: give 4 units BG 251–300: give 6 units BG 301–350: give 8 units BG <70 or >350: notify on-call physician	
		Diagnostic studies: Blood sugar q 4 hr (bedside monitor) CBC, electrolytes every morning BUN, creatinine every morning Flat and upright abdomen today	
		Salem sump to continuous suction—may irrigate prn	
		Accurate I&O. Record q 4 hr	
		Record daily weight	Dr. Morgan

Nursing Report

Report from previous shift nurse:

Mrs. Grace has had an uncomfortable night. Her pain has been from 6–8 on a scale of 0–10. She has had minimal relief with morphine. The pain seems to be worse this morning. Her husband has been with her tonight, and he is quite worried and frustrated. Mrs. Grace says her pain is in the upper abdomen with right side worse than left. The pain is intermittent and feels like bad labor pains. Her abdomen is distended and diffusely tender to palpation. Her abdomen seems more distended this morning. There are minimal, hypoactive bowel sounds present. The NG drained 600 mL dark brown green drainage this shift. Her urine output was 75 mL with dark yellow, thick urine.

Student Simulation Prep Assignments

1. Identify items and their purpose in the care of a patient with small bowel obstruction.

Item	Purpose
IV solution	
Emesis basin	
Gloves	
NG tube	
Suction control and tubing	
pH paper	
Irrigation set	

Item	Purpose
NS for irrigation	
Stethoscope	
BP cuff	
Thermometer	
Pulse oximeter	
Graduated cylinder	

2. Identify team members and their specific roles in the care of a patient with small bowel obstruction.

Team Member	Role
Primary RN	
Secondary RN	
CNA	
Physician (by telephone)	

3. Relevant Data Exercise: Fill in the columns below.

Relevant Data from Report	Relevant Data from Other Sources	Data Missing	Sources for Missing Data	Data Requiring Follow-Up

4. Initial Focused Assessment

After reviewing the client background and nursing report, you are ready to assess your client's current status. Under each category, identify how you would target your assessment, and what you would expect to find for the patient with small bowel obstruction

History

Are there any questions you need to ask the patient or family to obtain additional relevant data?

Physical Exam

- General appearance:
- Integumentary:
- HEENT:
- Respiratory:
- CV:
- Breasts:
- Abdominal:
- Neuro:
- Musculoskeletal:
- Additional:
- Developmental:

Considering the age of your client, are there any developmental issues you need to address?

Answers:

5. Diagnostic Tests

What diagnostic test results relevant to the patient's current problem are needed to plan care?

Complete the table using Van Leeuwen et al, *Davis's Comprehensive Handbook of Laboratory and Diagnostic Testing with Nursing Implications* 4e, or other diagnostic test reference.

Diagnostic Test	Significance to This Patient's Problem
CBC	
BUN	
Creatinine	
Electrolytes	
Glucose	
Flat plate abdomen	

6. Treatment

Identify drugs that may be used to treat a patient with a small bowel obstruction and a nasogastric tube.

Complete the table using Deglin et al, *Davis's Drug Guide for Nurses* 12e, or other drug reference.

Medication	Dose, Route, Frequency	Indications	Side Effect	Nasogastric Implications
Morphine	2 mg IV			
Ciprofloxacin	400 mg q 12 hr			
Metronidazole	1200 mg IV x 1 dose then 500 mg q 6 hr			
Acetaminophen	650 mg q 4 hr for temperature >100.3°F			
Promethazine HCl	10 mg IV q 4–6 prn			
Lisinopril	20 mg NG tube daily			
Regular insulin	Sliding scale			

7. Nursing Problems/Diagnoses

Identify three priority nursing problems/diagnoses.

Assessment Data	Priority Problem	Intervention	Expected Patient Outcome	Which Interventions Could Be Delegated to Unlicensed Personnel?
1.				
2.				

Continued

Assessment Data	Priority Problem	Intervention	Expected Patient Outcome	Which Interventions Could Be Delegated to Unlicensed Personnel?
3.				

References

Best, C. (2005). Caring for a patient with a nasogastric tube. *Nursing Standard, 20*(3), 59-67.

Deglin, J. H., & Vallerand, A. H. (2009). *Davis's drug guide for nurses* (11th ed.). Philadelphia: F. A. Davis.

Dillon, P. (2007). *Nursing health assessment: A critical thinking and case studies approach* (2nd ed.). Philadelphia: F. A. Davis.

Ellett, M. (2004). What is known about methods of correctly placing gastric tubes in adults and children? *Gastroenterology Nursing, 27*(6), 253-259.

Erikson, E. H. (1950). *Childhood and society*. New York: Norton.

Lagerquist, S. (2006). *NCLEX-RN success*. Philadelphia: F. A. Davis.

Sumar, S. (2005). Methods to check correct placement of a nasogastric tube: Beware of the pitfalls. *Age and Aging, 34*(3), 415.

Van Leeuwen, A. M. & Poelhuis-Leth, D.J., & Bladh, M.L. (2011). *Davis's comprehensive handbook of laboratory and diagnostic tests with nursing implications.* (4th ed.). Philadelphia: F. A. Davis.

5-2 Postoperative Hip

MEDICAL SURGICAL

STANDARD FORMS

These templates are included in the Appendix; copy before each use.

LEARNING OUTCOMES

Cognitive

The student will be able to:

1. Determine essential assessments for the postoperative client and correctly perform assessments specific to the client's priority needs in a coordinated and timely manner based on data and setting resources:
   - Focused postoperative assessment: neurological, cardiac, respiratory, mobility
   - Vital signs including pain
   - Intake and output
   - Dressing
   - Drain
2. Analyze assessment data and identify the appropriate interventions for the postoperative patient that will address priority actions specific to client's physiological status, age, culture, and setting resources.
3. Engage in purposeful, efficient information sharing and plan of care implementation and evaluation when necessary.

Psychomotor

The student will be able to:

1. Demonstrate timely and efficient integration of postoperative nursing interventions specific to health patterns to promote oxygenation, hydration, mobility, elimination, and skin integrity.
   - Administer oxygen—appropriate O_2 delivery device, positioning, and flow.
   - Assists client with incentive spirometer and turn, cough, and deep breathe (TCDB).
   - Monitors fluid balance.
     - Check IV fluid type and infusion rate.
     - Monitor urine output.
     - Jackson- Pratt (JP) drain output.
   - Administer medications with attention to The Joint Commission National Patient Safety goals for safe medication delivery:
     - Pain medication
     - Anticoagulant
     - Antibiotic
   - Assures abductor pillow placement.
2. Guide and support client and family through the illness experience with communication and learning strategies specific to learning readiness, culture, age, and education level. Provides client with explanation for the following:
   - Oxygen delivery
   - Abductor pillow placement
   - Medications
   - JP drain
3. TCDB and incentive spirometry (IS)
4. Document and evaluate care to support continuity of care and patient outcomes.

Affective

The student will be able to:

1. Critique own actions using a nursing framework in adapting a plan of care specific to the changing client story and setting resources.
2. Reflect upon performance in the care of a postoperative patient with hip replacement.
3. Identify own feelings in delivering care to a postoperative patient with hip replacement.
4. Discuss feelings related to working as a member of a team in the care of a postoperative patient with hip replacement.
5. Identify factors that worked well during the simulation.
6. Identify factors that needed improvement during the simulation.

Communication

The student will be able to:

1. Communicate effectively with healthcare team members utilizing the SBAR reporting format.
   - Dialogue with peers, faculty, and/or charge RN regarding client condition.
2. Communicate effectively with the patient in the care of a postoperative patient with hip replacement.
3. Will practice Transparent Thinking (thinking out loud) to facilitate group problem solving.
4. Use Directed Communication (directing a message to specific individual) when delegating tasks.
5. Employ Closed-Loop Communication (acknowledgment of receipt of the message and status) to acknowledge communications from others.

Safety

The student will be able to:

Administer and maintain specific protecting interventions with attention to safety of the client and healthcare professional.

1. Demonstrate a safe environment with attention to hazards to healthcare providers, visitors, and the client. Includes body mechanics, tripping hazards, and equipment issues.
2. Demonstrate attention to national patient safety goals. Includes patient identification standards, effective communication among healthcare providers, and safe medication administration.
3. Demonstrate attention to standard precautions. Includes hand washing, infection control measures, and use of personal protective equipment (PPE) as needed.

Leadership and Management/Delegation

The student will be able to:

1. Identify tasks that can be legally, ethically, and safely delegated to unlicensed assistive personnel (UAP) or LPN in the care of a postoperative patient with hip replacement.
2. Identify and prioritize patient's needs in care of a postoperative patient with hip replacement.

OVERVIEW OF THE PROBLEM

Total hip replacement

Definition

Femoral head and acetabulum are replaced by a prosthesis.

Pathophysiology

- Performed to replace a joint with limited and painful function due to bony alkalosis and deformity caused by degenerative joint disease or when vascular supply to the femoral head is compromised from a fracture.

Goal: To restore or improve function of the hip joint and prevent complications of immobilization.

Risk Factors

- Rheumatoid arthritis
- Osteoarthritis
- Fractures of the femoral head
- Congental hip disease

Assessment

Subjective

- Pain, sensation

Objective

- Movement, circulation

Diagnostic Tests

- CBC
- PT—if on warfarin
- Hip x-ray
- Duplex scan

Treatment

Medical management includes administration of:

- Antibiotics
- Pain management
- Anticoagulants
- Stool softeners
- IV therapy

Nursing Management—Postoperative

Goal: Prevent DVT or pulmonary emboli

- Sequential compression device (SCD) or TED hose
- Maintain fluid intake
- Administer anticoagulants as ordered

Goal: Prevent complications of shock or infection

- Antibiotics as ordered
- Sterile dressing change
- Check dressing and drains
- Monitor intake and output and vital signs

Goal: Prevent respiratory complications

- Turn, cough, deep breathe
- Incentive spirometry

Goal: Prevent contractures and muscle atrophy

- Initiate exercises

Goal: Promote mobility and early ambulation and prevent dislocation

  - Total hip precautions
  - Maintain abduction
  - Report signs of dislocation
  - Use trapeze
  - Transfer technique—pivot on unaffected leg
  - Progressive ambulation
  - Monitor side effects of medications
  - Safety and fall prevention

Goal: Maintain bowel and bladder function

- Increase fluid intake
- Use fracture bedpan
- Assess bowel sounds, abdominal distention, and I&O

Goal: promote comfort

- Skin care
- Pressure mattress
- PCA or analgesics as ordered

Goal: Health teaching

- Hip precautions
- Exercises
- Support hose

Evaluation/Outcome Criteria

- Participates in postoperative nursing care plan to prevent complications
- Reports decrease in pain
- Ambulates safely with assistive devices
- Complications of immobility are avoided
- Able to resume self-care activities

REVIEW QUESTIONS

1. What are the priority assessments for postoperative clients?
Answer:

2. What are the major complications associated with postoperative clients?
Answer:

3. Elderly clients are at higher risk for fluid and electrolyte imbalances. What essential assessments are required to monitor fluids and electrolytes?
Answer:

4. Your postoperative client's urinary output has been 25 mL/hr for the past 2 consecutive hours. Is this amount acceptable? Where else would you look to see if this client is developing fluid overload?
Answer:

5. Deep vein thrombosis is a complication associated with surgery. List interventions to prevent DVT.
Answer:

Related Evidence-Based Practice Guidelines

The Joint Commission National Patient Safety Goals Hospital Program. Retrieved from http://www.jointcommission.org/GeneralPublic/NPSG/10_npsgs.htm

National Guideline Clearing House. Postoperative Management in adults. A Practical Guide to Postoperative Care for Clinical Staff. Retrieved July 2007, www.guideline.gov

Topics to Review Prior to the Simulation

- Postoperative care: assessments, anticipated interventions, and expected outcomes.
- Hip replacement postfracture: pathophysiology associated with fracture, potential complications, and ORIF procedure.
- Atelectasis: pathophysiology and anticipated interventions.

SIMULATION

Client Background

Terry VanDyke is a 79-year-old, 5 ft 11 in, 210 lb white, English-speaking male. He is a retired physical education teacher from a local high school. Mr. VanDyke is married and has three grown children, all living nearby. Past medical history is positive for smoking for 30 years (1 pack/day) and mild hypertension that was diagnosed 4 years ago for which he takes metroprolol 12.5 mg po daily. Mr. VanDyke reports a family history of depression, but denies this for himself. He denies previous surgeries or hospital admissions. Mr. VanDyke was cleaning the garage yesterday when he fell approximately 3 ft from a ladder and broke his right hip. His wife called 911 and he was transported by ambulance to this hospital. He was admitted and underwent a total right hip replacement. He was transferred from the OR to this unit 3 hr ago.

Biographical Data

- Age: 79
- Gender: male
- Height: 5 ft 11 in
- Weight: 210 lb

Cultural Considerations

- Language: English
- Ethnicity: Dutch
- Nationality: American
- Culture: no significant cultural considerations identified

Demographic

- Marital status: married
- Educational level: college
- Religion: Christian
- Occupation: retired teacher

Current Health Status

- Was cleaning the garage yesterday when he fell approximately 3 ft from a ladder and broke his right hip. His wife called 911 and he was transported by ambulance to this hospital. He was admitted and underwent a total right hip replacement.

History

- Psychosocial history
  - Social support—wife, three grown children live nearby
- Past health history
  - Medical: smoked for 30 years (1 pack/day) and mild hypertension that was diagnosed 4 years ago for which he takes metroprolol 12.5 mg po daily. Denies previous hospital admissions.
  - Surgical: denies previous surgeries or hospital admissions.
- Family history: depression

Admission Sheet	
Name:	Terry VanDyke
Age:	79
Gender:	Male
Marital Status:	Married
Education Level:	Bachelors in Education
Religion:	Christian—nondenominational
Ethnicity:	Dutch
Nationality:	American
Language:	English
Occupation:	Retired physical education teacher—high school level

Diagnostic test	**Normal Range**	**Patient values**
CBC	WBC 5,000–10,000	WBC: 12,000
	Neutrophils 1,935–7,942	Neutrophils: 7,000
	RBC 4.5–5.3 million	RBC: 4 million
	Hgb: 13–18 g/100 mL	Hgb: 14
	Hct: 37–49%	Hct: 38%
	Platelet: 150,000– 400,000/mm^3	Platelets: 350,000 mm^3
Electrolytes	Na 136–145 mEq/L	Na 138 mEq/L
	K 3.5–5.1 mEq/L	K 5 mEq/L
	Cl 98–107 mEq/L	Cl 100 mEq/L
	Ca 8.6–10.2 mg/dL	Ca 9 mg/dL
Coagulation studies	APTT: 20–35 sec	APTT: 36 sec
	PTT: 60–70 sec	PTT: 77 se
	INR: 2–3	INR: 2.8

Hospital
Provider's Orders

Patient's Name: Terry VanDyke
Allergies: NKDA

Diagnosis: total right hip replacement

Date	**Time**	**Order**	**Signature**
		Vital signs: Vitals q 4 hr—include pulse oximetry	
		Diet: Clear liquid diet advance as tolerated	
		Activity: OOB to chair every shift with two-person assist	

Diagnosis: total right hip replacement—cont'd

Date	Time	Order	Signature
		Turn/position q 2 hr Abductor pillow while in bed	
		IV therapy: 0.9% NS 100 mL/hr Decrease IV fluid to 40 mL/hr when taking po well	
		Medications: Morphine sulfate 5 mg IV push q 2–4 hr prn Tylenol 1,000 mg po q 8 hr prn mild pain Ancef 1-g IV q 6 hr x 3 days Metoprolol 25.0 mg po daily, decrease to 12.5 mg daily when BP below 140/80 Lovenox 30 mg SQ bid	
		Diagnostic studies: PTT, PT/INR every AM CBC, CMP daily	
		Treatments: Oxygen 2–4 L prn via NC to keep O_2 sats >90%	
		JP drain—empty every shift, record amount	
		SCDs in place to lower legs	
		Foley bag to gravity drainage	
		PT consult	Dr. Chorpenning

Medication Administration Record

Name: Terry VanDyke DOB: 01/10/35

Allergies: NKDA

Diagnosis: ORIF right hip

Physician: Dr. Chorpenning

Comments:

Administration Period

Medication	Start	Stop	Shift 1 06:00–13:59	Shift 2 14:00–21:59	Shift 3 22:00–05:59
Lovenox 30 mg SQ bid	Today		0800	2100	
Ancef 1 g IV q 6 hr x 3 days	Today	3 days	0800	1500 2100	0300 —given lck
Metropolol 25 mg po daily; decrease to 12.5 mg daily when BP below 140/80	Today		0800		

Continued

Administration Period—cont'd

Medication	Start	Stop	Shift 1 06:00–13:59	Shift 2 14:00–21:59	Shift 3 22:00–05:59
Tylenol 1,000 mg po q 8 hr prn mild pain	Today				
Morphine sulfate 5 mg IV q 2 hr prn severe pain	Today		0130 5 mg IV lck 0530 5 mg IV lck		

Injection Sites	Initial	Signature	Initial	Signature	Initial	Signature
I. Right deltoid area	Lck	Lckrautscheid, RN				
II. Left deltoid						
III. Right gluteal area						
IV. Left gluteal						
V. Right abdomen						
VI. Left abdomen						
VII. Right thigh						
VIII. Left thigh						

Nursing Report

The time right now is 0700—it is the beginning of day shift.

- Situation: Mr. VanDyke was admitted to our unit 6 hr ago after right hip surgery. He is stable. He received 5 mg morphine IV at 0430. His pain at that time was 6/10; his acceptable level is less than 4.
- Background: He is a retired physical education teacher. Past medical history is positive for osteoarthritis, smoking for 30 years (1 pack/day), and mild hypertension. Mr. VanDyke reports a family history of depression but denies this of himself. Mr. VanDyke was cleaning the garage yesterday when he fell and broke his right hip. He was transported by ambulance to Providence St. Vincent's hospital where he underwent a total right hip replacement earlier this morning. He was transferred to your unit earlier today. Mr. VanDyke has a wife and three grown children, all living nearby. The client asks you, "When is physical therapy coming so I can get out of bed and move around?"
- Assessment: His lungs are clear, heart is normal sinus rhythm, he is afebrile, his dressing is clean, dry, intact. His JP drain is charged and working. His pain is under control now that I gave him morphine. He has in IV infusing, normal saline, at 100 mL/hr. Tolerating clear liquids. He is not passing gas yet. His abductor pillow is in place and he must be turned q 2 hr. I last turned him at 0630. He has had minimal urine output, but it has been at least 30 mL per hour.
- Recommendation: Complete your shift assessment. Double check his pain level. Keep an eye on his urine level; hopefully, he'll start diuresing

Student Simulation Prep Assignments

1. Identify items and their purpose in the care of a postoperative hip patient.

Item	Purpose
Clinical attire	
Watch with second hand	
Goggles	
Stethoscope	
Clinical worksheet	

2. *Identify team members and their specific roles in the care of a postoperative hip patient.*

Team Member	Role
Nurse	
Charge RN	
UAP	
Physician	
Respiratory therapy	
Physical therapy	
Pharmacist	

3. *Relevant Data Exercise:*
Fill in columns below.

Relevant Data from Report	Relevant Data from Other Sources	Data Missing	Sources for Missing Data	Data Requiring Follow-Up

4. *Initial Focused Assessment*

After reviewing the client background and nursing report, you are ready to assess your client's current status. Under each category, identify how you would target your assessment, and what you would expect to find for the patient with ORIF right hip replacement.

History
Are there any questions you need to ask the patient or family to obtain additional relevant data?

Physical Exam

- General appearance:
- Integumentary:
- HEENT:
- Respiratory:
- CV:
- Breasts.
- Abdominal:
- Neuro:
- Musculoskeletal:
- Reproductive:
- Additional:
- Developmental:

What are the nursing implications considering the developmental stage of your patient?

Answer:

5. *Diagnostic Tests*

What diagnostic test results relevant to the patient's current problem are needed to plan care?

Complete the table using Van Leeuwen et al, *Davis's Comprehensive Handbook of Laboratory and Diagnostic Testing with Nursing Implications* 4e, or other diagnostic test reference.

Diagnostic test	Significance to This Patient's Problem
CBC	
Electrolytes	
Coagulation studies	

6. Treatment

Identify drugs that are used to treat a patient with total right hip.

Complete the table using Deglin et al, *Davis's Drug Guide for Nurses* 12e, or other drug reference.

Medication	Dose, Route, Frequency	Action	Side Effect	Nursing. Implications
Morphine	5 mg IV push q 2-4 hr prn			
Tylenol	1,000 mg po q 8 hr prn mild pain			
Metoprolol	25 mg po daily, decrease to 12.5 mg daily when BP < 140/80			
Lovenox	30 mg SQ bid			
Ancef	1 g IV q 6 hr ×3 days			

7. Nursing Problems/Diagnoses

Identify three priority nursing problems/diagnoses.

Assessment Data	Priority Problem	Intervention	Expected Patient Outcome	Which Intervention Could be Delegated to Unlicensed Personnel?
1.				
2.				

Assessment Data	Priority Problem	Intervention	Expected Patient Outcome	Which Intervention Could be Delegated to Unlicensed Personnel?
3.				

References

Deglin, J. H., & Vallerand, A. H. (2009). *Davis's drug guide for nurses* (11th ed.). Philadelphia: F. A. Davis.

Dillon, P. (2007). *Nursing health assessment: A critical thinking and case studies approach* (2nd ed.). Philadelphia: F. A. Davis.

Erikson, E. H. (1950). *Childhood and society*. New York: Norton.

The Joint Commission National Patient Safety Goals Hospital Program. Retrieved from http://www.jointcommission.org/GeneralPublic/NPSG/10_npsgs.htm

Lagerquist, S. (2006). *NCLEX-RN success*. Philadelphia: F. A. Davis.

National Guideline Clearing House. *Postoperative management in adults. A practical guide to postoperative care for clinical staff.* Retrieved July 2007, www.guideline.gov

Smith, S. (2006) *Sandra Smith's review for NCLEX-RN* (11th ed.). Los Altos, CA: National Nursing Review.

Smith, S., Duell, D., & Martin, B. (2008). *Clinical nursing skills*. Upper Saddle River, NJ: Pearson Education.

Van Leeuwen, A. M., Poelhuis-Leth, D. J., & Bladh, M. L. (2011). *Davis's comprehensive handbook of laboratory and diagnostic tests with nursing implications.* (4th ed.). Philadelphia: F. A. Davis.

5-3 Pulseless Electrical Activity

MEDICAL-SURGICAL/ADULT HEALTH

STANDARD FORMS

These templates are included in the Appendix; copy before each use.

LEARNING OUTCOMES

Cognitive

The student will be able to:

1. Identify the etiology of PEA.
2. Recognize the importance of treating the patient and not the monitor.
3. Identify risk factors for PEA.
4. Discuss causes and treatments for PEA.

Psychomotor

The student will be able to:

1. Assess the airway, breathing, and circulation of a patient with PEA.
2. Initiate appropriate interventions (open airway, perform manual ventilation with a bag-valve mask, perform chest compressions) for a patient with PEA.
3. Work collaboratively as part of the healthcare team in the care of a patient with PEA.

Affective

The student will be able to:

1. Identify factors that worked well during the simulation of care of a patient with PEA.
2. Develop self-confidence in the care of a patient with PEA.
3. Reconcile that the monitor might not be truly reflecting the patient's condition.

Communication

The student will be able to:

1. Communicate effectively with healthcare team members in care of a patient with PEA.
2. Communicate effectively with the patient and family in the care of a patient with PEA.
3. Practice Transparent Thinking (thinking out loud) to facilitate group problem solving.
4. Use Directed Communication (directing a message to specific individual) when delegating tasks.
5. Employ Closed-Loop Communication (acknowledgment of receipt of the message and status) to acknowledge communications from others.

Safety

The student will be able to:

Administer and maintain specific protecting interventions with attention to safety of the client and healthcare professional.

1. Demonstrate a safe environment with attention to hazards to healthcare providers, visitors and the client. Includes body mechanics, tripping hazards, and equipment issues.
2. Demonstrate attention to national patient safety goals. Includes patient identification standards, effective communication among healthcare providers, and safe medication administration..
3. Demonstrate attention to standard precautions. Includes hand washing, infection control measures and use of personal protective equipment (PPE) as needed.

Leadership and Management/Delegation

The student will be able to:

1. The student will be able to identify tasks that can be legally, ethically, and safely delegated to unlicensed assistive personnel (UAP) or licensed practical nurse (LPN) in the care of a patient with PEA.
2. Identify and prioritize patient's needs in care of PEA.

OVERVIEW OF PROBLEM

DEFINITION

Pulseless electrical activity is a form of cardiac arrest in which the heart's electrical conduction system still works in PEA even though the heart is not effectively pumping oxygenated blood to the body. Because the electrical conduction system is intact, an organized ECG rhythm appears on the cardiac monitor, but the patient has no pulse and minimal or no perfusion.

Pathophysiology

- Electromechanical dissociation
- Escape rhythms

Risk Factors

Postoperative or trauma patient prone to blood loss which can lead to hypovolemia (one of the most common causes of PEA). This case focuses on hypovolemia, but other causes include cardiac tamponade, tension pneumothorax, acidosis, drug overdose, hypothermia, and hyperkalmia/hypokalemia.

Assessment

- Airway
- Breathing
- Circulation

Diagnostic Tests

None initially as this is a cardiac arrest. However, nurses should consider drawing labs on the patient to include ABG (for possible acidosis) and electrolytes (for out-of-range potassium levels).

Treatment

- Begin CPR
- Medications—oxygen, epinephrine
- Fluid challenge

Nursing Management

- CPR AHA ACLS algorithms
- Administer medications and fluid therapies as ordered
- Provide for physical, emotional and safety needs

Evaluation/Outcome Criteria

- Regular cardiac rhythm
- No complications
- Tolerates regular activity
- Reports reduced anxiety

Review Questions

1. What is one aspect of normal sinus rhythm?
   Answer:

   A. Appears as PQRST waves on the monitor.

   B. Is relatively uncommon

   C. Is always a perfusing rhythm

   D. Has a rate of over 100 beats per minute

2. List three common causes of hypovolemia.
   Answer:

3. The ultimate treatment for PEA is:
   Answer:

4. Three other rhythms commonly seen in cardiac arrest include:
   Answer:

5. What is the recommended use of epinephrine in cardiac arrest (dose and timing):
   Answer:

Related Evidence-Based Practice Guidelines

American Heart Association Advanced Cardiac Life Support, 2010 Guidelines, Cardiac Arrest Algorithm with emphasis on PEA

American Heart Association Basic Life Support, 2010 Guidelines, Adult CPR

The American Heart Association (as referenced above) provides evidence-based updates to its guidelines on a regular basis. The current guidelines are based on the 2005 updates.

The Joint Commission National Patient Safety Goals Hospital Program. Retrieved from http://www.jointcommission.org/GeneralPublic/NPSG/10_npsgs.htm

SBAR Technique for Communication: A situational briefing model published by The Institute for Healthcare Improvement was downloaded on December 19, 2008, fromhttp://www.ihi.org/IHI/Topics/PatientSafety/SafetyGeneral/Tools/SBARTechniqueforCommunicationASituationalBriefingModel.htm

Topics to Review Prior to the Simulation

- Review of basic adult CPR techniques
- Review of basic ECG rhythm interpretation (normal sinus rhythm will appear on the monitor— this will be the only rhythm that they will see).
- Review of causes of PEA (particularly hypovolemia as this is what will happen in this case, but also review other causes such as cardiac tamponade, tension pneumothorax, hypoxia, hypothermia, hyperkalemia/hypokalemia, myocardial infarction, and drug overdose).

SIMULATION

Client Background

Biographical Data

- Age: 55
- Gender: male
- Height: 6 ft
- Weight: 200 lb

Cultural Considerations

- Language: English
- Ethnicity: not known
- Nationality: American
- Culture: no significant cultural considerations identified

Demographic

- Marital status: married
- Educational level: Bachelors in Business
- Religion: Protestant
- Occupation: businessman

Current Health Status

- Patient complained of chest discomfort 1 week prior and saw primary care provider, who sent him for a cardiac catheterization. It showed 80% occlusion in right coronary artery. MDs elected to do a cardiac bypass. The surgery was uneventful. The patient is currently status post 24 hr and is on the cardiac progressive care (step-down) unit.

History

- Psychosocial history
  - Social support: supportive spouse
- Past health history
  - Medical: knee injury from football 20 years ago
  - Surgical: none prior to this current surgery
- Family history
  - Both parents died of heart disease in their 60s

Admission Sheet	
Name:	Joseph Thrower
Age:	55
Gender:	Male
Marital Status:	Married
Educational Level:	Bachelors in Business
Religion:	Protestant
Ethnicity:	Not known
Nationality:	American
Language:	English
Occupation:	Businessman

Hospital Provider's Orders

Patient's Name: Joseph Thrower
Allergies: NKDA

Diagnosis: S/p cardiac bypass surgery

Date	Time	Order	Signature
10/1	1200	Vital signs q 4 hr Cardiac monitor	
		Diet: Progress to normal diet	
		Activity: PT consult	
		IV therapy: IV NSS 40 mL/hr x 1 L	
		Medications: Percocet 5/325 2 tabs po for pain prn q 4 hr Atenolol 50 mg po once daily Plavix 75 mg po daily Oxygen nasal cannula 2–4 L; keep O_2 sats >95%	
		Diagnostic studies: CBC and CMP every other day	
		Treatments: Incentive spirometer 2/hr while awake	
		Intake and output	
		Post Code Labs: ABGs CBC, CMP CK, troponin levels	Dr. Sussman

Nursing Report

1400

Patient complained of chest discomfort 1 week prior and saw primary care provider, who sent him for a cardiac catheterization. It showed 80% occlusion in right coronary artery. MDs elected to do a cardiac bypass. The surgery was uneventful. The patient is currently status post 4 days and is on the cardiac progressive care (step-down) unit. He walked briefly before noon. For intake and output, he has had two small cups (100 mL each) of apple juice, and voided 150 mL since being transferred to the progressive care unit at 10 AM. 1300 VS: HR 80 normal sinus rhythm, BP 130/70, respirations 18, temperature 37°C, pulse ox 93% on 2 L oxygen. He has no reported problems. His spouse is with him. She went outside for a break about 20 min ago and has not returned.

Student Simulation Prep Assignments

1. Identify items and their purpose for a patient with PEA?

Item	Purpose
Bag valve mask	
Epinephrine bristojets	
Code cart with CPR backboard	
IV pump	

2. Identify team members and specific roles in the care of a patient with PEA.

Team Member	Role
Respiratory therapist	
MD	
Nursing assistant	

Identify team members and specific roles in the care of a patient with cardiac arrest/PEA.

Team Member	Role
Respiratory therapist	
MD	
Primary nurse	
Critical care nurse	
Secondary nurse	
Anesthesia	
Nursing supervisor	
UAP	

3. Relevant Data Exercise: Fill in columns below.

Relevant Data from Report	Relevant Data from Other Sources	Data Missing	Sources for Missing Data	Data Requiring Follow-Up

4. *Initial Focused Assessment*

After reviewing the client background and nursing report, you are ready to assess your client's current status. Under each category, identify how you would target your assessment, and what you would expect to find for the patient with PEA.

History

Are there any questions you need to ask the patient or family to obtain additional relevant data?

Physical Exam

- General appearance:
- Integumentary:
- HEENT:
- Respiratory:
- CV:
- Breasts:
- Abdominal:
- Neuro:
- Musculoskeletal:
- Reproductive:
- Additional:
- Developmental:

What are the nursing implications considering the developmental stage of your patient?

Answer:

5. *Diagnostic Tests*

What diagnostic test results relevant to the patient's current problem are needed to plan care?

Complete the table using Van Leeuwen et al, *Davis's Comprehensive Handbook of Laboratory and Diagnostic Testing with Nursing Implications* 4e, or other diagnostic test reference.

MD might order ABG as one of the causes of PEA is acidosis. Chemistry would also be appropriate to check electrolyte levels.

Diagnostic Test	Significance to This Patient's Problem
ABG	
CMP	
Serum potassium	
CBC	
CK and troponin	

6. *Treatment*

Identify drugs that are used to treat a patient with PEA.

Complete the table using Deglin et al, *Davis's Drug Guide for Nurses* 12e, or other drug reference.

Medication	Dose, Route, Frequency	Indications	Side Effect	Nursing Implications
Epinephrine	1 mg IV push q 3–5 min			

7. Nursing Problem/Diagnoses

Identify three priority nursing problems/diagnoses.

Assessment Data	Priority Problem	Intervention	Expected Patient Outcome	Which Interventions Could be Delegated to Unlicensed Personnel?
1.				
2.				
3.				

References

American Heart Association Advanced Cardiac Life Support, 2005 Guidelines.

American Heart Association Basic Life Support, 2005 Guidelines.

Deglin, J. H., & Vallerand, A. H. (2009). *Davis's drug guide for nurses* (11th ed.). Philadelphia: F. A. Davis.

Dillon, P. (2007). *Nursing health assessment: A critical thinking and case studies approach* (2nd ed.). Philadelphia: F. A. Davis.

Erikson, E. H. (1950). *Childhood and society*. New York: Norton.

Lagerquist, S. L. (2006). *Davis's NCLEX-RN success* (2nd ed). Philadelphia: F. A. Davis.

Van Leeuwen, A. M., Poelhuis-Leth, D.J., & Bladh, M.L. (2011). *Davis's comprehensive handbook of laboratory and diagnostic tests with nursing implications.* (4th ed.). Philadelphia: F. A. Davis.

5-4 Uncontrolled Atrial Fibrillation

MEDICAL-SURGICAL

STANDARD FORMS

These templates are included in the Appendix; copy before each use.

LEARNING OUTCOMES

Cognitive

The student will be able to:

1. Describe effects of uncontrolled atrial fibrillation.
2. Differentiate atrial fibrillation from normal sinus rhythm (NSR).
3. Differentiate controlled vs uncontrolled atrial fibrillation.
4. Identify the signs and symptoms of atrial fibrillation.
5. Correlate the signs and symptoms of atrial fibrillation to the underlying pathophysiology.
6. Identify appropriate treatment for atrial fibrillation.
7. Interpret rhythm strips.

Psychomotor

The student will be able to:

1. Perform cardiac assessment on patient with uncontrolled atrial fibrillation.
2. Initiate appropriate interventions, such as start IV, ECG, administer medications.
3. Assist with possible cardioversion.

Affective

The student will be able:

1. Reflect upon performance in caring for a patient with uncontrolled atrial fibrillation.
2. Identify factors that worked will during the simulation.
3. Identify factors that needed improvement during the simulation.
4. Reflect on overall feelings about the scenario.
5. Discuss feeling related to working as a member of a healthcare team.
6. Develop confidence in caring for patients with cardiac arrhythmias.

Communication

The student will be able to:

1. Communicate effectively with the patient.
2. Communicate effectively with healthcare team members.
3. Use SBAR when communicating with healthcare team members.
4. Work collaboratively as a member of the healthcare team.
5. Accurately and succinctly document assessments, interventions. and patient response to treatment.
6. Practice Transparent Thinking (thinking out loud) to facilitate group problem solving.
7. Use Directed Communication (directing a message to specific individual) when delegating tasks.
8. Employ Closed-Loop Communication (acknowledgment of receipt of the message and status) to acknowledge communications from others.

Safety

The student will be able to:

Administer and maintain specific protecting interventions with attention to safety of the client and healthcare professional.

1. Demonstrate a safe environment with attention to hazards to healthcare providers, visitors, and the client. Includes body mechanics, tripping hazards, and equipment issues.
2. Demonstrate attention to national patient safety goals. Includes patient identification standards, effective communication among healthcare providers, and safe medication administration.
3. Demonstrate attention to standard precautions. Includes hand washing, infection control measures, and use of personal protective equipment (PPE) as needed.

Leadership and Management/Delegation

The student will be able to:

1. Identify tasks that can be legally, ethically, and safely delegated to unlicensed assistive personnel (UAP) or licensed practical nurse (LPN) in the care of a patient with uncontrolled atrial fibrillation.
2. Prioritize care for a patient with uncontrolled atrial fibrillation.

OVERVIEW OF PROBLEM

Definition

Cardiac arrhythmias (dysrhythmias) include any variation in normal rate, rhythm, or configuration of waves on the ECG. Types of arrhythmias are sinus, atrial, junctional, ventricular, and conduction deficits (blocks). Arrythmias are caused by dysfunction of SA node, atria, AV node or ventricles, and may be primary or secondary due to a systemic problem.

Pathophysiology

Atrial fibrillation is the most common arrhythmia in older adults. It is characterized by rapid irregular waves (>350/min) with irregular ventricular response . The ventricular rate varies, and may increase to 120–150/min if untreated. Complications include the promotion of thrombus formation in the atria.

Risk Factors

- CAD
- Rheumatic heart disease
- MI–atrial infarction
- Mitral valve disease (stenosis)
- Hypertension
- Digitalis toxicity
- Hyperthyroidism

Assessment

Subjective

- Confused
- Fatigue
- Palpitations

Objective

- Pulse: tachycardia
- Pulse deficit
- Decreased cardiac output if rate is rapid
- Respirations: SOB, crackles if in heart failure
- NVD (neck vein distention)
- Temperature: may be slightly elevated
- BP: hypotensive
- Skin: pale, clammy
- MS/Neuro: weakness, confusion, syncope

Diagnostic Tests

- ECG
- TEE (transesophageal echocardiogram)
- Clottting studies

Treatment

- Cardioversion
- Treat underlying cause
- Digitalis
- Cardizem
- Amiodarone
- Anticoagulation

Nursing Management

- Prepare for cardioversion
- Administer medications as ordered
- Prevent thromboemboli
- Provide for physical, emotional, safety, and learning needs

Evaluation/outcome Managemnent

- Regular cardiac rhythm
- Monitors own radial pulse
- No complications
- Tolerates activity
- Reports reduction of anxiety
- Understands treatment plan and precautions

REVIEW QUESTIONS

1. How would you differentiate controlled vs uncontrolled atrial fibrillation?
Answer:

2. Interpret the following rhythm strips:

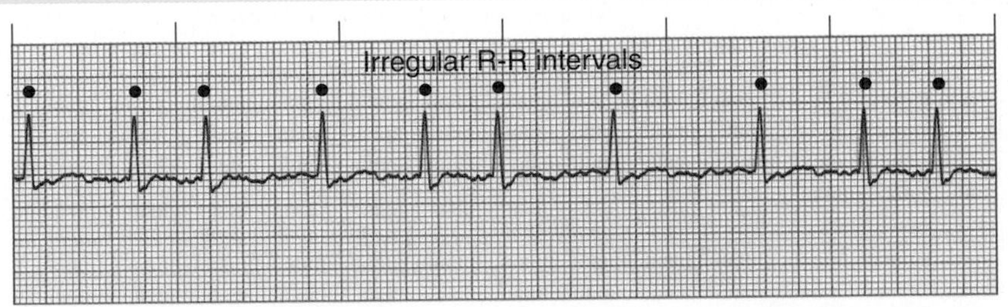

Answer:

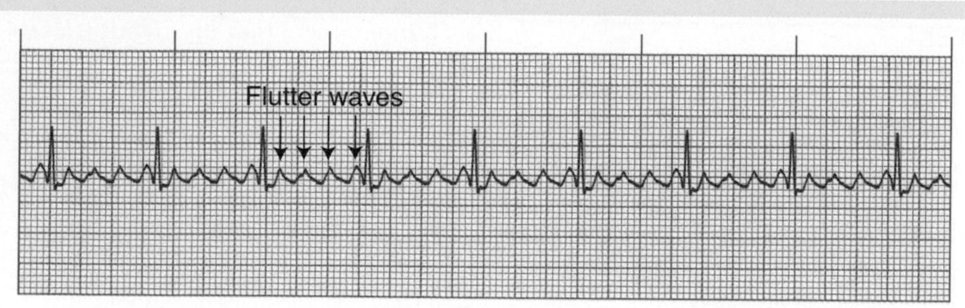

Answer:

3. Name a major complication of uncontrolled atrial fibrillation and explain the pathophysiology.
Answer:

4. Why is the patient with atrial fibrillation at greater risk for stroke?
Answer:

5. What effect does atrial fibrillation have on cardiac output?
Answer:

Related Evidenced-Based Guidelines

http://www.guidelines.gov/search/search.aspx?term=atrial+fibrillation

The Joint Commission National Patient Safety Goals Hospital Program. Retrieved from http://www.jointcommission.org/GeneralPublic/NPSG/10_npsgs.htm

SBAR Technique for Communication: A situational briefing model published by The Institute for Healthcare Improvement was downloaded on December 19, 2008, from http://www.ihi.org/IHI/Topics/PatientSafety/SafetyGeneral/Tools/SBARTechniqueforCommunicationASituationalBriefingModel.htm

Topics to Review Prior to the Simulation

- Cardiac dysrhythmias
- Medications used to treat dysrhythmias

SIMULATION

Client Background

Biographical Data

- Age: 90
- Gender: female
- Height: 5 ft 2 in
- Weight: 155 lb

Cultural Considerations

- Language: English
- Ethnicity: Irish
- Nationality: American
- Culture: no significant cultural considerations identified

Demographic

- Marital status: single
- Educational level: high school
- Religion: Catholic
- Occupation: retired

Current Health Status

Sudden onset of SOB

History

- Psychosocial history
  - Social support: lives at longterm care facility and has family members (sister, niece and nephew) who help
- Past health history
  - Medical: DJD, CHF, hypothyroidism, and ovarian cancer
  - Surgical: TAH
- Family history: + CVD, + ovarian cancer

Admission Sheet

Name:	Helen McCloskey
Age:	90
Gender:	Female
Marital Status:	Single
Educational Level:	High school
Religion:	Catholic
Ethnicity:	Irish
Nationality:	American
Language:	English
Occupation:	Retired

Hospital
Provider's Orders

Patient's Name: Helen McCloskey
Allergies: NKDA

Diagnosis: Uncontrolled atrial firillation

Date	Time	Order	Signature
7/8/07	5:45 PM	Admit to CCU	
		Vital signs: q 15 min	
		Diet: cardiac diet	
		Activity: Bed rest	
		IV therapy: 1,000 mL 5% D/0.45 NSS 100 mL/hr x 3	
		Medications: Heparin 5,000 U bolus then heparin 15 U/kg/hr Cardizem 0.25 mg/kg IV push Repeat in 15 min with cardizem gtt 0.35 mg/kg (paremeters if systolic BP >100 and HR >130)	
		Diagnostic studies: Serum electrolytes, BUN, creatinine, CBC, PTT, PT, BNP, cardiac enzymes, troponin level Repeat PTT q 4 hr ECG	
		Treatments: O_2 2 L via NC I&O monitor	Dr. L. Brown

Nursing Report

Helen McCloskey is a 90-year-old white female. She resides in an assisted living long-term care center. Even though frail, she is in relatively good health. She has a history of DJD, CHF, hypothyroidism, and ovarian cancer. Her medications include Lasix, Valium, Inderal, and Synthyroid. While making rounds, you note that Ms McCloskey becomes very SOB while walking to the bathroom. You assist her back to bed.

Student Simulation Prep Assignments

1. Identify items and their purpose in the care of a patient with uncontrolled atrial fibrillation.

Equipment	Purpose
IV with pump	
O_2 cannula	
Cardiac monitor	

2. Identify team members and their specific roles in the care of the patient with uncontrolled atrial fibrillation.

Team Member	Role
Primary nurse	
Secondary nurse	
Physician	

3. Relevant Data Assignment: Fill in columns below.

Relevant Data from Report	Relevant Data from Other Sources	Data Missing	Sources for Missing Data	Data Requiring Follow-Up

4. Initial Focused Assessment

After reviewing the client background and nursing report, you are ready to assess your client's current status. Under each category, identify how you would target your assessment and what you would expect to find for the patient with uncontrolled atrial fibrillation.

History

Are there any questions you need to ask the patient or family to obtain additional relevant data?

Physical Exam

- General appearance:
- Integumentary:
- HEENT:
- Respiratory:
- CV:
- Breasts:
- Neuro:
- Musculoskeletal:
- Reproductive:
- Additional:
- Developmental:

What are the nursing implications considering the developmental stage of your patient?

Answer:

5. Diagnostic Tests

What diagnostic test results relevant to the patient's current problem are needed to plan care?

Complete the table using Van Leeuwen et al, *Davis's Comprehensive Handbook of Laboratory and Diagnostic Testing with Nursing Implications* 4e, or other diagnostic test reference.

Diagnostic Test	Significance to This Patient's Problem
CBC • RBC • Hematocrit • Hemoglobin • WBC • Platelets	

Diagnostic	Significance
PT	
aPTT	
Electrolytes	
BUN and creatinine	
BNP	
Cardiac enzymes	
CK-MB	
CRP	
Myoglobin	
Troponin	

6. Treatment

Identify drugs that are used to treat a patient with uncontrolled atrial fibrillation.

Complete the table using Deglin et al, *Davis's Drug Guide for Nurses* 12e, or other drug reference.

Medication	Dose	Action	Side Effect	Nursing Implications
Heparin	IV regular heparin drip @ 35–70 U/kg 5,000 U bolus then 15 U/kg/hr			
Cardizem	IV 0.25 mg/kg may repeat in 15 min 0.35 mg/kg			

7. Nursing Problems/Diagnoses

Identify three priority nursing problems/diagnoses.

Assessment Data	Priority Problem	Intervention	Expected Outcome	Delegation (which intervention could be delegated to UAP?)
1.				
2.				

Continued

Assessment Data	Priority Problem	Intervention	Expected Outcome	Delegation (which intervention could be delegated to UAP?)
3.				

References

Deglin, J. H., & Vallerand, A. H. (2009). *Davis's drug guide for nurses* (11th ed.). Philadelphia: F. A. Davis.

Dillon, P. (2007). *Nursing health assessment: A critical thinking and case studies approach* (2nd ed.). Philadelphia: F. A. Davis.

Erikson, E. H. (1950). *Childhood and society*. New York: Norton.

Lagerquist, S. L. (2006). *Davis's NCLEX-RN success* (2nd ed). Philadelphia: F. A. Davis.

Ouimet Perrin, K. (2009). *Understanding the essentials of critical care nursing*. Upper Saddle River, NJ: Pearson.

Van Leeuwen, A. M., Poelhuis-Leth, D. J., & Bladh, M. L. (2011). *Davis's comprehensive handbook of laboratory and diagnostic tests with nursing implications.* (4th ed.). Philadelphia: F. A. Davis.

5-5 Cardiopulmonary Arrest

MEDICAL-SURGICAL/ADULT HEALTH

STANDARD FORMS

These templates are included in the Appendix; copy before each use.

LEARNING OUTCOMES

Cognitive

The student will be able to:

1. Identify conditions that are high risk for cardiopulmonary arrest.
2. Describe the pathophysiological effects of cardiopulmonary arrest.
3. Identify appropriate interventions for the patient in cardiopulmonary arrest.
4. Differentiate the roles of the code team.

Psychomotor

The student will be able to:

1. Perform appropriate assessment for a patient in cardiopulmonary arrest.
2. Initiate appropriate interventions for a patient in cardiopulmonary arrest.
3. Work collaboratively as part of the healthcare team.

Affective

The student will be able to:

1. Reflect upon performance in emergency situation.
2. Identify feelings in emergency situation.
3. Discuss feelings related to working as a member of a team.
4. Identify factors that worked well.
5. Identify factors that needed improvement.

Communication

The student will be able to:

1. Communicate effectively with members of the healthcare team.
2. Communicate effectively with the patient and family members.
3. Practice Transparent Thinking (thinking out loud) to facilitate group problem solving.
4. Use Directed Communication (directing a message to specific individual) when delegating tasks.
5. Employ Closed-Loop Communication (acknowledgment of receipt of the message and status) to acknowledge communications from others.

Safety

The student will be able to:

Administer and maintain specific protecting interventions with attention to safety of the client and healthcare professional.

1. Demonstrate a safe environment with attention to hazards to healthcare providers, visitors, and the client. Includes body mechanics, tripping hazards, and equipment issues.
2. Demonstrate attention to national patient safety goals. Includes patient identification standards, effective communication among healthcare providers, and safe medication administration.
3. Demonstrate attention to standard precautions. Includes hand washing, infection control measures, and use of personal protective equipment (PPE) as needed.

Leadership and Management/Delegation

1. The student should be able to identify tasks that can be legally, ethically, and safely delegated to unlicensed assistive personnel (UAP) or licensed practical nurse (LPN) in the care of a patient with cardiopulmonary arrest.
2. Identify and prioritize patient's needs in the care of of a patient with cardiopulmonary arrest.

OVERVIEW OF PROBLEM

Myocardial Infarction

Definition

Ischemia and necrosis of cardiac muscle.

Pathophysiology

Infarctions result from inadequate or obstructed coronary blood flow. Atherosclerosis causes loss of elasticity, thickening, and hardening of arterial walls. Coronary heart disease precedes angina pectoris and myocardial infarction.

Risk Factors

- Increased serum cholesterol
- Hypertension
- Smoking
- Diabetes
- Family history of premature coronary heart disease

Assessment

Subjective

- c/o chest pain unrelieved by nitroglycerin; may have nausea and breathing problems

Objective

- Skin: ashen, clammy, cold
- Vital signs: pulse rapid weak and thready; increased respirations, BP decreased
- Respiratory: bibasilar crackles
- CV: may have S_3 or S_4
- Neuro: restless, anxious

Diagnostic Tests

- ECG: Q wave associated with tissue necrosis; ST segment elevation d/t tissue injury
- Elevated CPK-MB, troponin

Treatment

- Cardiac monitor
- Oxygen
- Start IV for emergency drug treatment if needed
- Relieve pain: nitroglycerin, morphine
- ASA
- Draw labs: electrolytes, enzymes, and other tests per orders
- 12-lead ECG
- Transfer to CCU

Cardiac Arrest

Definition

Cardiac standstill or ventricular fibrillation due to rapid administration or overdose of anesthetics or narcotics, toxins, obstructed airway (mucus, vomitus, foreign object), tension pneumothorax, cardiac disease (acute coronary syndrome, cardiac tamponade), dehydration and electrolyte imbalance, shock, electric shock or embolism.

Assessment

Subjective

- Unresponsive

Objective

- Skin: cold, clammy, cyanotic
- Respirations: agonal or none
- Pulse: weak, thready, rapid or none
- Neuro/MS: unresponsive, sizures, twitching, flaccid
- Pupils: dilated

Treatment

- Begin CPR 30 compressions to two ventilations
- Immediate countershock (defibrillate) if pulseless V-tach or V-fib
- ACLS protocols

Nursing Management

Goals:

- Prevent irreversible cerebral anoxic damage
- Establish effective circulation and respiration

Evaluation/Outcome Criteria

- Carotid pulse present
- Responds to verbal stimuli
- Direct and consensual pupillary light response
- Return of spontaneous respiration with adequate ventilation

REVIEW QUESTIONS

1. Describe five conditions that may result in cardiopulmonary arrest.
   Answer:

2. Identify five drugs that are used to treat a patient in cardiopulmonary arrest.
   Answer:

3. What would you expect to find on a crash cart? Name five items.
   Answer:

4. Identify the members of a code team (at least five) and their roles.
   Answer:

5. Your patient is in cardiopulmonary arrest. After you determine unresponsiveness, what should be done next?
   Answer:

Related Evidence-Based Guidelines

AHA ACLS Standards 2010

American Heart Association BCLS for Healthcare Providers

The Joint Commission National Patient Safety Goals Hospital Program. Retrieved from http://www.jointcommission.org/GeneralPublic/NPSG/10_npsgs.htm

National Guidelines Clearing House—Search Cardiac Arrest http://www.guideline.gov/browse/browsecondition.aspx

SBAR Technique for Communication: A situational briefing model published by The Institute for Healthcare Improvement was downloaded on December 19, 2008, from http://www.ihi.org/IHI/Topics/PatientSafety/SafetyGeneral/Tools/SBARTechniqueforCommunicationASituationalBriefingModel.htm

Topics to Rreview Prior to the Simulation

- Cardiopulomonary arrest
- Basic cardiac life support for healthcare providers
- Drugs used in a cardiopulmonary arrest

SIMULATION

Client Background

Biographical Data

- Age; 65
- Gender: male
- Height: 6 ft
- Weight: 255 lb

Cultural Considerations

- Language: English
- Ethnicity: German heritage
- Nationality: American
- Culture: no cultural considerations identified

Demographic

- Marital status: married
- Educational level: MBA
- Religion: Protestant
- Occupation: executive

Current Health Status

- DJD, total right knee replacement

History

- Psychosocial history
  - Social support: lives with wife, children all grown, but live nearby
- Past health history
  - Medical: HTN
  - Surgical: none
- Family history - + HTN, CVD, DJD

Admission Sheet

Name:	Stephen Johnson
Age:	65
Gender:	Male
Marital status:	Married
Education level:	MBA
Religion:	Protestant
Ethnicity:	German heritage
Nationality:	American
Language:	English
Occupation:	Executive

Hospital
Provider's Orders

Patient's Name: Steven Johnson
Allergies: NKDA

Diagnosis: DJD , total right knee replacement

Date	Time	Order	Signature
		Admit: Dx total right knee replacement	
		Vital signs: VS q 4 hr	
		Diet: House diet	
		Activity: OOB in AM PT in AM CPM (Continuous passive motion machine)	
		IV therapy: 1,000 mL %5 dextrose/1/2 NSS q 10 hr	
		PCA morphine as per protocol	

Continued

Diagnosis: DJD , total right knee replacement—cont'd

Date	Time	Order	Signature
		Medications:	
		Percocet 2 tabs. Q 4 hr prn pain; start postoperative day 2	
		Lovenox 40 mg subq q 12 hr	
		Colace 100 mg po daily	
		Ancef 1 g IVPB q 6 hr x 4 doses	
		$FeSO_4$ 325 mg po daily	
		Cardizem SR 60 mg po bid	
		Diagnostic studies:	
		Repeat CBC in AM	
		BMP in AM	
		Telemetry	
		Repeat ECG in AM	
			Dr. Butler

Nursing Report

Mr. Johnson, a 65-year-old patient, had total right knee replacement yesterday for DJD.

- Anesthesia spinal duramorph
- Estimated blood loss: 1,000 mL
- IV fluid replacement: 2000 mL
- Postoperative H&H 8

In PACU, Mr. Johnson complained of chest pain. Monitor revealed NSR with occasional PVCs. Transfuse with 2 U of PRBCs (750 mL). ECG revealed ischemic changes; cardiac enzymes pending. He slept on and off during night. Complained of right knee pain 8/10, using PCA morphine with relief 4/10. Dressings dry and intact. Assessment includes VS: T 99.8°F, P 87 and regular, monitor NSR with occasional PVC, no chest pain, R 24, pulse ox 93% on RA, BP 130/88, AAOx3, lungs clear, heart RRR with occasional skipped beat, dressings on right knee dry and intact, Hemovac drained 10 mL bloody drainage, + pedal pulses, toes warm and movable, + sensation, slight edema right foot, c/o nausea, hypoactive bowel sounds, abdomen soft, non-tender, voiding quantity sufficient (qs) (400 mL).

Student Simulation Prep Assignments

1. Identify items and their purpose in care of patient with cardiopulmonary arrest.

Item	Purpose
Crash cart Contains equipment and medication needed to manage a cardiopulmonary arrest • Airways/oxygen, ET tubes, laryngescope, tubing, CO_2 detector • Medications • IVs, tubing, catheters • Defibrillator	

Item	Purpose
• External pacer • Specimen tubes • Suction catheters • Cardiac board	
IV pump	
ECG machine and monitor	
BP cuff, pulse ox, thermometer	
O_2 cannula	

2. Identify team members and their specific roles in the care of a patient with cardiac arrest.

Team Member	Role
Primary nurse	
Secondary nurse	
Physician	
Anesthetist	
Respiratory	
Medication nurse/pharmacy	
IV nurse	
Intern/medical student	
Recorder	
Third nurse "gofer"	
CNS/supervisor	

3. Relevant Data Assignment: Fill in columns below.

Relevant Data from Report	Relevant Data from Other Sources	Data Missing	Sources for Missing Data	Data Requiring Follow-Up
		Labs	Lab	

4. Initial Focused Assessment

After reviewing the client background and nursing report, you are ready to assess your client's current status. Under each category, identify how you would target your assessment and what you would expect to find for the patient with total right knee replacement.

What findings would you expect in a patient in cardiopulmonary arrest?

History
- Unresponsive
  What questions would you want to ask his family members?

Physical Exam
- General appearance:
- Integumentary:
- Respiratory:
- CV:
- MS/Neuro:
- Developmental
  Considering the age of your patient, are there any developmental issues to consider?
  Answer:

5. Diagnostic Tests

What diagnostic test results relevant to the patient's current problem are needed to plan care?

Complete the table using Van Leeuwen et al, *Davis's Comprehensive Handbook of Laboratory and Diagnostic Testing with Nursing Implications* 4e, or other diagnostic test reference.

Diagnostic Test	Significance to This Patient's Problem
CBC	
Cardiac enzymes	
Troponin level	
ECG	
BUN and creatinine	
Electrolytes	
ABG's	

6. Treatment

Identify drugs that are used to treat a patient with cardiac arrest.

Complete the table using Deglin et al, *Davis's Drug Guide for Nurses* 12e, or other drug reference.

Medication	Dose, Route, Frequency	Indication	Side Effect	Nursing Implications
Vasopressin	40 U once			
Epinephrine	1 mg q 5 min			
Amiodarone	300 mg IV then 150 mg IV			
Percocet	2 tabs			
Lovenox	40 mg			

Medication	Dose, Route, Frequency	Indication	Side Effect	Nursing Implications
Colace	1 tab			
Ancef	1 g			
Feosol	1 tab			
Cardizem SR	60 mg			
Morphine	PCA			

7. Nursing Problems/Diagnoses

Identify three priority nursing problems/diagnoses.

Assessment Data	Priority Problem	Intervention	Expected Outcome	Which Intervention could be Delegated to Unlicensed Personnel?
1.				
2.				
3.				

References

American Heart Association. (2010). *BLS for healthcare providers*. Dallas, TX: American heart association.org

American Heart Association. (2010). *ACLS for healthcare providers*. Dallas, TX: American heart association.org

Deglin, J. H., & Vallerand, A. H. (2009). *Davis's drug guide for nurses* (11th ed.). Philadelphia: F. A. Davis.

Dillon, P. (2007). *Nursing health assessment: A critical thinking and case studies approach* (2nd ed.). Philadelphia: F. A. Davis.

Erikson, E. H. (1950). *Childhood and society*. New York: Norton.

Lagerquist, S. L. (2006). *Davis's NCLEX-RN success* (2nd ed). Philadelphia: F. A. Davis.

Van Leeuwen, A. M. & Poelhuis-Leth, D. J., & Bladh, M. L. (2011). *Davis's comprehensive handbook of laboratory and diagnostic tests with nursing implications* (4th ed.). Philadelphia: F. A. Davis.

5-6 Cardiac Arrhythmia Rapid Response

ADVANCED MEDICAL-SURGICAL

STANDARD FORMS

These templates are included in the Appendix; copy before each use.

LEARNING OUTCOMES

Cognitive

The student will be able to:

1. Identify conditions that warrant a rapid response call.
2. Differentiate tachycardiac arrhythmias.
3. Understand the pathophysiology of tachycardiac arrhythymias.
4. Correlate the signs and symptoms of tachycardiac arrhythmias.
5. Identify the appropriate interventions for the patient with a tachyarrhythmia.
6. Differentiate the roles of team members in response to a patient with a tachyarrhythmia.

Psychomotor

The student will be able to:

1. Perform assessment for a patient with a tachyarrhythmia.
2. Initiate appropriate interventions for a patient with a tachyarrhythmia.
   - Call Rapid Response
   - Start IV
   - Administer medications per physician's orders
3. Work collaboratively as part of the healthcare team in the care of a patient with a tachyarrhythmia.

Affective

The student will be able to:

1. Reflect upon performance in the care of a patient with a tachyarrhythmia.
2. Identify own feelings in delivering care to a patient with a tachyarrhythmia.
3. Discuss feelings related to working as a member of a team in the care of a patient with a tachyarrhythmia.
4. Identify factors that worked well during the simulation of care of a patient with a tachyarrhythmia.
5. Identify factors that needed improvement during the simulation of care of a patient with a tachyarrhythmia.
6. Develop self-confidence in the care of a patient with a tachyarrhythmia.

Communication

The student will be able to:

1. Communicate effectively with healthcare team members in care of a patient with a tachyarrhythmia.
2. Communicate effectively with the patient with a tachyarrhythmia.
3. Use SBAR when communication with team members in the care of a patient with a tachyarrhythmia.
4. Practice Transparent Thinking (thinking out loud) to facilitate group problem solving
5. Use Directed Communication (directing a message to specific individual) when delegating tasks.
6. Employ Closed-Loop Communication (acknowledgment of receipt of the message and status) to acknowledge communications from others.

Safety

The student will be able to:

Administer and maintain specific protecting interventions with attention to safety of the client and healthcare professional.

1. Demonstrate a safe environment with attention to hazards to healthcare providers, visitors and the client. Includes body mechanics, tripping hazards, and equipment issues.
2. Demonstrate attention to national patient safety goals. Includes patient identification standards, effective communication among healthcare providers, and safe medication administration.
3. Demonstrate attention to standard precautions. Includes hand washing, infection control measures and use of personal protective equipment (PPE) as needed.

Leadership and Management/Delegation

The student will be able to:

1. Identify tasks that can be legally, ethically, and safely delegated to unlicensed assistive personnel (UAP) or licensed practical nurse (LPN) in the care of a patient with a tachyarrhythmia.
2. Identify and prioritize patient's needs in care of a patient with a tachyarrhythmia.

OVERVIEW OF PROBLEM

- Tachyarrhythmias
- Rapid response
- Cardiac arrhythmias: any variation in normal rate, rhythm, or configuration of waves on ECG
- Sinus tachycardia

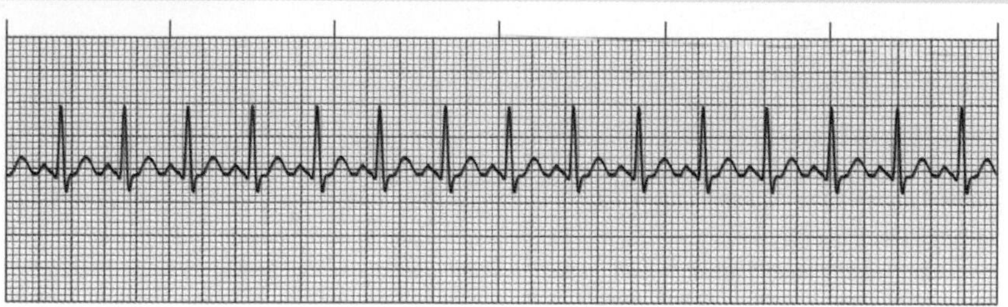

- Atrial tachycardia (PAT)

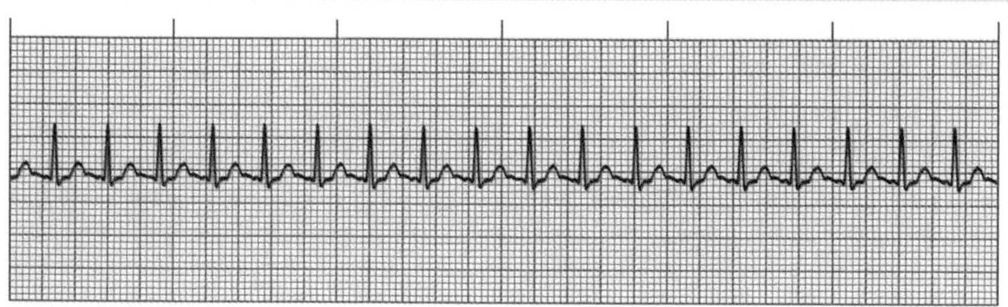

- Atrial fibrillation

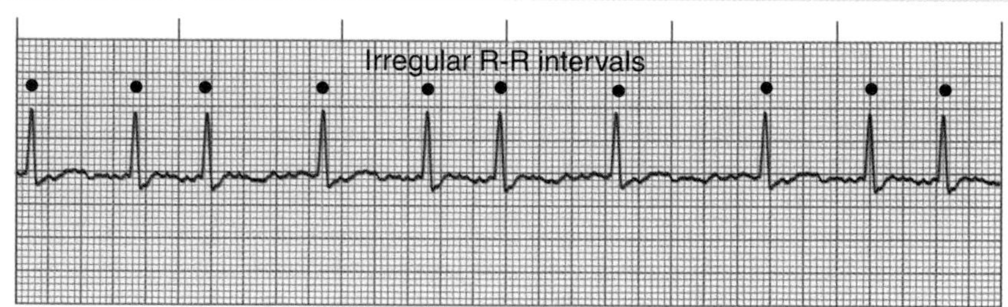

- Atrial flutter

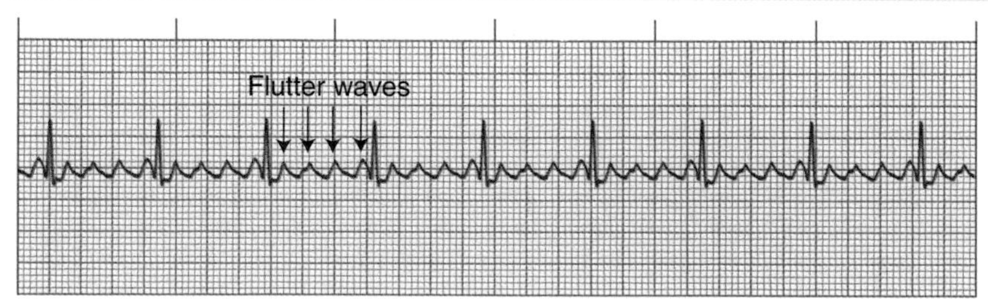

- Multifocal atrial tachyardia

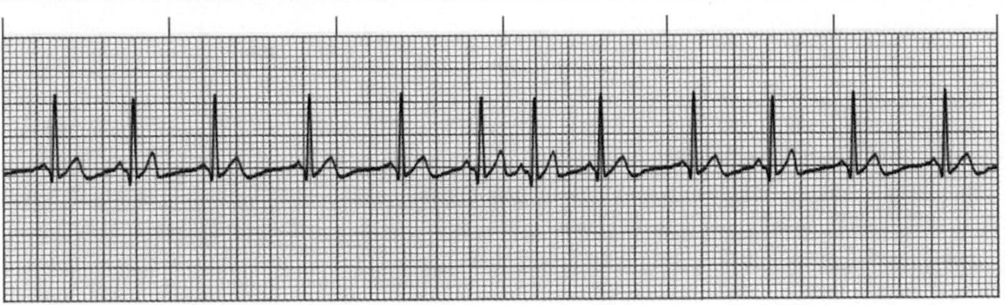

- Junctional tachycardia

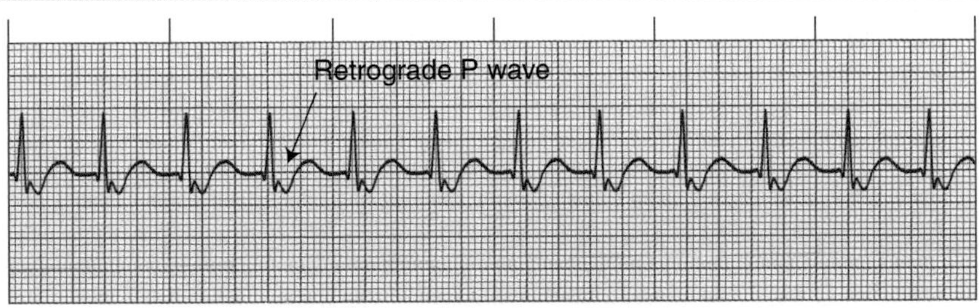

- Supraventricular tachycardia

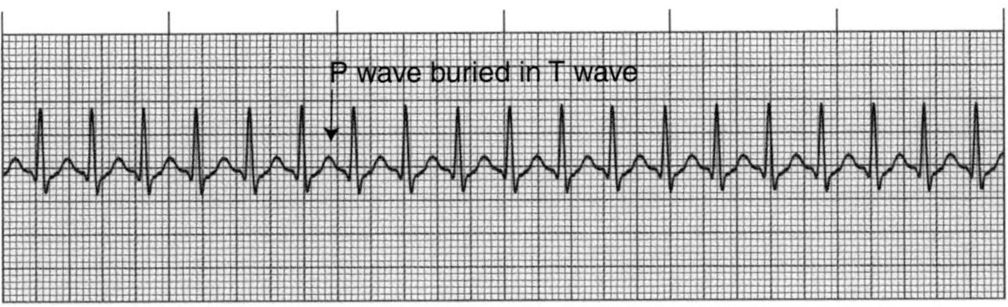

- Ventricular tachycardia

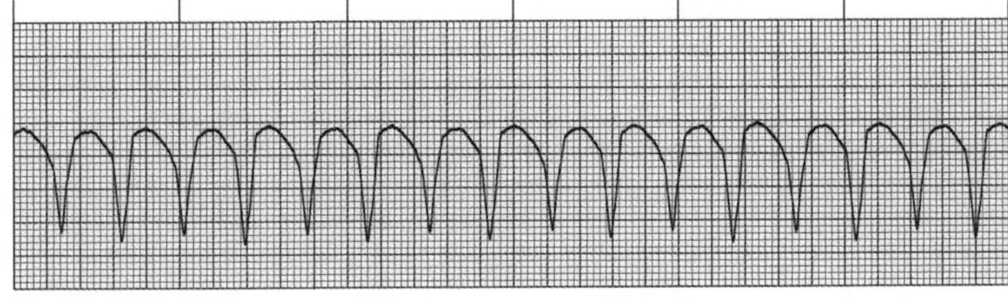

Tachyarrhythmias

Tachyarrhythmia	Rhythm	Rate	P wave	PR interval	QRS
Sinus tachycardia	Regular	>100 100–160	Normal	Normal	Normal
Atrial tachycardia PAT (paroxysmal atrial tachycardia)	Regular	160–250	Abnormal	Normal, but may be buried in T wave	Normal
Atrial tachycardia nonparoxsymal	Regular	>150	May be buried in T wave	Difficult to measure	Normal
Atrial fibrillation	Irregular	Controlled <100 Uncontrolled >100	Absent P F waves	Not measurable	Normal
Atrial flutter	Atrial regular Ventricular dependent	Atrial 250–400	Flutter waves	Not measurable	Normal
Multifocal atrial tachycardia	Irregular	100–250	3 different P waves	Varies	Normal

QT Interval	Pacemaker Site	Causes	Clinical s/s	Treatment
Normal	Sinus	Normal response to exercise, fever Stimulants Medications	Benign	Treat underlying cause
Normal	Atria	Rheumatic heart disease CAD/MI Stimulants Caused by reentry mechanism	Starts and stops suddenly Decreased CO leads to change in mental status, dizziness, syncope, dyspnea	Adenosine Verapamil Digoxin Beta blockers Diltiazem Cardioversion
Normal	Atria	Caused by increased automaticity Gradual onset and stop	Palpitations Anxiety Hypotension	Vagal stimulation Verapamil Digitalis Beta blockers Calcium channel blockers
Not measurable	Atria	Rheumatic heart disease/mitral stenosis Ischemic heart disease/MI Stimulants Stress	Decreased cardiac output related s/s thrombi	Diltiazem Beta blockers Verapamil Digoxin Procainamide or quinidine Anticoagulants Unstable patient cardioversion
Not measurable	Atria	Mitral/tricuspid valve disease CAD, MI Cor pulmonale	Decreased cardiac output related s/s 1:1 flutter Medical emergency	Diltiazem Beta blockers Verapamil Digoxin Procainamide or quinidine Anticoagulants Unstable patient cardioversion
Normal	Ectopic atrial sites	COPD and CHF Digitalis toxicity Hypokalemia	Decrease CO leads to change in mental status, dizziness, syncope, angina, MI, and CHF in patients with CAD	Treat cause Verapamil

Continued

Tachyarrhythmias—cont'd

Tachyarrhythmia	Rhythm	Rate	P wave	PR interval	QRS
Supraventricular tachycardia	Regular	150–200	Difficult to see	Not measurable	Narrow ≤0.1
Junctional tachycardia	Regular	>100	No P wave, inverted P wave before, after, or in QRS	No PR interval Unless P wave precedes QRS, then <0.12	Normal
Ventricular tachycardia	Regular	110–250	None	None	Widen >0.12

Rapid Response

Purpose: Intervene before patient is in crisis.

Role:

- Assess
- Stabilize
- Assist with communication
- Educate and support
- Assist with transfer, if necessary

Team members:

- Critical care nurse
- Respiratory therapist
- Intensivist, resident, hospitalist, or physician

Calling a Rapid Response:

- Worried about a patient
- Acute change in heart rate <40 or >130 bpm
- Acute change in BP systolic <90 mm Hg
- Acute change in respiratory rate <8 or >28/min
- Acute change in oxygen saturation <90% despite oxygen
- Acute change in mental status
- Acute change in urinary output to <50 mL in 4 hr

SBAR Communication

S = Situation
B= Background
A = Assessment
R = Recommendation

Benefits of Rapid Response teams:

- Better patient outcomes
- Improved relationships
- Improved satisfaction for:
  - Nursing
  - Physicians
  - Patients
- Impact on nursing retention
- Financial benefits

REVIEW QUESTIONS

1. What effect does tachycardia have on cardiac output?
   Answer:

2. What signs and symptoms would you expect to see in a patient with tachyarrhythmias?
   Answer:

3. How would you differentiate a benign sinus tachycardia from uncontrolled atrial fibrillation?
   Answer:

QT Interval	Pacemaker Site	Causes	Clinical s/s	Treatment
Usually normal	Anything above ventricles	Same as PAT, Atrial tachycardia	s/s relate to cause	Treatment depends on cause
Normal	AV junction	Nonparoxsymal junctional tachycardia Enhanced automaticity Digitalis toxicity Paroxsymal junctional tachycardia: Reentry mechanism increase sympathetic tone stimulants	Decreased cardiac output related s/s, chest pain, dyspnea Can lead to MI, CHF	Adenosine Verapamil Digoxin Beta blockers Diltiazem Unstable patient cardioversion
Not measurable	Ventricles	AMI , CAD, digitalis toxicity, CHF, MVP	May be conscious and stable or unconscious and pulseless	Amiodarone Lidocaine Procainamide Unstable, no pulse defibrillate

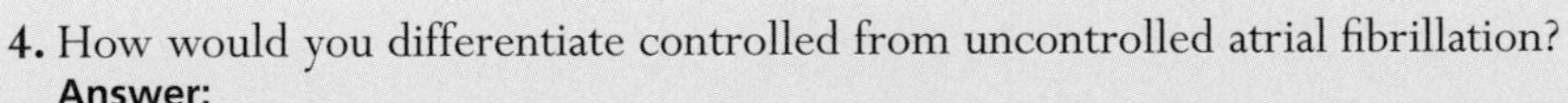

4. How would you differentiate controlled from uncontrolled atrial fibrillation?
Answer:

5. Interpret the following rhythm.

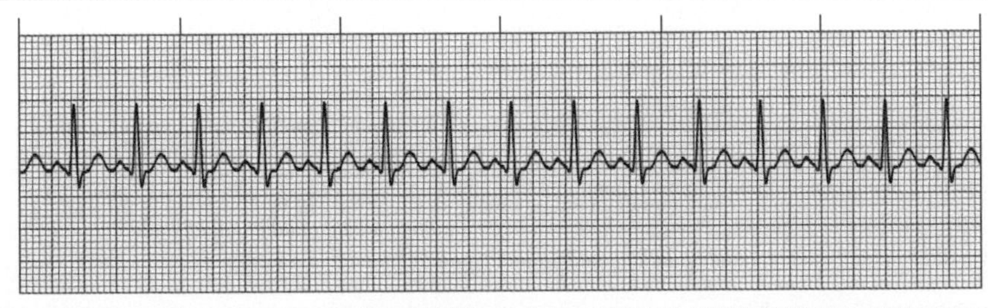

Answer:

6. Interpret the following rhythm.

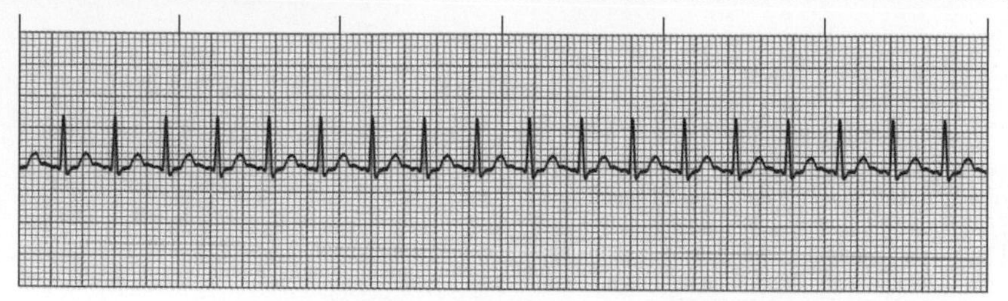

Answer:

7. Interpret the following rhythm.

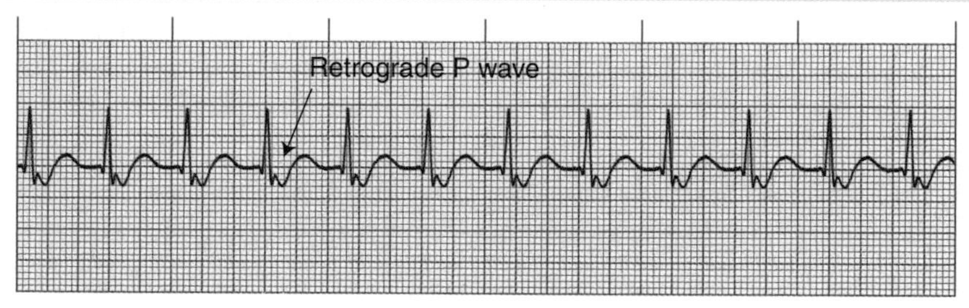

Answer:

8. Interpret the following rhythm.

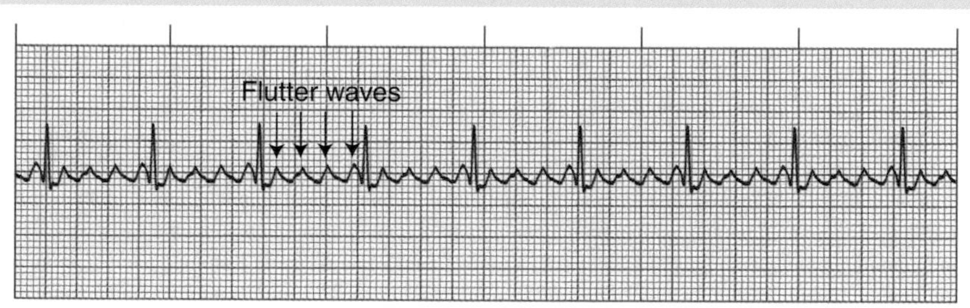

Answer:

9. Interpret the following rhythm.

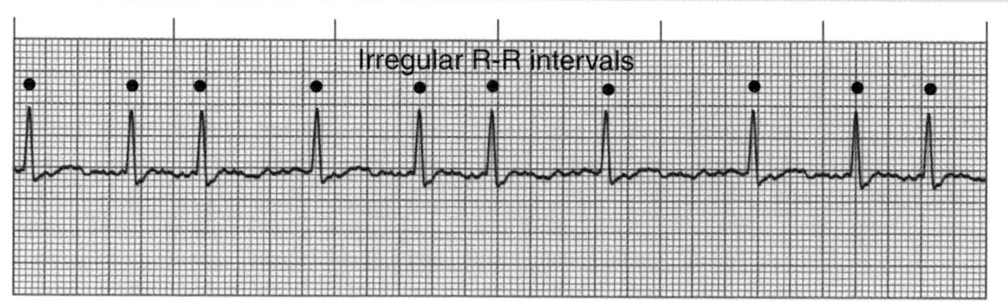

Answer:

10. Interpret the following rhythm.

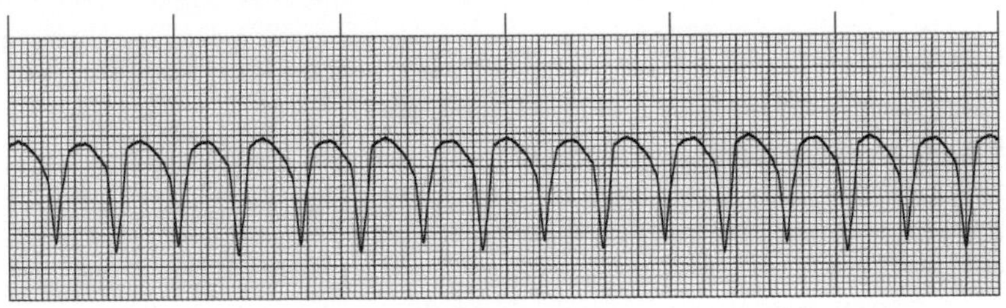

Answer:

Related Evidence-Based Practice Guidelines

Getting Started Kit: Rapid Response Teams. http://www.100kliveswashington.org/resources/RRT-bibliography-050217.pdf

Institute for Healthcare Improvement, 100,000 Lives Campaign. http://www.ihi.org/IHI/Programs/Campaign/Campaign.htm

The Joint Commission National Patient Safety Goals Hospital Program. Retrieved from http://www.jointcommission.org/GeneralPublic/NPSG/10_npsgs.htm

SBAR Technique for Communication: A situational briefing model published by The Institute for Healthcare Improvement was downloaded on December 19, 2008, from http://www.ihi.org/IHI/Topics/PatientSafety/SafetyGeneral/Tools/SBARTechniqueforCommunicationASituationalBriefingModel.htm

Topics to Review Prior to the Simulation

- Cardiac arrhythmias
- COPD
- Rapid response

SIMULATION

Client Background

Biographical Data

- Age: 71
- Gender: male
- Height: 6 ft
- Weight: 220 lb

Cultural Considerations

- Language: English
- Ethnicity: African American
- Nationality: American
- Culture: no significant cultural considerations identified

Demographic

- Marital status: married
- Educational level: high school + trade school
- Religion: Baptist
- Occupation: retired

Current Health Status

Acute exacerbation COPD secondary to pneumonia

History

- Psychosocial history
  - Social support: family
- Past health history
  - Medical : + HTN, +COPD
  - Surgical: none
- Family history: + CVD, COPD, DM

Admission Sheet	
Name:	Fredrick Hankins
Age:	71
Gender:	Male
Marital Status:	Married
Educational Level:	High school + trade school
Religion:	Baptist

Continued

Admission Sheet—cont'd

Ethnicity:	African American
Nationality:	American
Language:	English
Occupation:	Retired

Hospital Provider's Orders

Patient's Name: Fredrick Hankins

Allergies: NKDA

Diagnosis: Acute exacerbation COPD

Date	Time	Order	Signature
		Admit to Respiratory Unit Dx acute exacerbation COPD, pneumonia	
		Vital signs: q 4 hr	
		Diet: Regular NAS	
		Activity: OOB	
		IV therapy: INT with routine flush	
		Medications: Atrovent inhaler 1 puff q 8 hr Lasix 40 mg po daily Lovenox 40 mg subq q 12 hr Protonix 40 mg po daily Rocephin 1 g IVPB daily Zithromax 500 mg IVPB daily SoluMedrol 40 mg IV push q 8 hr	
		Diagnostic studies: Repeat CXR in AM CBC, BMP	
		Treatments: Oxygen 2 L via NC Neb treatment q 6 h with ipratropium/albuterol 3 mL	
			Dr. Schuman

Nursing Report

Mr. Hankins, a 71-year-old patient of Dr. Schuman, was admitted yesterday with the diagnosis of acute exacerbation COPD/pneumonia. Hx of HTN. AAOx3, slept most of night; had one neb treatment at 4 AM. VS stable BP 148/90, pulse 90 HRRR, respirations 24, pulse ox 94% on 2 L via nasal cannula, lungs crackles, occasional expiratory wheeze, + productive cough, yellow sputum. Voiding qs INT #22 in left hand. For repeat CXR, CBC, and BMP today.

Student Simulation Prep Assignments

1. Identify items and their purpose in the care of a patient with tachyarrhythmia.

Item	Purpose
IV with pump	
O_2 cannula	
ECG	
Neb treatment	

2. Identify team members and their specific roles in the care of a patient with tachyarrhythmia.

Team Member	Role
Night nurse	
Primary nurse	
Secondary nurse	
Physician	
Nurse manager/supervisor	

3. Relevant Data Assignment: Fill in columns below.

Relevant Data from Report	Relevant Data from Other Sources	Data Missing	Sources for Missing Data	Data Requiring Follow-Up

4. Initial Focused Assessment

After reviewing the client background and nursing report, you are ready to assess your client's current status. Under each category, identify how you would target your assessment and what you would expect to find for the patient with tachyarrhythmia

History

Are there any questions you need to ask the patient or family to obtain additional relevant data?

Physical Exam

- General appearance:
- Integumentary:
- HEENT:
- Respiratory:
- CV:
- Breasts:
- Abdominal:
- Neuro:
- Musculoskeletal:
- Reproductive:
- Additional:
- Developmental:

What are the nursing implications considering the developmental stage of your patient?

Answer:

5. Diagnostic Tests

What diagnostic test results relevant to the patient's current problem are needed to plan care?

Complete the table using Van Leeuwen et al, *Davis's Comprehensive Handbook of Laboratory and Diagnostic Testing with Nursing Implications* 4e, or other diagnostic test reference.

Diagnostic Test	Significance to This Patient's Problem
ABG	
CBC	
BMP	
CXR	

6. Treatment

Identify drugs that are used to treat a patient with tachyarrythmia.

Complete the table using Deglin et al, *Davis's Drug Guide for Nurses* 12e, or other drug reference.

Medication	Dose, Route, Frequency	Indications	Side Effect	Nursing Implications
Atrovent inhaler	1 puff q 8 hr			
Lasix	40 mg po daily			
Protonix	40 mg po daily			
SoluMedrol	40 mg IV push q 8 hr			
Rocephin	1 g IVPB daily			
Zithromax	500 mg IVPB daily			

7. Nursing Problems/Diagnoses

Identify three priority nursing problems/diagnoses.

Assessment Data	Priority Problem	Intervention	Expected Patient Outcome	Which Intervention could be Delegated to Unlicensed Personnel?
1.				
2.				
3.				

References

Deglin, J. H., & Vallerand, A. H. (2009). *Davis's drug guide for nurses* (11th ed.). Philadelphia: F. A. Davis.

Dillon, P. (2007). *Nursing health assessment: A critical thinking and case studies approach* (2nd ed.). Philadelphia: F. A. Davis.

Erikson, E. H. (1950). *Childhood and society*. New York: Norton.

Jones, S. (2005). *ECG notes*. Philadelphia: F. A. Davis.

Lagerquist, S. L. (2006). *Davis's NCLEX-RN success* (2nd ed). Philadelphia: F. A. Davis.

Ouimet Perrin, K. (2009). *Understanding the essentials of critical care nursing*. Upper Saddle River, NJ: Pearson Education.

Van Leeuwen, A. M. & Poelhuis-Leth, D. J., & Bladh, M. L. (2011). *Davis's comprehensive handbook of laboratory and diagnostic tests with nursing implications* (4th ed.). Philadelphia: F. A. Davis.

5-7 CHF/COPD

ADULT/MEDICAL-SURGICAL

STANDARD FORMS

These templates are included in the Appendix; copy before each use.

LEARNING OUTCOMES

Cognitive

The student will be able to:

1. Identify pertinent history question relevant a patient with COPD/CHF.
2. Differentiate the signs and symptoms of COPD/CHF.
3. Differentiate the pathophysiology of COPD/CHF.
4. Identify appropriate diagnostic studies for a patient with COPD/CHF.
5. Describe appropriate treatment for COPD/CHF.

Psychomotor

The student will be able to:

1. Obtain a pertinent health history from a patient with COPD/CHF.
2. Perform appropriate assessment for a patient with COPD/CHF.
3. Implement patient safety standards for a patient with COPD/CHF.

Affective

The student will be able to:

1. Reflect upon performance in performing an assessment on a patient with COPD/CHF.
2. Identify factors that worked well during the simulation of care of a patient with COPD/CHF.
3. Identify factors that needed improvement during the simulation of care of a patient with COPD/CHF.
4. Develop self-confidence in performing an assessment on a patient with COPD/CHF.

Communication

The student will be able to:

1. Communicate effectively with the patient while performing an assessment on a patient with COPD/CHF.
2. Use SBAR when communication assessment findings.
3. Accurately and succinctly document assessment findings.
4. Practice Transparent Thinking (thinking out loud) to facilitate group problem solving
5. Use Directed Communication (directing a message to specific individual) when delegating tasks.
6. Employ Closed-loop Communication (acknowledgment of receipt of the message and status) to acknowledge communications from others.

Safety

The student will be able to:

Administer and maintain specific protecting interventions with attention to safety of the client and healthcare professional.

1. Demonstrate a safe environment with attention to hazards to healthcare providers, visitors and the client. Includes body mechanics, tripping hazards, and equipment issues.
2. Demonstrate attention to national patient safety goals. Includes patient identification standards, effective communication among healthcare providers, and safe medication administration.
3. Demonstrate attention to standard precautions. Includes hand washing, infection control measures, and use of personal protective equipment (PPE) as needed.

Leadership and Management/Delegation

The student will be able to:

1. Identify tasks that can be legally, ethically, and safely delegated to unlicensed assistive personnel (UAP) or licensed practical nurse (LPN) in the care of a patient with COPD/CHF.
2. Identify and prioritize patient's needs in care of a patient with a COPD/CHF.

Teaching

The student will be able to:

1. Develop a discharge plan for a patient with COPD/CHF.
2. Develop a teaching plan for the patient with COPD/CHF.
3. Make appropriate referrals for the patient with COPD/CHF.
4. Implement an effective teaching plan for the patient with COPD/CHF.
5. Evaluate the discharge and teaching plan for the patient with COPD/CHF.

OVERVIEW OF PROBLEM

COPD/CHF

COPD

Definition

- **Emphysema:** Chronic disease with excessive inflation of the air spaces distal to the terminal bronchioles, alveolar ducts, and alveoli; characterized by increased airway resistance and decreased diffusing capacity.
- **Chronic Bronchitis**: Chronic inflammation of the bronchi characterized by hypersecretion of mucus and chronic cough for 3 months per year for 2 consecutive years. Emphysema and chronic bronchitis constitute COPD.

Pathophysiology

- **Emphysema**: Imbalance between proteases which break down lung tissue, and alpha-antitrypsin, which inhibits the breakdown. Increased airway resistance during expiration results in air trapping and hyperinflation leads to increased residual volumes. Increased dead space leads to unequal ventilation leading to perfusion of poorly ventilated alveoli resulting in hypoxia and carbon dioxide retention (hypercapnia). Chronic hypercapnia reduces sensitivity of respiratory center; chemorecpetors in aortic arch and carotid sinus become principal regulators of respiratory drive (respond to hypoxia).
- **Chronic Bronchitis**: Bronchial walls are infiltrated with lymphocytes and macrophages; lumen becomes obstructed due to decreased ciliary action and repeated bronchospasm. Hyperventilation of alveolar sacs occurs. Long-term condition results in respiratory acidosis, recurrent pneuminitis, emphysema, or cor pulmonale.

Risk Factors

- Smoking
- Air pollution
- Alpha-antitrypsin deficiency
- Destruction of lung parenchyma
- Family history and increased age
- Repeated respiratory infections

Assessment

Subjective

- **Emphysema**
  - Weakness, lethargy
  - Shortness of breath
  - History of repeated respiratory infections
  - Long-term smoking
  - Irritability
  - Dyspnea on exertion (DOE)
- **Bronchitis**
  - Shortness of breath
  - Recurrent productive cough
  - Anorexia

Objective

- **Emphysema**
  - Increased BP, pulse
  - Nasal flaring
  - Nonproductive cough
  - Wheezing, crackles
  - Increased AP: Lateral diameter (barrel chest)
  - Decreased excursion
  - Use of accessory muscles
  - Position: tripod, orthopnea
  - Pursed lip breathing
  - Ruddy skin color, or cyanosis
  - Clubbing
- **Bronchitis**
  - Use of accessory muscles
  - Dusky, cyanosis
  - Productive cough
  - Wheezing, rhonchi
  - Weight loss
  - Fever

Diagnostic Tests

- **Emphysema**
  - CXR reveals hyperinflation and flattened diaphragm
  - Lung scan differentiates between ventilation/perfusion
  - Pulmonary functions:
    - Prolonged rapid, forced exhalation
    - Decreased vital capacity (<4000 mL) forced expiratory volume
    - Increased residual volume (may be 200%), total lung capacity
    - ABG pH < 7.35, PaO_2 <80 mm Hg, $PaCO_2$ >45 mm Hg
- **Bronchitis**
  - Pulmonary functions:
    - Decreased forced expiratory volume
    - ABG PaO_2 , >90 mm Hg, $PaCO_2$ >40 mm Hg
    - RBC elevated (polycythemia)
    - WBCs elevated

Treatment

- Oxygen with humidification: low flow no more than 2 L
- Nebulizer treatment
- Medication:
  - Bronchodilators
  - Antimicrobials
  - Steroids
  - Expectorants
  - Bronchial detergents
  - Immunotherapy: Flu and pneumonia vaccines

Nursing Management

Goal: Improved ventilation

- Fowler's or leaning forward
- Chest PT, postural drainage
- Administer oxygen and medication as ordered

Goal: Promote comfort and support body systems

- Oral hygiene
- Skin care
- Active/passive ROM
- Adequate rest

Goal: Improve nutrition

- High protein, high calorie
- Small frequent meals
- Fluids

Goal: Minimize bronchial irritants

- Avoid irritants, such as smoke
- Air conditioning

Goal: Family support

- Measures to identify and decrease anxiety
- Assist family coping

Goal: Health teaching

- Breathing exercises
- Stress management
- Smoking cessation
- Avoidance of respiratory infection
- Desired and side effects of medications
- Bronchial hygiene therapy
- Rest/activity
- Nutrition and fluid
- Medical follow-up

Evaluation/Outcome Criteria

- Takes prescribed medications
- Participates in rest/activity schedule
- Improves nutritional and fluid intake
- No complications
- No respiratory infections
- Acid-base balance maintained

Complications

- Early—respiratory alkalosis; late—respiratory acidosis
- Cor pulmonale, acute right side heart failure d/t increased pulmonary artery pressure
- Respiratory failure

CHF

Definition

Inability of the heart to meet peripheral circulatory demands of the body; cardiac decompensation, combined right and left failure.

Pathophysiology

Increased cardiac workload or decreased effective myocardial contractility leads to decreased cardiac output (forward effects). Left ventricular failure leads to pulmonary congestion. Right atrial and ventricular failure leads to systemic congestion and peripheral edema (backward effects). Compensatory mechanisms in heart failure include tachycardia, ventricular dilation and hypertrophy.

Risk Factors

- Decreased contractility
- Increased workload

Assessment

Subjective

- Shortness of breath
  - Orthopnea
  - Dyspnea on exertion (DOE)
  - Paroxsymal nocturnal dyspnea (PND)
- Apprehension
- Fatigue
- Feeling of puffiness

Objective

- Vital signs:
  - BP decreasing systolic and narrowing pulse pressure
  - Pulsus alternans
  - Cheyne-Stokes respirations
- Left ventricular failure:
  - Crackles
  - Tachycardia
  - S_3
  - Cardiac murmurs
  - Paradoxical splitting of S_2
- Right ventricular failure:
  - Jugular venous distention
  - Peripheral edema
  - Ascities
  - + Hepatojugular efflux
  - Congestion hepatomegaly

Diagnostic Tests

- CXR:
  - Cardiac enlargement
  - Dilated pulmonary vessels
  - Diffuse interstitial lung edema
- Labs:
  - CBC
  - CK, MB, troponin
  - BUN, creatinine
  - Electrolytes
  - PT/INR
  - B-type natriuretic peptide (BNP)
- ECG

Treatment

Medications

- Digitalis
- ACE inhibitors
- Inotropic agents
- Diuretics
- Tranquilizers
- Vasodilators

Nursing Management

Goal: Promote rest and reduce stimuli

- Position: semi-Fowler's
- Planned rest periods
- Sedatives as ordered
- Measures to decrease anxiety
- Family support

Goal: Prevent or treat respiratory distress
- Oxygen
- Elevate HOB

Goal: Promote safety
- Skin care
- ROM
- Side rails if confused from hypoxia
- Monitor vital signs
- TEDS

Goal: Maintain fluid/electrolyte balance and nutrition
- Monitor urinary output
- Check bun and electrolytes
- Daily weights
- Low sodium diet
- Small, frequent meals

Goal: Health teaching
- Diet and meal preparation
- Activity restrictions
- Medications
- Community resources

Evaluation/Outcome Criteria

- Fatigue decreased, increased activity tolerance
- No complications
- Reduction in edema

REVIEW QUESTIONS

1. How would you differentiate the s/s of CHF from COPD?
   Answer:

2. Patients with COPD may have cardiac involvement. Which side of the heart is most likely to be affected?
   Answer:

3. Differentiate right and left CHF.
   Answer:

4. Chronic bronchitis and emphysema are categorized as COPD. How would you differentiate chronic bronchitis from emphysema?
   Answer:

5. What should be included in a health teaching plan for a patient with COPD and CHF?
   Answer:

Related Evidenced-Based Practice Guidelines

Search http://www.guideline.gov CHF and COPD

The Joint Commission National Patient Safety Goals Hospital Program. Retrieved from http://www.jointcommission.org/GeneralPublic/NPSG/10_npsgs.htm

SBAR Technique for Communication: A situational briefing model published by The Institute for Healthcare Improvement was downloaded on December 19, 2008, from http://www.ihi.org/IHI/Topics/PatientSafety/SafetyGeneral/Tools/SBARTechniqueforCommunicationASituationalBriefingModel.htm

Topics to Review Prior to the Simulation

- Health assessment: cardiac and respiratory
- COPD/CHF/pulmonary edema

SIMULATION

Client Background

Biographical Data

- Age: 64
- Gender: male
- Height: 5 ft 2 in
- Weight: 189 lb

Cultural Considerations:

- Language: Spanish
- Ethnicity: Hispanic
- Nationality: American
- Culture: may require interpreter

Demographic

- Marital status: married
- Educational level: technical school
- Religion: Catholic
- Occupation: construction worker

Current Health Status

- Increasing tiredness, foot and ankle swelling

History

- Past medical history
  - History of COPD stage II
  - Surgery: T&A and hernia repair
- Psychosocial history
  - Social support: family
  - \+ smoking 20 pack years
- Family history: + CVD, HTN, COPD

Admission Sheet	
Name:	Juan Manuel
Age:	64
Gender:	Male
Marital Status:	Married
Educational Level:	Technical school
Religion:	Catholic
Ethnicity:	Hispanic
Nationality:	American
Language:	Spanish
Occupation:	Construction worker

Hospital **Patient's Name: Juan Manuel**
Provider's Orders **Allergies: NKDA**

Diagnosis: Exacerbation COPD/CHF

Date	Time	Order	Signature
		Admit to telemetry	
		Cardiac monitor	
		Vital signs: q 4 hr	
		Diet: low-sodium, cardiac diet	
		Activity: BRP	
		IV therapy: Intermittent infusion device, flush q shift with 3 mL NSS	
		TEDS, pneumatic stockings	
		Medications: Lasix 40 mg IVP x 1 dose stat Vasotec 3 mg po daily Aspirin 81 mg po daily Singulair 10 mg po daily Advair 1 disk bid Zithromax 500 mg IV daily Lovenox 40 mg subq daily Protonix 40 mg IVP daily Tylenol 650 mg po q 4 hr prn for pain or fever Nebulizer treatment: Ventolin 2.5/Atrovent 0.5 q 4 hr	
		Diagnostic studies: ECG Pulmonary functions Repeat CBC, BMP, BNP in AM	

Diagnosis:	Exacerbation COPD/CHF—cont'd		
Date	**Time**	**Order**	**Signature**
		Routine UA	
		ABGs x 1 stat	
		Treatments:	
		Oxygen 2 L via NC	
		Strict I&O	
			Dr Dooner

Nursing Report

Juan Manuel, age 64, a patient of Dr. Dooner, admitted yesterday with CHF and exacerbation COPD stage II. Has had COPD for several years, but recently diagnosed with CHF. He has become increasingly weak and tired, and has ankle swelling. His daughter brought him in when he could no longer get his shoes on. The patient is AAOx3, and speaks little English. VS: T 99°F, P 95 and regular, R 26, pulse ox on 2 L 93%, SOB with activity, BP 154/90. Lungs decreased breath sounds at bases, scattered wheezes and crackles, + productive cough with green sputum. HRRR, no extra sounds, monitor NSR + 1 pedal pulses, + 2 pedal edema, abdomen large and round, + BS, soft, nontender, voiding qs. Weak bilateral handgrip and decreased strength in lower extremities.

Student Simulation Prep Assignments

1. Identify items and their purpose in the care of a patient with COPD/CHF.

Item	Purpose
IV with pump	
O_2 cannula	
Monitor	
Nebulizer	

2. Identify team members and their specific roles in the care of a patient with COPD/CHF.

Team Member	Role
Primary nurse	
Physician	
Secondary nurse	

3. Relevant Data Assignment: Fill in the columns below.

Relevant Data from Report	Relevant Data from Other Sources	Data Missing	Sources for Missing Data	Data Requiring Follow-Up

Continued

Relevant Data from Report	Relevant Data from Other Sources	Data Missing	Sources for Missing Data	Data Requiring Follow-Up

4. *Initial Focused Assessment*

After reviewing the client background and nursing report, you are ready to assess your client's current status. Under each category, identify how you would target your assessment and what you would expect to find for the patient with COPD/CHF.

History

Are there any questions you need to ask the patient or family to obtain additional relevant data?

Physical Exam

- General appearance:
- Integumentary:
- HEENT:
- Respiratory:
- CV:
- Breasts:
- Abdominal:
- Neuro:
- Musculoskeletal:
- Reproductive:
- Additional:
- Developmental:

What are the nursing implications considering the developmental stage of your patient?

Answer:

5. *Diagnostic Tests*

What diagnostic test results relevant to the patient's current problem are needed to plan care?

Complete the table using Van Leeuwen et al, *Davis's Comprehensive Handbook of Laboratory and Diagnostic Testing with Nursing Implications* 4e, or other diagnostic test reference.

Diagnostic Test	Significance to This Patient's Problem
ECG	
CBC	
BMP • Glucose • Lytes • BUN • Creatinine	
UA	
BNP	
Pulmonary functions	
ABGs	
CXR	

6. Treatments

Identify drugs that are used to treat a patient with COPD/CHF.

Complete the table using Deglin et al, *Davis's Drug Guide for Nurses* 12e, or other drug reference.

Medication	Dose, Route, Frequency	Indications	Side Effect	Nursing Implications
Vasotec	5 mg daily			
Aspirin	81 mg daily			
Singulair	10 mg daily			
Protonix	40 mg IVP daily			
Tylenol	2 tabs q 4 hr prn pain or fever			

Continued

Medication	Dose, Route, Frequency	Indications	Side Effect	Nursing Implications
Advair	1 disk			
Zithromax	500 mg IVPB			
Lovenox	40 mg subq daily			
Lasix	40 mg IV stat			

7. Nursing Problems/Diagnoses

Identify three priority nursing problems/diagnoses.

Assessment Data	Priority Problem	Intervention	Expected Patient Outcome	Which Intervention Could Be Delegated to Unlicensed Personnel?
1.				
2.				

Assessment Data	Priority Problem	Intervention	Expected Patient Outcome	Which Intervention Could Be Delegated to Unlicensed Personnel?
3.				

References

Deglin, J. H., & Vallerand, A. H. (2009). *Davis's drug guide for nurses* (11th ed.). Philadelphia: F. A. Davis.

Dillon, P. (2007). *Nursing health assessment: A critical thinking and case studies approach* (2nd ed.). Philadelphia: F. A. Davis.

Erikson, E. H. (1950). *Childhood and society*. New York: Norton.

Lagerquist, S. L. (2006). *Davis's NCLEX-RN success* (2nd ed.). Philadelphia: F. A. Davis.

Ouimet Perrin, K. (2009). *Understanding the essentials of critical care nursing*. Upper Saddle River, NJ: Pearson Education.

Van Leeuwen, A. M., Poelhuis-Leth, D. J., & Bladh, M. L. (2011). *Davis's comprehensive handbook of laboratory and diagnostic tests with nursing implications* (4th ed.). Philadelphia: F. A. Davis.

5-8 Complications of Cardiac Catheterization

CARDIAC CARE

STANDARD FORMS

These templates are included in the Appendix; copy before each use.

LEARNING OUTCOMES

Cognitive

The student will be able to:

1. Describe the routine assessment for postcardiac catheterization safety.
2. Describe signs and symptoms of retroperitoneal hemorrhage.
3. Correlate signs and symptoms of retroperitoneal hemorrhage to the pathophysiology of hyperanticoagulation and invasive vascular catheterization.
4. Identify factors in a patient's history that increase risk for delayed clotting and vascular rupture.
5. Identify factors in a patient's current condition that increase risk for delayed clotting and vascular rupture.
6. Identify the appropriate interventions for the patient with comorbid hypertension, diabetes, and atherosclerosis.
7. Differentiate the roles of team members in response to a patient with emergent hemorrhage and hypotension.

Psychomotor

The student will be able to:

1. Perform a routine assessment postcardiac catheterization.
2. Perform appropriate assessment for a patient with multiple comorbidities, declining hemodynamic status, declining respiratory status, declining mental status, and pain.
3. Initiate appropriate interventions including BCLS, application of oxygen, IV insertion and fluid delivery, blood product delivery, preparation for emergent diagnostic tests and emergency surgery for a patient with pain, tachypnea, tachycardia, hypertension, hypotension, oliguria, disorientation, and anxiety.
4. Work collaboratively as part of the healthcare team in the care of a patient with emergently declining homeostasis postinvasive procedure.

Affective

The student will be able to:

1. Reflect upon performance in the care of a patient returning from cardiac catheterization with multiple comorbidities, declining hemodynamic status, declining respiratory status, declining mental status, and pain.
2. Reflect upon knowledge needs to improve care of a patient with complex underlying medical problems and emergent care requirements.
3. Identify own feelings in delivering care to a patient with rapidly declining homeostasis and potential death.
4. Discuss feelings related to working as a member of a team in the care of a patient with rapidly declining homeostasis and potential death.
5. Identify factors that worked well during the simulation of care of a patient with complex underlying medical problems and emergent care requirements.
6. Identify factors that needed improvement during the simulation of care of a patient with complex underlying medical problems and emergent care requirements.
7. Develop self-confidence in the care of a patient with complex underlying medical problems and emergent care requirements.

Communication

The student will be able to:

1. Communicate effectively with healthcare team members in care of a patient with multiple comorbidities, declining hemodynamic status, declining respiratory status, declining mental status, and pain.
2. Communicate effectively with the patient and family in the care of a patient with rapidly declining homeostasis and potential death.
3. Use SBAR when communication with team members in the care of a patient with rapidly declining homeostasis and potential death.
4. Practice Transparent Thinking (thinking out loud) to facilitate group problem solving.
5. Use Directed Communication (directing a message to specific individual) when delegating tasks
6. Employ Closed-Loop Communication (acknowledgment of receipt of the message and status) to acknowledge communications from others

Safety

The student will be able to:

Administer and maintain specific protecting interventions with attention to safety of the client and healthcare professional.

1. Demonstrate a safe environment with attention to hazards to healthcare providers, visitors, and the client. Includes body mechanics, tripping hazards, and equipment issues.
2. Demonstrate attention to national patient safety goals. Includes patient identification standards, effective communication among healthcare providers, and safe medication administration.

3. Demonstrate attention to standard precautions. Includes hand washing, infection control measures, and use of personal protective equipment (PPE) as needed.

Leadership and Management/Delegation

The student will be able to:

1. Identify tasks that can be legally, ethically, and safely delegated to unlicensed assistive personnel (UAP) in the care of a patient returning from a cardiac catheterization with multiple comorbidities, declining hemodynamic status, declining respiratory status, declining mental status, and pain.
2. Identify when care of the patient is beyond the scope of unlicensed assistive personnel.
3. Identify when care of a patient is beyond the scope of a student nurse.
4. Identify when care of a patient is beyond the scope of a registered nurse.
5. Identify who in the healthcare team is most qualified to direct care of the client.

Spiritual

The student will be able to:

1. Discuss role of family during patient's decline.
2. Identify characteristics of nursing diagnoses requiring spiritual support (risk for powerlessness, anticipatory grieving, and fear).

OVERVIEW OF PROBLEM

Cardiac Catheterization

Definition

A diagnostic procedure to evaluate cardiac status. Introduces a catheter into the heart and blood vessels: analyzes blood samples.

Assessment

Subjective

- Allergies
  - Iodine
  - Seafood

Objective

- Vital signs, baseline data
- Distal pulses
- Mark for reference after catheterization

Nursing Management

Goal: provide for safety and comfort

- Signed informed consent
- NPO
- Urinate prior to going to cath lab
- Administer sedatives as ordered

Goal: Health Teaching

- Explain procedure length, expectations, sensations
- Alert physician to unusual sensations

Postcathertization

Assessment

Subjective

- Puncture site: increasing pain, tenderness
- Palpitations
- Affected extremity: tingling, numbness, pain from hematoma or nerve damage
- Lightheaded, weakness, generalized anxiety, back pain

Objective

- Vital signs: shock, respiratory distress (pulmonary emboli, allergic reaction)
- LOC, orientation
- Puncture site: bleeding, hematoma
- ECG: arrhythmias, signs of MI
- Affected extremity: color, temperature, peripheral pulses
- Abdomen: mild distention, Grey Turner's sign, bruit, dull to percussion, flank pain

Diagnostic Tests

- Diagnostic blood tests: HGB, HCT, PTT, PT, Chem 7, bedside blood glucose assessment, type and cross match for blood replacement
- Arterial blood gasses to identify acid-base imbalance
- Emergent diagnostic exams: ultrasound, computerized tomography

Treatment

Hypovolemia

- Application of oxygen
- IV insertion and fluid delivery
- Blood product delivery
- Analgesia
- Preparation for emergent diagnostic tests and emergency surgery for a patient with pain, tachypnea, tachycardia, hypertension, hypotension, oliguria, disorientation, and anxiety

BLS treatments

- Positioning of patient for profusion
- Maintain airway

Emergent treatments

- Application of oxygen for confusion/deteriorating mental status
- Insertion of large-bore IV angiocatheters
- Administration of 0.9% sodium chloride
- Administration of blood products: PRBC, platelets, fresh frozen plasma
- Insertion of indwelling bladder catheter to measure urine

Medications:

- Pain relieving analgesics: IV morphine
- Vasopressor agents: Dopamine (Intropin), Norepinephrine (Levophed) and epinephrine (adrenalin), Vasopressin (Pitressin)

Nursing Management

Goal: prevent complications

- Bed rest
- Vital signs
- Observe puncture site
- ECG: monitor and document rhythm
- Give medications as ordered

Goal: provide emotional support

- Brief accurate explanations
- Referrals as indicated

Goal: provide for safety and comfort

- Signed informed consent
- NPO
- Urinate prior to going to cath lab
- Administer sedatives as ordered

Goal: health teaching

- Potential complications
- Prepare for surgery if indicated
- Follow-up medical care
- Limitations of activity
- Explain procedure length, expectations, sensations
- Alert physician to unusual sensations

Evaluation/Outcome Criteria

- No complications

REVIEW QUESTIONS

1. Cardiac catheterization can be performed with or without radiological dye to enhance the image. Which is one of the major concerns with the use of the dye?
A. Potential for renal failure due to the dye.
B. Potential for venous scaring due to the dye.
C. Potential for hepatic failure due to the dye.
D. Potential for bluish discoloration due to the dye.
Answer:

2. Cardiac catheterization is most commonly performed via access through the right femoral artery. After catheterization the nurse conducts a routine pulse assessment. Which pulses are typically checked?
A. Right popliteal & right femoral
B. Right & left politeal
C. Right dorsalis pedis & left posterior tibial
D. Right & left dorsalis pedis & posterior tibial
Answer:

3. Patient is scheduled for cardiac catheterization. Pre-catheterization VS include: T 98.6°, P 80, R-20, pulse ox 94% on RA, BP 130/70. Post-catheterization VS include: T 97.6°, P 115, R-24, pulse ox 90% on RA, BP 90/50. These findings suggest:
A. Normal findings
B. Hypovolemia
C. Pain
D. DVT
Answer:

4. Certain blood products must be delivered via a cannula gauge 20 or greater. The rationale for this requirement is:
A. The size of the red blood cells
B. To allow frozen plasma to mix with warm blood
C. Blood transfusion reduces venous elasticity
D. To decrease the need for heparin
Answer:

5. The student nurse is aware that the aorta and iliac arteries lie:
A. Anterior to the peritoneal lining
B. Superior to the peritoneal lining
C. Posterior to the peritoneal lining
D. Inferior to the peritoneal lining
Answer:

Related Evidence-Based Practice Guidelines

Hirsch, A.T., Haskal, Z.J., Hertzer, N.R., Bakal, C.W., Creager, M.A., Halperin, J. L, Riegel B. (2006). Peripheral arterial disease: ACC/AHA 2005 Guidelines for the Management of Patients With Peripheral Arterial Disease (Lower Extremity, Renal, Mesenteric, and Abdominal Aortic): A Collaborative Report From the American Association for Vascular Surgery/Society for Vascular Surgery, Society for Cardiovascular Angiography and Interventions, Society for Vascular Medicine and Biology, Society of Interventional Radiology, and the ACC/AHA Task Force on Practice Guidelines (Writing Committee to Develop Guidelines for the Management of Patients With Peripheral Arterial Disease). Journal of the American College of Cardiology, *47*, 1239-312. The full-text guidelines are available at http://www.acc.org/clinical/guidelines/pad/index.pdf, and an executive summary is available at http://www.acc.org/clinical/guidelines/pad/index.pdf

Clinical Policy: Procedural Sedation and Analgesia in the Emergency Department from the American College of Emergency Physicians Clinical Policies Subcommittee (Writing Committee) on Procedural Sedation and Analgesia:

Steven A. Godwin, MD, Chair, David A. Caro, MD, Stephen J. Wolf, MD, Andy S. Jagoda, MD, Ronald Charles, MD, Benjamin E. Marett, RN, MSN, CEN, CNA, COHN-S (ENA Representative 2002-2003), Jessie Moore, RN, MSN, CEN (ENA Representative 2001-2002). *Annals of Emergency Medicine, 45*(2), February 2005.

Smith, S.C., Jr., Feldman, T.E., Hirshfeld, J.W., Jr.,

Jacobs, A.K., Kern, M.J., King, S.B. III, Williams, D.O. (2005). ACC/AHA/SCAI 2005 guideline update for percutaneous coronary intervention: a report of the American College of Cardiology/American Heart Association Task Force on Practice Guidelines (ACC/AHA/SCAI Writing Committee to Update the 2001 Guidelines for © 2005 by the American College of Cardiology Foundation and the American Heart Association, Inc. Percutaneous Coronary Intervention). American Heart Association Web Site. Available at: http://www.americanheart.org.

The Joint Commission National Patient Safety Goals Hospital Program. Retrieved from http://www.jointcommission.org/GeneralPublic/NPSG/10_npsgs.htm

SBAR Technique for Communication: A situational briefing model published by The Institute for Healthcare Improvement was downloaded on December 19, 2008, from http://www.ihi.org/IHI/Topics/PatientSafety/SafetyGeneral/Tools/SBARTechniqueforCommunicationASituationalBriefingModel

Summary of Practice Guidelines

Patients who present to the emergency department with chest pain should rapidly be evaluated for acute ischemia (Ryan & Reeder, 2008). The ED staff should consider the possibility of "atypical" chest pain that is not uncommon in women, diabetics, and the elderly (Ryan & Reeder, 2008). For initial assessment, which includes an ECG, the goal is completion within 10 min from presentation in the ED (Ryan & Reeder, 2008). Initial assessment would include assessment for the "ABCs," cardiac monitor attached, resuscitation equipment nearby, oxygen provided (to keep saturation above 90%), lab work obtained (electrolytes, PT/INR, PTT, cardiac markers, lipid profile), and IV started (Ryan & Reeder, 2008). Aspirin, nitrates, and morphin should also be provided if not contraindicated (Ryan & Reeder, 2008). Caution must exercised in using nitrates in the presence of hypotension or possible right ventricle involvement as it may cause severe hypotension (Ryan & Reeder, 2008). The 12-Lead ECG should be assessed by an experienced provider immediately (Ryan & Reeder, 2008). A focused history and physical exam is important in helping the clinician differentiate potential causes of the chest pain including noncardiac causes (pulmonary embolism, aortic dissection, tension pneumothorax, perforating peptic ulcer) (Ryan & Reeder, 2008). Description of the pain, including factors which aggravate or alleviate the pain are important (Ryan & Reeder, 2008). The patient should be questioned regarding any medications they may have taken for the pain. The patient should be asked if they have a history of similar symptoms, a history of cardiovascular disease, any history of risk factors for cardiovascular disease (atherosclerosis, hyperlipidemia, hypertension, smoking, diabetes mellitus, obesity, family history) (Ryan & Reeder, 2008). Additionally, contraindications for thrombolytic therapy should also be assessed (Ryan & Reeder, 2008).

The 12-lead ECG helps to determine the location of the ischemia. Thrombolytic therapy is an option (if not contraindicated) with elevated troponin levels and with persistent ST segment elevations (Ryan & Reeder, 2008).

Topics to Review Prior to the Simulation

- Cardiac catheterization
- Hemodynamic instability
- Chronic diabetic client
- Assessment techniques

SIMULATION

Client Background

Biographical Data

- Age: 52
- Gender: female
- Height: 5 ft 2 in
- Weight: 200 lb

Cultural Considerations

- Language: English
- Ethnicity: Irish heritage
- Nationality: American
- Culture: Roman Catholic, evaluate spiritual needs

Demographic

- Marital status: married
- Educational level: high school graduate
- Religion: Roman Catholic
- Occupation: school bus driver

Current Health Status

- Arrived at the ED via EMS 48 hr ago with vague cardiac symptoms of headache, nausea, a blood pressure of 210/100, sinus tachycardia in the 120s, and chest pain of 2/10, persisting until time of catheterization.

History

- Psychosocial history
  - Social support: husband and teenaged son, lives in own townhome, has work-related insurance.
  - No history of mental illness
- Past health history
  - Medical: obesity, hypertension, smoker (quit x 5 years, 20 ppd history), insulin-controlled diabetes mellitus (x 20 years), atherosclerosis, one child
  - Surgical: hysterectomy x 5 years, appendectomy x 10 years
- Family history
  - Mother deceased at 68 from MI
  - Father with stroke at 63, surviving

Admission Sheet

Name:	Agnes McCarthy
Age:	52
Gender:	Female
Marital Status:	Married
Educational Level:	High school graduate
Religion:	Roman Catholic
Ethnicity:	Irish
Nationality:	American
Language:	English
Occupation:	School bus driver

Hospital
Provider's Orders

Patient's Name: Agnes McCarthy
Allergies: NKDA

Diagnosis: Coronary Artery Disease

Date	Time	Order	Signature
	14:00 PM	Vital signs: vital signs and vascular checks initially on arrival to unit then q 15 min for 1 hr, then q 30 min for 2 hr, and then q 4 hr until stable	
		Diet: cardiac prudent, 2,000 calorie, encourage po fluids	
		Activity: bed rest with R leg immobilized x 6 hr	
		IV therapy: maintain IV intermittent infusion device(INT) flush q 8 hr with 2 cc NSS and cap	
		Medications: Lipitor (Atorvastatin) 10 mg po daily Metoprolol 25 mg po bid Metformin 500 mg po bid ON HOLD Aspart insulin 15 units subq with meals Lispro insulin 25 units subq q AM Warfarin sodium 2.5 mg q daily ON HOLD Nitroglycerin SL 0.3 mg q 5 min for 15 min prn for chest pain Morphine sulfate 4 mg IV q 4 hr prn chest pain, may repeat x 1	
		Diagnostic studies: Nonexercise stress test Echocardiogram ECG q AM Place on telemetry monitoring	
			Dr. Albright

SECONDARY ORDER SHEET

Hospital **Patient's Name:** Agnes McCarthy
Physician Orders **Allergies:** NKDA

Diagnosis: Coronary Artery Disease

Date	Time	Order	Signature
	15:57 PM	O_2 NRB at 15 Lpm	
		Diet: cardiac prudent, 2,000 calorie, encourage po fluids	
		Activity: bed rest with R leg immobilized x 6 hr	
		Blood therapy: transfuse 2 units fresh frozen plasma stat	
		IV therapy: NSS 1 L IV wide open stat	
		LABS: type and cross for 2 units PRBC stat PT/PTT/INR, CBC, Chem 7, ABG	
		Medications: Morphine 2 mg IV Dopamine 10/mcg/kg/min	
			Dr. Albright

Nursing Report

Given by Cath Lab RN to staff RN and student nurse: Agnes McCarthy, a 52-year-old female with a history of obesity, hypertension, a 20-ppd history of smoking (quit x 5 years), insulin-controlled diabetes mellitus (20 years), atherosclerosis, gravida 1, para 1, a surgical history of hysterectomy (5 years ago), appendectomy (10 years ago) arrived at the ED via EMS 48 hr ago with vague cardiac symptoms of headache, nausea, a blood pressure of 210/100, sinus tachycardia in the 120s, and chest pain of 2/10, persisting until time of cath. ECG and cardiac enzymes ruled out for MI. Pain and HTN resolved by IV nitroglycerin, morphine, and heparin drips (due to patient's medication history of warfarin sodium use, which was held on arrival at ED). FFP administered prior to cardiac cath. All drips were DC'd prior to cardiac catheterization, at which time all symptoms were also resolved. Conscious sedation with IV Versed and Fentanyl. Cath shows mild narrowing of coronary arteries that will be treated by medication. Cath via right femoral artery. Catheter withdrawn at 1400. Fem-stop device removed at 1500 with scant oozing of blood and a pressure dressing and sandbag applied. All pulses equal, bilaterally and a "2/3." No hematoma. No pain at site. Decreased bilateral LE sensation. Patient states this is due to chronic diabetic neuropathy. #22 IV INT in right arm. Orders are for cardiac-prudent diet. Foley in place, 90 cc out during cath, clear amber. Precath vital signs: temp 36.8°C, HR NSR 78, BP 132/68, resp 21, pulse ox 99% on 2 L via nasal cannula. Postcath vital signs: temp 37°C, HR NSR 92, BP148/70, esp 24, pulse ox 99% on 2 L via nasal cannula.

Student Simulation Prep Assignments

1. Identify items and their purpose in the care of a postcardiac catheterization patient.

Item	Purpose
Standard assessment equipment: stethoscope, penlight, watch	
Blood pressure sphygmomanometer, manual and electronic	

Continued

Item	Purpose
Cardiac monitor (if available)	
Pulse ox monitor	
IV and blood tubing and equipment and products, IV pump	
Simulated morphine	
Simulated dopamine	
IV insertion and blood-drawing devices and kits	
Blood glucose fingerstick measuring devices	
Indwelling bladder catheterization	
Sterile and clean gloves	
Materials for a pressure dressing and sandbag	
O_2 nasal canual and face mask	

2. Identify team members and their specific roles in the care of a patient with postcardiac catheterization complications.

Team Member	Role
Cardiac catheterization lab RN	
Cardiac catheterization lab MD	
Postcatheterization unit RN	
Postcatheterization unit (House Officer) MD	
Nursing student	
Unlicensed nursing care assistant (UAP)	
Family members	
Social worker or pastoral care	

3. Relevant Data Assignment: Fill in columns below.

Relevant Data from Report	Relevant Data from Other Sources	Data Missing	Sources for Missing Data	Data Requiring Follow-Up

Relevant Data from Report	Relevant Data from Other Sources	Data Missing	Sources for Missing Data	Data Requiring Follow-Up

4. *Initial Focused Assessment*

After reviewing the client background and nursing report, you are ready to assess your client's current status. Under each category, identify how you would target your assessment, and what you would expect to find for the patient postcardiac catheterization complications.

History

Are there any questions you need to ask the patient or family to obtain additional relevant data?

Physical Exam

- General appearance:
- Integumentary:
- HEENT:
- Respiratory:
- CV:
- Breasts:
- Abdominal:
- Neuro:
- Musculoskeletal:
- Reproductive:
- Additional:
  - GU:
  - Psychosocial:
- Developmental:

What are the nursing implications considering the developmental stage of your patient?

Answer:

5. *Diagnostic Tests*

What diagnostic test results relevant to the patient's current problem are needed to plan care?

Complete the table using Van Leeuwen et al, *Davis's Comprehensive Handbook of Laboratory and Diagnostic Testing with Nursing Implications* 4e, or other diagnostic test reference.

Diagnostic Test	Significance To This Patient's Problem
CBC	
Basic chemistry	
PT/PTT/INR	
ECG	

6. *Treatment*

Identify drugs that are used to treat a patient with postcardiac catheterization complications.

Complete the table using Deglin et al, *Davis's Drug Guide for Nurses* 12e, or other drug reference.

Medication	Drug, Dose, Frequency	Indications	Side Effect	Nsg Implications
Lipitor (Atorvastatin)	10 mg po daily			

Medication	Drug, Dose, Frequency	Indications	Side Effect	Nsg Implications
Metoprolol	25 mg po bid			
Metformin	500 mg po bid			
Aspart insulin	15 units subq with meals			
Lispro insulin	25 units subq q AM			
Warfarin sodium	2.5 mg q daily			
Nitroglycerin SL	0.3 mg q 5 min for 15 min prn for chest pain			
Morphine sulfate	4 mg IV 2 mg IV			
Dopamine				

7. Nursing Problems/Diagnoses

Identify three priority nursing problems/diagnoses.

Assessment Data	Priority Problem	Intervention	Expected Patient Outcome	Which Intervention Could Be Delegated to Unlicensed Personnel?
1.				

Continued

Assessment Data	Priority Problem	Intervention	Expected Patient Outcome	Which Intervention Could Be Delegated to Unlicensed Personnel?
2.				
3.				

References

Arthur, H. (2003). *Final Report: Reducing anxiety in patients awaiting elective cardiac catheterization*. The Heart and Stroke Foundation (Ontario) and The Canadian Nurses Foundation. Retrieved July 24, 2007 from http://www.canadiannursesfoundation.com/documents/ArthurNov2003reportEng.pdf

Balasubramanian, V. P. (2007). Cullen's sign. *Resident & Staff Physician*, 53(2), 10.

Blank-Reid, C. (2004). Abdominal trauma: Dealing with the damage. *Nursing 2004*, *34*(9), 36-41

Deglin, J. H., & Vallerand, A. H. (2009). *Davis's drug guide for nurses* (11th ed.). Philadelphia: F. A. Davis.

Dillon, P. (2007). *Nursing health assessment: A critical thinking and case studies approach* (2nd ed.). Philadelphia: F. A. Davis.

Emergency Nurses Association (2005). Emergency Nurses Association position statement: Family presence at the bedside during invasive procedures and cardiopulmonary resuscitation. Retrieved July 23, 2007 from www.ena.org/about/position/PDFs/4E6C256B26994E319F66C65748BFBDBF.pdf

Erikson, E. H. (1950). *Childhood and society*. New York: Norton.

Ernits, M., Mohan, P. S., Fares, L. G., & Hardy, H. (2005). A retroperitoneal bleed induced by enoxaparin therapy. *American Surgeon*, *71*(5), 430-433.

Gilmartin, K. (2006). Gaining access: Arterial intervention techniques and special patient needs. *Cath Lab Digest*, *14*(3), 12-14.

Ignatavicius, D., & Workman, L. D. (2006). *Medical-surgical nursing: Critical thinking for collaborative care* (5th ed.) (p. 698). St. Louis: Elsevier Saunders.

Lagerquist, S. L. (2006). *Davis's NCLEX-RN success* (2nd ed). Philadelphia: F. A. Davis.

Ryan, T. J. & Reeder, G. S., (2008). *Management of suspected acute coronary syndrome in the emergency department.* Retrieved from www.uptodate.com/online/content/topic.do?topickey=ad_emer/2821&selectedTitle=3150&source=search_result.

Tang, T., Lee, J., & Dickinson, R. (2003). Retroperitoneal haemorrhage during warfarin therapy. *Journal of the Royal Society of Medicine*, *96*(6), 294-295.

Van Leeuwen, A. M., Poelhuis-Leth, D. J., & Bladh, M. L. (2011). *Davis's comprehensive handbook of laboratory and diagnostic tests with nursing implications* (4th ed.). Philadelphia: F. A. Davis.

5-9 Atypical Chest Pain

MEDICAL-SURGICAL

STANDARD FORMS

These templates are included in the Appendix; copy before each use.

LEARNING OUTCOMES

Cognitive

The student will be able to:

1. Describe signs and symptoms of typical and atypical chest pain.
2. Correlate signs and symptoms of angina to the pathophysiology of cardiac ischemia.
3. Identify factors in a patient's history that increase risk for angina and myocardial infarction.
4. Identify factors in a patient's current condition that increase risk for myocardial infarction.
5. Identify the appropriate interventions for the patient with angina and myocardial infarction.
6. Differentiate the roles of team members in response to a patient with angina and myocardial infarction.

Psychomotor

The student will be able to:

1. Perform appropriate assessment and establish a treatment plan for a patient with chest pain.
2. Initiate appropriate interventions including diagnostics such as a 12-lead ECG, electrolytes, troponin I and CPK levels.
3. Initiate appropriate medical interventions including establishing an IV, application of oxygen, nitroglycerin, morphine, aspirin for a patient with suspected myocardial infarction.
4. Work collaboratively as part of the healthcare team (secondary RN, respiratory therapist, physician) in the care of a patient with chest pain.

Affective

The student will be able to:

1. Reflect upon performance in the care of a patient with suspected myocardial infarction.
2. Identify own feelings in delivering care to a patient with suspected myocardial infarction.
3. Discuss feelings related to working as a member of a team in the care of a patient with for a patient with suspected myocardial infarction.
4. Identify factors that worked well during the simulation.
5. Identify factors that needed improvement during the simulation.
6. Develop self-confidence in the care of a patient with chest pain.

Communication

The student will be able to:

1. Communicate effectively with healthcare team members.
2. Communicate effectively with the patient and family regarding signs, symptoms, and treatment of myocardial infarction.
3. Use SBAR when communication with team members.
4. Work in collaboration as part of the healthcare team.
5. Practice Transparent Thinking (thinking out loud) to facilitate group problem solving.
6. Use Directed Communication (directing a message to specific individual) when delegating tasks.
7. Employ Closed-Loop Communication (acknowledgment of receipt of the message and status) to acknowledge communications from others.

Safety

The student will be able to:

Administer and maintain specific protecting interventions with attention to safety of the client and healthcare professional.

1. Demonstrate a safe environment with attention to hazards to healthcare providers, visitors, and the client. Includes body mechanics, tripping hazards, and equipment issues.
2. Demonstrate attention to national patient safety goals. Includes patient identification standards, effective communication among healthcare providers, and safe medication administration.
3. Demonstrate attention to standard precautions. Includes hand washing, infection control measures, and use of personal protective equipment (PPE) as needed.

Leadership and Management/Delegation

The student will be able to:

1. Identify tasks that can be legally, ethically, and safely delegated to unlicensed assistive personnel (UAP) or licensed practical nurse (LPN) in the care of a patient with myocardial infarction.
2. Identify and prioritize patient's needs in care of a patient with myocardial infarction.

Pharmacology

The student will be able to:

1. Identify the indications for drugs used in the treatment of a patient with myocardial infarction.
2. Identify adverse reactions or contraindications for drugs in this scenario.

OVERVIEW OF PROBLEM

Angina

Definition

Angina pectoris is classified as stable (follows an event with the same amount of severity), unstable (at rest or with minimal exertion, recent onset, increasing severity), or Prinzmetal's variant (at rest and caused by coronary artery spasm).

Pathophysiology

The pain is caused by insufficient blood flow to the cardiac muscle through the coronary arteries. This imbalance causes myocardial ischemia. The ischemia can progress to infarction if the blood flow is not reestablished. Coronary occlusion can occur as a result of a thrombus, an embolism, or a hemorrhage in the adjacent atherosclerotic plaque.

Risk factors

- Age (35–70 years)
- Men and women after menopause
- High cholesterol, low-density lipoproteins, high serum triglycerides
- Cardiovascular
  - Atherosclerosis
  - Thromboangiitis obliterans
  - Aortic regurgitation
- Hypertension
- Hormonal
  - Hypothyroidism
  - Diabetes
- Blood disorders
  - Anemia
  - Polycythemia vera
- Lifestyle factors
  - Smoking
  - Obesity
  - Cocaine use
  - Inactivity
  - Stress
  - Diet

Assessment

Subjective

- Pain
  - Type: squeezing, burning, pressing
  - Location retrosternal region, substernal, or left of the sternum and possibly radiating to the left arm.
  - Duration usually 3–5 min; less than 30 min
  - Cause emotional stress, overeating, physical exertion, exposure to cold; may occur at rest
  - Relief: rest or nitroglycerin

Note: Atypical chest pain symptoms in women are described as jaw or upper back pain or persistent gastric upset. In contrast to angina, the pain of an MI is severe, sudden, crushing, heaviness, or tightness. These signs, however, may be absent in those who are elderly, female, or diabetic. The duration of MI pain is >30 min and is not relieved with nitroglycerin or rest. SOB, nausea, apprehension, and a fear of impending death may also accompany MI chest pain. Signs of shock may be evident (tachycardia, hypotension, S_3 gallop, tachypnea, shallow respiration, elevated temperature, cold and clammy skin, restlessness)

- Dyspnea
- Palpitations
- Dizziness, faintness
- Epigastric distress, indigestion, belching

Objective

- Diaphoresis
- Tachycardia
- Pallor
- ECG changes during attack

Diagnostic Tests

- Lab data: elevated troponin levels, CKMB, myoglobin
- ECG: may indicate ST elevation, ST depression, new-onset Q waves
- Blood gases may indicate acidosis
- Electrolytes: decreased potassium; magnesium may cause arrhythmias
- Cardiac catheterization and possibly percutaneous coronary intervention
- Pulmonary artery catheter to trend levels and note changes with heart failure

Treatment

- Narcotics
- Oxygen
- Nitroglycerin or amyl nitrate
- Beta-adrenergic blockers
- Antiarrythmics
- IV fluids
- Thrombolytic agents as appropriate.

Nursing Management

Goals

- Reduce pain and provide rest
- Identify and avoid precipitating factors.
- Maintain adequate circulation. Decrease oxygen demand by providing oxygen and maintaining bed rest
- Monitor for response to treatments by assessing vital signs
- Promote safety: Assist with ambulation
- Provide emotional support
  - Encourage verbalization of feelings
  - Provide reassurance
  - Promote positive self-concept
  - Promote acceptance of limitations
- Health teaching
  - Pain: Identify precipitating factors, alleviation, differentiation from MI

- Medication regimen
- Diet
- Diagnostic tests
- Rest and activity
- Prepare for surgery if indicated
- Behavior modification to assist with lifestyle change

Evaluation/Outcome Criteria

- Pain relieved
- Fewer attacks
- No MI
- Alters lifestyle and complies with modifications
- No smoking

REVIEW QUESTIONS

1. Compare and contrast stable angina and unstable angina including its presentation and treatment.
   Answer:

2. Compare and contrast the symptoms of right- and left-sided heart failure.
   Answer:

3. Explain the importance of cardiac markers (troponin I, CKMB, myoglobin) in evaluating a patient's chest pain.
   Answer:

4. Name five risk factors for acute coronary syndrome.
   Answer:

5. Describe classic and "atypical" chest pain presentations and which patients usually present with "atypical" pain.
   Answer:

Related Evidence-Based Practice Guidelines

http://www.guideline.gov Acute Coronary Syndrome

The Joint Commission National Patient Safety Goals Hospital Program. Retrieved from http://www.jointcommission.org/GeneralPublic/NPSG/10_npsgs.htm

SBAR Technique for Communication: A situational briefing model published by The Institute for Healthcare Improvement was downloaded on December 19, 2008, from http://www.ihi.org/IHI/Topics/PatientSafety/SafetyGeneral/Tools/SBARTechniqueforCommunicationASituationalBriefingModel.htm

Summary of Practice Guidelines

Patients who present to the emergency department with chest pain should rapidly be evaluated for acute ischemia. The ED staff should consider the possibility of "atypical" chest pain that is not uncommon in women, diabetics, and the elderly. For initial assessment, which includes an ECG, the goal is completion within 10 min from presentation in the ED. Initial assessment would include assessment of the "ABCs," cardiac monitor attached, resuscitation equipment nearby, oxygen provided (to keep saturation above 90%), lab work obtained (electrolytes, PT/INR, PTT, cardiac markers, lipid profile), and IV started. Aspirin, nitrates, and morphine should also be provided if not contraindicated. Caution must exercised in using nitrates in the presence of hypotension or possible right ventricle involvement as it may cause severe hypotension. The 12-lead ECG should be assessed by an experienced provider immediately. A focused history and physical exam is important in helping the clinician differentiate potential causes of the chest pain including noncardiac causes (pulmonary embolism, aortic dissection, tension pneumothorax, perforating peptic ulcer). Description of the pain, including factors which aggravate or alleviate the pain are important. The patient should be questioned regarding any medications they may have taken for the pain. The patient should be asked if they have a history of similar symptoms, a history of cardiovascular disease, any history of risk factors for cardiovascular disease (atherosclerosis, hyperlipidemia, hypertension, smoking, diabetes mellitus, obesity, family history). Additionally, contraindications for thrombolytic therapy should also be assessed.

The 12-lead ECG helps to determine the location of the ischemia. Thrombolytic therapy is an option (if not contraindicated) with elevated troponin levels and with persistent ST segment elevations (Ryan & Reeder, 2008).

Topics to Review Prior to the Simulation

- Cardiac history and physical examination.
- Signs and symptoms of right-sided heart failure vs left-sided heart failure.
- Abnormal heart sounds.
- Cardiac enzymes and markers (troponin I, CKMB, myoglobin) and their value in assessing cardiac damage.

- Echocardiogram, cardiac catheterization and angiography —use in diagnostics with patients with ACS.
- 12-lead ECG and what you need to know when your patient is experiencing ACS.
- Pathophysiology of ACS, etiology, signs and symptoms, diagnostic study findings, goals of care and management of the patient.

SIMULATION

Client Background

Biographical Data

- Age: 68
- Gender: female
- Height: 5 ft 2 in
- Weight: 170 lb

Cultural Considerations

- Language: English
- Ethnicity: Northern European heritage
- Nationality: American
- Culture: no significant cultural considerations identified

Demographic

- Marital status: widowed
- Educational level: college
- Religion: Catholic
- Occupation: retired elementary school teacher

Current Health Status

- Awoke this morning at 0615 diaphoretic, very weak, and with neck pain (up the left side of the neck and into her jaw). Decided she just had a "flu bug," but has gotten progressively worse this morning. She has had this problem before but never this bad. Her breathing and the pain gets worse with walking and a little better when she rests. She has not taken any medication for it since she states she "doesn't like to take too many medicines."

History

- Psychosocial history
  - Social support: has one daughter who lives in town
  - No ETOH
  - Stopped smoking 10 years ago.
- Past health history
  - Medical: type 2 diabetes for 10 years, takes Metformin and Glyburide, HTN—takes HCTZ 50 mg a day.and Lasix 40 mg daily.
  - She had an echocardiogram about 5 years ago that showed an ejection fraction of 60%.
  - Surgical: hysterectomy 25 years ago, laser eye surgery 2 years ago.
- Family history: mother deceased from stroke, father deceased from MI.

Admission Sheet

Name:	Carmela Smythe
Age:	68
Gender:	Female
Marital Status:	Widowed
Educational Level:	College
Religion:	Catholic
Ethnicity:	Northern European heritage
Nationality:	American
Language:	English
Occupation:	Retired high school english teacher

Hospital
Provider Orders

Patient's Name: **Carmela Smythe**
Allergies: **Duracef**

Diagnosis: **Chest pain**

Date	Time	Order	Signature
	1230	Vital signs: q 30 min, bedside monitor	
		Diet: NPO	
		Activity: Bed rest	
		IV therapy: NSS at 100 mL/hr	
		Medications: Aspirin 325 mg po x 1 Morphine sulfate 2 mg IV q 5 min prn for pain	
*		Nitroglycerin 0.4 mcg SL x 3 for chest pain q 5 min if systolic BP <90	
		Diagnostic studies: STAT 12-lead ECG, BMP, CBC, troponin, CK, myoglobin, PT/INR, PTT, Hgb A1C, CXR	
		Treatments: Titrate O_2 to keep sats > 92%	
		Call orders: HR <60 >140, SBP <90 >160, RR <10 >30, O_2 sat < 92%, temp > 101.5°F, blood glucose <60 >120, pain uncontrolled with morphine, changes in LOC: concerns please call	
			Dr. M. Kendall

Nursing Report

Report from the triage nurse:

Mrs. Smythe has arrived with her daughter at the ER. She states that she is feeling "very low." She awakened at 0615 diaphoretic, extremely weak, and with a painful neck and jaw –7/10. She has had this happen before but this is the worst it has ever been. She thinks she may have hurt her neck yesterday as she has been trying to pack up her house to move into a smaller apartment. It gets worse with ambulation and a little better with rest. She called her daughter, who came immediately and noted that she appeared "gray," and decided that her mother's situation was serious enough to bring her to the ER. She has just had a chest x-ray taken and has been brought into room 3 in the ER. You have some initial orders that have not been completed. VS in triage: HR 70, BP 110/60, RR 28, O_2 sat 90% on RA.

History: DM controlled with Metformin and Glyburide; HTN for which she takes Lasix 40 mg daily and HCTZ 50 mg a day. Her blood pressures at home are usually in the 120s.

Student Simulation Prep Assignments

1. Identify items and their purpose in the care of a patient with MI.

Item	Purpose
IV with pump	
O_2 via nasal cannula	

Item	Purpose
Monitor	
12-lead ECG	
Specimen tubes	

2. Identify team members and their specific roles in the care of a patient with MI.

Team Member	Role
Primary nurse	
Secondary nurse	
RT	
Physician	

3. Relevant Data Exercise: Fill in columns below.

Relevant Data from Report	Relevant Data from Other Sources	Data Missing	Sources for Missing Data	Data Requiring Follow-Up

4. Initial Focused Assessment

After reviewing the client background and nursing report, you are ready to assess your client's current status. Under each category, identify how you would target your assessment and what you would expect to find for the patient with MI.

History

Are there any questions you need to ask the patient or family to obtain additional relevant data?

Physical Exam

- General appearance:
- Integumentary:
- HEENT:
- Respiratory:
- CV:
- Breasts:
- Abdominal:
- Neuro:
- Musculoskeletal:
- Reproductive:
- Additional:
- Developmental:

What are the nursing implications considering the developments stages of your patients.

Answer:

5. *Diagnostic Tests*

What diagnostic test results relevant to the patient's current problem are needed to plan care?

Complete the table using Van Leeuwen et al, *Davis's Comprehensive Handbook of Laboratory and Diagnostic Testing with Nursing Implications* 4e, or other diagnostic test reference.

Diagnostic Test	Significance to This Patient's Problem
12-lead ECG	
BMP	
CBC	
Cardiac enzymes and troponin	
PT/INR	
PTT	
Hgb A_{1C}	
CXR	

6. *Treatment*

Identify drugs that are used to treat a patient with MI.

Complete the table using Deglin et al, *Davis's Drug Guide for Nurses* 12e, or other drug reference.

Medication	Dose, Route, Frequency	Indications	Side Effect	Nursing Implications
Morphine	2 mg IVP q 5–30 min			
Nitroglycerin	0.4-mg tablets sublingual/ sublingual spray			
Aspirin	Chew 325 mg po once			

Medication	Dose, Route, Frequency	Indications	Side Effect	Nursing Implications
Normal saline 1-L bags (0.9% NaCl)	IV infusion at 100 mL/hr			
TNKase (tenecteplase recombinant)	45 mg IVP over 5 sec once			

7. Nursing Problems/Diagnoses

Identify three priority nursing problems/diagnoses.

Assessment Data	Priority Problem	Intervention	Expected Patient Outcome	Which Interventions Could Be Delegated to Unlicensed Personnel?
1.				
2.				
3.				

References

Deglin, J. H., & Vallerand, A. H. (2003). *Davis's drug guide for nurses*. Philadelphia: F. A. Davis.

Dillon, P. (2007). *Nursing health assessment: A critical thinking and case studies approach* (2nd ed.). Philadelphia: F. A. Davis.

Erikson, E. H. (1950). *Childhood and society*. New York: Norton.

Lagerquist, S. L. (2006). *Davis's NCLEX-RN success* (2nd ed.). Philadelphia: F. A. Davis.

Meisel, J. (2008). Differential diagnosis of chest pain in adults. Retrieved June 21, 2008 from http://www.uptodate.com

Ryan, T., & Reeder, G. (2008). Management of suspected acute coronary syndrome in the emergency department. Retrieved June 21, 2008 from http://www.uptodate.com

Van Leeuwen, A. M., Poelhuis-Leth, D.J., & Bladh, M.L. (2011). *Davis's comprehensive handbook of laboratory and diagnostic tests with nursing implications.* (4th ed.). Philadelphia: F. A. Davis.

5-10 Subdural Hematoma/Alcohol Withdrawal

ADULT HEALTH

STANDARD FORMS

These templates are included in the Appendix; copy before each use.

LEARNING OUTCOMES

Cognitive

The student will be able to:

1. Describe signs and symptoms of chronic subdural hematoma and alcohol withdrawal.
2. Correlate signs and symptoms of a chronic subdural hematoma and alcohol withdrawal to the pathophysiology of these processes.
3. Identify factors in a patient's current condition that increase risk for chronic subdural hematoma.
4. Identify the appropriate interventions for the patient with alcohol withdrawal.
5. Differentiate the roles of team members in response to a patient with alcohol withdrawal.

Psychomotor

The student will be able to:

1. Perform appropriate assessment and establish a treatment plan for a patient with a subdural hematoma and alcohol withdrawal.
2. Initiate appropriate interventions including frequent monitoring, reorientation, intiate seizure precautions, protecting the patient from self-harm, providing a calming atmosphere, establishing an IV, and providing sedation.
3. Work collaboratively as part of the healthcare team (secondary RN, respiratory therapist, physician) in the care of a patient with alcohol withdrawal.

Affective

The student will be able to:

1. Reflect upon performance in the care of a patient with alcohol withdrawal.
2. Identify own feelings in delivering care to a patient with alcohol withdrawal.
3. Discuss feelings related to working as a member of a team in the care of a patient with for a patient with alcohol withdrawal.
4. Identify factors that worked well during the simulation.
5. Identify factors that needed improvement during the simulation.
6. Develop self-confidence in the care of a patient with chest pain.

Communication

The student will be able to:

1. Communicate effectively with healthcare team members.
2. Communicate effectively with the patient and family regarding signs, symptoms, and treatment of alcohol withdrawal.
3. Use SBAR when communication with team members.
4. Work in collaboration as part of the healthcare team.
5. Understand the importance of maintaining patient confidentiality and measures that attempt to do so.
6. Practice Transparent Thinking (thinking out loud) to facilitate group problem solving.
7. Use Directed Communication (directing a message to specific individual) when delegating tasks.
8. Employ-Closed Loop Communication (acknowledgment of receipt of the message and status) to acknowledge communications from others.

Safety

The student will be able to:

Administer and maintain specific protecting interventions with attention to safety of the client and healthcare professional

1. Demonstrate a safe environment with attention to hazards to healthcare providers, visitors, and the client. Includes body mechanics, tripping hazards, and equipment issues.
2. Demonstrate attention to national patient safety goals. Includes patient identification standards, effective communication among healthcare providers, and safe medication administration.
3. Demonstrate attention to standard precautions. Includes hand washing, infection control measures, and use of personal protective equipment (PPE) as needed.

Leadership and Management/Delegation

The student will be able to:

1. Identify tasks that can be legally, ethically, and safely delegated to unlicensed assistive personnel (UAP) or licensed practical nurse (LPN) in the care of a patient with patient with alcohol withdrawal.
2. Identify and prioritize patient's needs in care of a patient with alcohol withdrawal.

Pharmacology

The student will be able to:

1. Identify the indications for drugs used in the treatment of a patient with alcohol withdrawal.
2. Identify adverse reactions or contraindications for drugs used in the treatment of a patient with alcohol withdrawal.

OVERVIEW OF PROBLEM

Subdural Hematoma

Definition

A subdural hematoma is considered a secondary trauma in response to a primary traumatic brain injury (a concussion, contusion, laceration, or fracture). Blood accumulates between the arachnoid and dura from a ruptured or torn vein. These collections can be acute, subacute, or chronic.

Pathophysiology

The mechanism for the primary injury can be a deformation (blow to head), acceleration-deceleration, or rotational injury.

As a result of the accumulation of blood, CNS functioning can be affected. A depressed level of consciousness is a result of depressed neuronal activity in the reticular activating system. When the lower brain stem and spinal cord are depressed, this can result in reduction of reflex activity, unequal pupils, reduced pupilary response to light, and possibly fixed and dilated pupils.

Risk Factors

Risk factors for traumatic brain injury include accidents such as automobile, industrial, or home accidents and motorcycle accidents. The risk for accidents increases when substance abuse or intoxication is a factor as coordination is impaired, the client can become disoriented, and judgment is altered.

Assessment

Subjective

- Headache
- Dizziness
- Loss of balance
- Double vision
- Nausea

Objective

- Lacerations or abrasions may be noted around face or head
- Drainage from ears or nose
- Projectile vomiting or hematemesis
- Vital sign changes with increased intracranial pressure (Cushing's triad)
- Altered level of consciousness
- Pupils may be unequal, dilated, or unresponsive to light
- Paresis or paralysis may be evident in extremities
- Hypotonia or hypertonia evident in reflexes

Diagnostic Tests

CT scan will show evidence of subdural hematoma and any resulting shifting of intracranial contents. A subdural hematoma will appear crescent shaped on CT scan. Skull and spinal radiographs would be completed initially to rule out any additional injury.

Treatment

Craniotomy may be indicated to evacuate hematomas or control hemorrhage.

Nursing Management

Goal: Maintain vital functions and prevent or minimize complications

- Maintain a patent airway
- Oxygen to prevent hypoxia and an exacerbation of cerebral edema
- Position prone or semiprone with head of bed elevated to prevent aspiration
- Vital signs as ordered to detect changes in baseline
- Neurological checks to detect changes in baseline
  - Seizure precautions
  - Medications as ordered might include:
    - Steroids
    - Anticonvulsants
    - Analgesics (morphine contraindicated)
    - Cooling measures if elevated temperature
    - Assist with diagnostic tests
  - Diet: NPO, progress as tolerated
  - Fluids: IV therapy, NG tube feedings, intake and output
  - Monitor blood work

Goal: Provide emotional support and comfort measures

- Skin care, oral hygiene, wrinkle-free linen
- Eye care
- ROM
- Avoid restraints
- Encourage verbalization and family communication

Evaluation/Outcome Criteria

- Alert and oriented
- No signs of increased ICP
- No paralysis
- Resumes self-care

Alcohol Dependence

Definition

Alcohol dependence is a primary and chronic disorder that is progressive and often fatal in which the individual is unable, for physical or psychological reasons or both, to refrain from frequent consumption of alcohol in quantities that produce intoxication and disrupt health and ability to perform daily functions.

Pathophysiology

Alcohol affects memory, judgment, and reasoning. It is a depressant that relaxes, lessens repression and inhibition, and releases hostility and primitive drives. Alcohol dependence is a disease and not a symptom. Often fear and anxiety motivate the alcoholic to drink. The spouse of the alcoholic can function as a codependent or coalcoholic and can contribute to the drinking behavior.

Signs of intoxication (blood alcohol level >0.08%) include incoordination, slurred speech, and dulled perception. Tolerance occurs with chronic drinking where larger amounts of alcohol must be consumed to obtain the desired effect.

All patients need a careful history and physical exam if there is any suspicion of chronic alcohol consumption and a risk for alcohol withdrawal. Any history of seizures or delirium tremens should be noted. Medications should be given based on the patient's tolerance of the withdrawal syndrome. Different dosing schedules can be used including a fixed schedule despite the absence of symptoms (may be required if the patient is at high risk for major withdrawal symptoms such as seizures) or a schedule based on symptom assessment or also called "symptom-triggered treatment". An alcohol assessment tool such as the Clinical Institute Withdrawal Assessment for Alcohol Scale is recommended for evaluating the patient's symptoms (nausea and vomiting, tremors, diaphoresis, auditory disturbance, agitation, anxiety, etc.). Patients require close monitoring to assess for tolerance, need for additional medication, aspiration risk, and respiratory compromise (Weinhouse, 2008).

Assessment

Complications of abuse include alcohol withdrawal delirium, or delirium tremens (DTs). This syndrome develops as a result of nutritional deficiencies and toxins.

Early signs of alcohol withdrawal include:

- Restlessness
- Irritability
- Tremors of hands and feet
- Increased BP
- Tachycardia
- Diaphoresis
- Dysrhythmias
- Nausea, vomiting, and anorexia

Actual signs of delirium tremens include:

- Confusion
- Hallucinations
- Seizures
- Death is possible if left untreated as a result of cardiac dysrhythmias, respiratory arrest, dehydration or infection

Diagnostic Tests

- Blood alcohol level
- CBC
- Glucose
- Electrolytes
- Liver function tests
- Nutritional tests
- Urinalysis
- CXR
- ECG
- Other screening tests dependent on condition (hepatitis, HIV, TB)

Treatment

- Sedation and anxiety control
- Anticonvulsants to prevent seizures
- Control of nausea and vomiting
- Assess vital signs to note change from baseline and treat appropriately
- Proper nutrition and supplements
- Promote client safety

Nursing Management

Detoxification phase:

- Administer sedation and anticonvulsants as ordered
- Control nausea and vomiting
- Assess for complications
- Promote client safety

Recovery phase:

- Refer to community resources for follow-up
- Provide health teaching

Evaluation/Outcome Criteria

- No complications
- Living patterns restructured without alcohol use
- Demonstrates feelings of self-worth, confidence, and resilience

REVIEW QUESTIONS

1. Define the difference between acute, subacute, and chronic subdural hematomas (SDHs).
   Answer:

2. Describe the Monroe-Kellie hypothesis.
   Answer:

3. List five early signs of alcohol withdrawal.
   Answer:

4. Describe alcohol delirium/delirium tremens.
   Answer:

5. Describe pharmacological and nonpharmacological treatment of alcohol withdrawal.
   Answer:

Related Evidence-Based Practice Guidelines

National Guideline Clearing House—Alcohol Withdrawal http://www.guideline.gov/browse/browsecondition.aspx

Management of alcohol withdrawal delirium. An evidence-based practice guideline. American Society of Addiction

Medicine—Medical Specialty Society, 2004 Jul 12. 8 pages. NGC:004109

EFNS guideline on the diagnosis and management of alcohol-related seizures: Report of an EFNS task force. European Federation of Neurological Societies—Medical Specialty Society, 2005. 30 pages. NGC:005164

The Joint Commission National Patient Safety Goals Hospital Program. Retrieved from http://www.jointcommission.org/GeneralPublic/NPSG/10_npsgs.htm

SBAR Technique for Communication: A situational briefing model published by The Institute for Healthcare Improvement was downloaded on December 19, 2008, from http://www.ihi.org/IHI/Topics/PatientSafety/SafetyGeneral/Tools/SBARTechniqueforCommunicationASituationalBriefingModel.htm

Topics to Review Prior to the Simulation

- Pathophysiology of subdural hematoma, etiology, signs and symptoms, diagnostic study findings, goals of care, and management of the patient
- Pathophysiology of alcohol withdrawal, etiology, signs and symptoms, diagnostic study findings, goals of care, and management of the patient
- Pharmacology of labetolol, clonidine, lorazepam

SIMULATION

Client Background

Biographical Data

- Age: 75
- Gender: female
- Height: 5 ft 5 in
- Weight: 110 lb

Cultural Considerations

- Language: English
- Ethnicity: European heritage
- Nationality: American
- Culture: no significant cultural considerations identified

Demographic

- Marital status: married
- Educational level: college
- Religion: Presbyterian
- Occupation: philanthropist

Current Health Status

- She was admitted 2 days ago after being difficult to arouse from a nap. A CT scan revealed a chronic subdural hematoma. The follow-up CT scan this morning showed some improvement. Patient recalled falling and hitting head on coffee table over 2 weeks prior. She has some old ecchymoses to her right temporal region from the fall over 2 weeks ago.

History

- Psychosocial history
  - Social support: lives with husband/daughter
  - States social drinker only
  - Smokes 2 ppd
- Past health history
  - Patient states she is "perfectly healthy"
  - Has not been to PCP in over 10 years
- Family history
  - Mother deceased from liver failure
  - Father deceased from lung cancer

Admission Sheet

Name:	Theodora Phillips
Age:	75
Gender:	Female
Marital Status:	Married
Educational Level:	College
Religion:	Presbyterian
Ethnicity:	European heritage
Nationality:	American
Language:	English
Occupation:	Philanthropist

Hospital Provider's Orders		Patient's Name: Theodora Phillips Allergies: None	
Diagnosis: Subdural hematoma, ETOH withdrawal			
Date	**Time**	**Order**	**Signature**
	1230	Vital signs: q 4 hr, telemetry.	
		Diet: Mechanical soft diet	
		Activity: Up with assistance, chair bid	
		IV therapy: Saline lock, flush with 3 cc N/S q 8 hr	
		Medications: Multivitamin tablet po Magnesium 4 g IV in 250 mL D5W infused over 1 hr Labetolol 10 mg IV q 10 min over 2 min prn SBP >140 Nicotine patch 21 mg apply daily and remove old patch Dimenhydrinate 50 mg IV push q 6 hr prn nausea Acetaminophen 650 mg po q 4 hr prn pain	
		Diagnostic studies: BMP, CBC, INR, PTT daily	
		Treatments: Titrate O_2 to keep sats >92%	
		Call orders: HR <60 >120, SBP <90 >200, RR <10 >30, O_2 sat <92%, temp >101.5°F Blood glucose <60 >120, changes in LOC, or concerns please call	
			Dr. M. Kendall @ 555-1234

Nursing Report

Report from the night shift nurse:

Mrs. Theodora Phillips is a 75-year-old female. She and her husband are well known in the local community as philanthropists. The local media have been calling the hospital for updates on the situation. We are not to provide any information regarding her situation.

She was admitted 2 days ago after being difficult to arouse from a nap. A CT scan revealed a chronic subdural hematoma. The follow-up CT scan this morning showed some improvement. Patient recalled falling and hitting head on coffee table over 2 weeks prior. She has some old ecchymoses to her right temporal region from the fall. She is a 2-ppd smoker, drinks socially. She has not been to her PCP in over 10 years.

Neurologically she has improved from her original GCS of 12 to a score of 14 today. She requires frequent orientation to place and time. She initially was lethargic on admission but now can hardly sleep at all. She is pleasant and is able to ambulate with assistance. She does have ataxia, tremors, and there is apparent mild left-sided hemiparesis, so her husband/daughter helps with feeding her. Her right pupil is slightly larger than the left.

Her chest has crackles to mid and lower lobes with a productive cough. She sats at 92% on 2 L nasal cannula. RR is in the 20s. She is on a nicotine patch. She requests cigarettes frequently and has to be reminded that she is in the hospital on oxygen.

She has normal heart sounds, no peripheral edema, and cap refill is <3 sec. She is on telemetry, and reports indicate that she is in a sinus rhythm to a sinus tachycardia with a rate of 80–110. Her BP is 130–180/80–90. We are treating her blood pressures with labetolol prn. I last gave that to her 2 hr ago.

She has bowel sounds and her abdomen is soft and flat. She is cachectic in appearance. She had a BM yesterday. She doesn't have much of an appetite and claims the food is "horrible." She is on a mechanical soft diet. She had some nausea last evening and vomited. She got Zofran at 2100.

She has a Foley in for clear yellow urine. I&O was 2100/1900 mL.

She has a peripheral saline lock that flushes well.

Her lab work from this morning is WNL except her Hgb is low (7.8), her magnesium is low (1.7), and liver enzymes are elevated. We just got an order to treat her magnesium but it has not arrived from pharmacy yet. Mrs. Theodora Phillips is in her bed awaiting breakfast. Her husband/daughter is with her in the room.

Student Simulation Prep Assignments

1. Identify items and their purpose in the care of a patient with SDH and alcohol withdrawal.

Item	Purpose
IV with pump	
O_2 via nasal cannula	
Monitor	
BP cuff, thermometer, stethoscope	
Soft wrist restraints	

2. Identify team members and their specific roles in the care of a patient with SDH and alcohol withdrawal.

Team Member	Role
Primary nurse	
Secondary nurse	
Physician	

3. Relevant Data Exercise: Fill in columns below.

Relevant Data from Report	Relevant Data from Other Sources	Data Missing	Sources for Missing Data	Data Requiring Follow-Up

Continued

Relevant Data from Report	Relevant Data from Other Sources	Data Missing	Sources for Missing Data	Data Requiring Follow-Up

4. Initial Focused Assessment

After reviewing the client background and nursing report, you are ready to assess your client's current status. Under each category, identify how you would target your assessment and what you would expect to find for the patient with a chronic SDH and alcohol withdrawal.

History

Are there any questions you need to ask the patient or family to obtain additional relevant data?

Physical Exam

- General appearance:
- Integumentary:
- HEENT:
- Respiratory:
- CV:
- Breasts:
- Abdominal:
- Neuro:
- Musculoskeletal:
- Reproductive:
- Additional:
- Developmental:

What are the nursing implications considering the developmental stage of your patient?

Answer:

5. *Diagnostic Tests*

What diagnostic test results relevant to the patient's current problem are needed to plan care?

Complete the table using Van Leeuwen et al, *Davis's Comprehensive Handbook of Laboratory and Diagnostic Testing with Nursing Implications* 4e, or other diagnostic test reference.

Diagnostic Test	Significance to This Patient's Problem
Blood alcohol level	
Liver enzymes	
Magnesium	
Calcium	
Phosphorus	
Potassium	
Hbg	
Albumin	

6. *Treatment*

Identify drugs that are used to treat a patient with SDH and alcohol withdrawal.

Complete the table using Deglin et al, *Davis's Drug Guide for Nurses* 12e, or other drug reference.

Medication	Dose, Route, Frequency	Indications	Side Effect	Nursing Implications
Magnesium	4 g IV in 250 mL D5W infused over 1 hr			
Labetolol	10 mg IV q 10 min over 2 min prn SBP >140			
Clonidine	0.1-mg tablet po/NG tube BID			
Normal saline 1-L bags (0.9% NaCl)	IV infusion at 100 mL/hr			
Nicotine patch	21 mg apply daily and remove old patch			

Continued

Medication	Dose, Route, Frequency	Indications	Side Effect	Nursing Implications
Dimenhydrinate	50 mg IV push q 6 hr prn nausea			
Lorazepam	1 mg IV push q 4 hr prn agitation			
Acetaminophen	650 mg po q 4 hr prn pain			

7. Nursing Problems/Diagnoses

Identify three priority nursing problems/diagnoses.

Assessment Data	Priority Problem	Intervention	Expected Patient Outcome	Which Intervention Could Be Delegated to Unlicensed Personnel?
1.				
2.				
3.				

References

Deglin, J. H., & Vallerand, A. H. (2003). *Davis's drug guide for nurses.* Philadelphia: F. A. Davis.

Dillon, P. (2007). *Nursing health assessment: A critical thinking and case studies approach* (2nd ed.). Philadelphia: F. A. Davis.

Erikson, E. H. (1950). *Childhood and society*. New York: Norton.

Gold, M., & Aronson, M. (2008). Screening for and diagnosis of patients with alcohol problems. Retrieved June 25, 2008 from http://www.uptodate.com

Lagerquist, S. L. (2006). *Davis's NCLEX-RN success* (2nd ed). Philadelphia: F. A. Davis.

Smith, E., & Amin-Hanjan, S. (2008). Evaluation and management of elevated intracranial pressure in adults. Retrieved June 25, 2008 from http://www.uptodate.com

Van Leeuwen, A. M., Poelhuis-Leth, D. J., & Bladh, M. L. (2011). *Davis's comprehensive handbook of laboratory and diagnostic tests with nursing implications.* (4th ed.). Philadelphia: F. A. Davis.

Weinhouse, G. (2008). Alcohol withdrawal syndromes. Retrieved June 24, 2008 from http://www.uptodate.com

5-11 Spinal Cord Injury

ADULT/FUNDAMENTALS

STANDARD FORMS

These templates are included in the Appendix; copy before each use.

LEARNING OUTCOMES

Cognitive

The student will be able to:

1. Recognize autonomic dysreflexia as a medical emergency.
2. Identify pertinent history question relevant to a patient with autonomic dysreflexia.
3. Identify appropriate physical assessment techniques for a patient with autonomic dysreflexia.
4. Analyzes assessment data to make appropriate clinical decisions.
5. Identify appropriate nursing interventions for a patient with autonomic dysreflexia.

Psychomotor

The student will be able to:

1. Perform focused symptom analysis for a patient with autonomic dysreflexia.
2. Perform focused physical assessment for a patient with autonomic dysreflexia.
3. Implement appropriate interventions for a patient with autonomic dysreflexia.

Affective

The student will be able to:

1. Reflect upon performance in performing an assessment on a patient with autonomic dysreflexia.
2. Identify factors that worked well during the simulation of care of a patient.
3. Identify factors that needed improvement during the simulation of care of a patient with autonomic dysreflexia.
4. Develop self-confidence in assessing a patient with autonomic dysreflexia.

Communication

The student will be able to:

1. Communicate effectively with the patient with autonomic dysreflexia.
2. Utilize SBAR to communicate with members of healthcare team.
3. Accurately and succinctly document assessment findings.
4. Practice Transparent Thinking (thinking out loud) to facilitate group problem solving.
5. Use Directed Communication (directing a message to specific individual) when delegating tasks.
6. Employ Closed-Loop Communication (acknowledgment of receipt of the message and status) to acknowledge communications from others.

Safety

The student will be able to:

Administer and maintain specific protecting interventions with attention to safety of the client and healthcare professional.

1. Demonstrate a safe environment with attention to hazards to healthcare providers, visitors, and the client. Includes body mechanics, tripping hazards, and equipment issues.
2. Demonstrate attention to national patient safety goals. Includes patient identification standards, effective communication among healthcare providers, and safe medication administration.
3. Demonstrate attention to standard precautions. Includes hand washing, infection control measures, and use of personal protective equipment (PPE) as needed.

Leadership and Management/Delegation

The student will be able to:

1. Identify tasks that can be legally, ethically, and safely delegated to unlicensed assistive personnel (UAP) or licensed practical nurse (LPN) in the care of a patient with spinal cord injury.
2. Identify and prioritize patient's needs in care of a patient with spinal cord injury.

OVERVIEW OF PROBLEM

Autonomic Dysreflexia (Hyperreflexia)

Definition

Autonomic dysreflexia is a group of symptoms characterized by uninhibited sympathetic response. It occurs with injuries above 6th thoracic vertebrae, most commonly with cervical or high thoracic injuries. It usually occurs after spinal shock up to 6 years after injury.

Pathophysiology

Autonomic dysreflexia is a pathological reflex condition which is an acute medical emergency characterized by extreme hypertension and autonomic response.

Risk Factors

- Distended bladder
- Distended rectum
- Pain
- Stimulation of the skin
  - Tight clothing
  - Pressure ulcers
  - Cool temperature/drafts
  - Wrinkled clothes or bedding

Assessment

Subjective

- Severe, throbbing headache
- Blurred vision
- Nausea
- Restlessness
- Feel flushed

Objective

- Hypertension (may be as high as a systolic of 300 mm Hg)
- Bradycardia (30–40 bpm)
- Diaphoresis above level of injury
- Flushing above level of injury
- Pale skin below level of injury
- Goose flesh
- Nasal congestion
- Distended bowel, bladder
- Skin breakdown
- Seizures

Treatment

- Nitrates
- Nifedipine (Procardia)
- Hydralazine (Apresoline)
- Suppositories, enemas, or laxatives

Nursing Management

Goal: Decrease symptoms and prevent side effects
- Elevate head of bed (high Fowler's position)
- Identify and correct source of stimulation
- Call physician
- Loosen clothes or sheets
- Monitor vital signs
- Give medications as ordered such as nitrates, nifedipinde, or hydralazine

Goal: Maintain patency of catheter
- If Foley catheter present, check urinary catheter for kinks and irrigate with small amount of saline
- Insert new catheter immediately if blocked
- If Foley catheter not present, monitor output, check for distended bladder
- Do not Crede or tap the bladder

Goal: Promote bowel elimination
- Check for fecal impaction, use topical anesthetic

Goal: Prevent pressure ulcers
- Meticulous skin care
- Assess for skin breakdown
- Position change q 1–2 hr
- Flotation pads, alternating pressure mattress

Goal: Identify source of stimulation
- Check room temperature; make sure not too cold or drafty (chills, pilomotor spasms, goose bumps)

Goal: Health teaching
- Recognition of precipitating factors
- Methods to prevent stimulation

Evaluation/Outcome Criteria

- BP remains within normal limits
- No complications

REVIEW QUESTIONS

1. How would you differentiate spinal shock from autonomic dysreflexia?
   Answer:

2. What possible complications may occur from autonomic dysreflexia?
   Answer:

3. How can you explain the s/s associated with autonomic dysreflexia?
   Answer:

4. Name three possible nursing diagnoses related to autonomic dysreflexia.
   Answer:

5. Identify appropriate nursing interventions for each risk factor for autonomic dysreflexia.
   Answer:

Related Evidence-Based Practice Guidelines

Search http://www.guidelines.gov autonomic dysreflexia

The Joint Commission National Patient Safety Goals Hospital Program. Retrieved from http://www.jointcommission.org/GeneralPublic/NPSG/10_npsgs.htm

SBAR Technique for Communication: A situational briefing model published by The Institute for Healthcare

Improvement was downloaded on December 19, 2008, from http://www.ihi.org/IHI/Topics/PatientSafety/SafetyGeneral/Tools/SBARTechniqueforCommunicationASituationalBriefingModel.htm

Topics to Review Prior to the Simulation

- Spinal cord injury

SIMULATION

Client Background

Biographical Data

- Age: 23
- Gender: male
- Height: 6 ft
- Weight: 185 lb

Cultural Considerations

- Language: English
- Ethnicity: Scottish and Italian descent
- Nationality: American
- Culture: no significant cultural considerations identified

Demographic

- Marital status: single
- Educational level: college
- Religion: none
- Occupation: unemployed

Current Health Status

- Patient quadriplegic s/p spinal cord injury

History

- Psychosocial history
  - Social support: family, lives with family
- Past health history
  - Medical: healthy adult
  - Surgical: none
- Family history: + for CV disease

Admission Sheet

Name:	Tom Brucker
Age:	23
Gender:	Male
Marital Status:	Single
Educational Level:	College
Religion:	None
Ethnicity:	Scottish and Italian descent
Nationality:	American
Language:	English
Occupation:	Unemployed

Hospital
Provider's Orders

Patient's Name: Tom_Brucker
Allergies: NKDA

Diagnosis: s/p spinal cord injury C5 quadriplegic

Date	Time	Order	Signature
3/10/09	6 PM	Admit to spinal cord injury rehabilitation Dx quadriplegic	

Continued

Diagnosis: s/p spinal cord injury C5 quadriplegic—cont'd

Date	Time	Order	Signature
		Vital signs: q 8 hr	
		Diet: Regular	
		Physical therapy consult	
		Occupational therapy consult	
		Activity: As per PT orders	
		Medications: Tylenol 325 mg po q 4 hr prn temp >101°F or pain Colace 100 mg po daily Baclofin 10 mg po tid Ducolax 1 PR prn	
			Dr. Stanley

Nursing Report

Mr. Tom Bruker, age 23, was admitted yesterday for rehab. He is quadriplegic at C5 from a motorcycle accident. His assessment findings include:

- VS: BP 100/58, pulse 58, resp 20, pulse ox 96% on RA, pain scale 0/0
- General: AAOx3, affect pleasant considering what he's been through
- Skin: cool and dry below injury, skin intact, no breakdown
- CV: HRRR, no extra sounds
- Resp: lungs clear, but decreased at the bases
- Abdomen: soft nontender, started on bowel training program while in hospital LBM yesterday, Foley indwelling catheter drained 300 mL clear yellow urine
- Neuro/MS: quadriplegic, no movement forearms and lower extremities, has sensation in shoulders and upper arms, no sensation chest on down
- PT and OT will evaluate today to begin therapy

Student Simulation Prep Assignments

1. Identify items and their purpose in the care of a patient with autonomic dysreflexia.

Item	Purpose
IV with pump	
Urinary catheter	
Gloves	
BP cuff, thermometer	

2. Identify team members and their specific roles in the care of a patient with autonomic dysreflexia.

Team Member	Role
Primary nurse	
Secondary nurse	
Physician	

3. ***Relevant Data Exercise:*** Fill in columns below.

Relevant Data from Report	Relevant Data from Other Sources	Data Missing	Sources for Missing Data	Data Requiring Follow-Up

4. ***Initial Focused Assessment***

After reviewing the client background and nursing report, you are ready to assess your client's current status. Under each category, identify how you would target your assessment and what you would expect to find for the patient with autonomic dysreflexia.

History

Are there any questions you need to ask the patient or family to obtain additional relevant data?

Physical Exam

- General appearance:
- Integumentary:
- HEENT:
- Respiratory:
- CV:
- Breasts:
- Abdominal:
- Neuro:
- Musculoskeletal:
- Reproductive:
- Additional:
- Developmental:

What are the nursing implications considering the developmental stage of your patient?

Answer:

5. ***Diagnostic Tests***

Not applicable

6. Treatment

Identify drugs that are used to treat a patient with autonomic dysreflexia.

Complete the table using Deglin et al, *Davis's Drug Guide for Nurses* 12e, or other drug reference.

Medication	Dose, Route, Frequency	Indications	Side Effect	Nursing Implications
Tylenol	2 tab po q 4 hr prn			
Colace	100 mg po daily			
Baclofen	10 mg po tid			
Dulcolax	1 suppository PR prn			

7. Nursing Problems/Diagnoses

Identify three priority nursing problems/diagnoses.

Assessment Data	Priority Problem	Intervention	Expected Patient Outcome	Which Intervention Could Be Delegated to Unlicensed Personnel?
1.				
2.				
3.				

References

Deglin, J. H., & Vallerand, A. H. (2009). *Davis's drug guide for nurses* (11th ed.). Philadelphia: F. A. Davis.

Dillon, P. (2007). *Nursing health assessment: A critical thinking case studies approach* (2nd ed.). Philadelphia: F. A. Davis.

Erikson, E. H. (1950). *Childhood and society*. New York: Norton.

Lagerquist, S. L. (2006). *Davis's NCLEX-RN success* (2nd ed). Philadelphia: F. A. Davis.

Van Leeuwen, A. M., Poelhuis-Leth, D. J., & Bladh, M. L. (2011). *Davis's comprehensive handbook of laboratory and diagnostic tests with nursing implications* (4th ed.). Philadelphia: F. A. Davis.

Geriatric Nursing 6

6-1 Elder Abuse/Thoracic trauma

GERIATRICS

STANDARD FORMS

These templates are included in the Appendix; copy before each use.

LEARNING OUTCOMES

Cognitive

The student will be able to:

1. Describe the steps in the primary and secondary trauma assessment.
2. Identify priority intervention for each step of primary and secondary trauma assessment.
3. Correlate risk factors for trauma and abuse in the elderly client.
4. Identify priority nursing assessments for the patient with thoracic trauma.
5. Identify priority nursing interventions for the patient with thoracic trauma.
6. Identify appropriate nursing interventions for a patient with a chest drainage system.

Psychomotor

The student will be able to:

1. Demonstrate an accurate primary and secondary assessment for the patient with thoracic trauma.
2. Initiate appropriate priority interventions for the patient with thoracic trauma by

- Immobilizing C spine
- Applying oxygen and pulse ox
- Assisting with chest tube insertion
- Establishing IV access
- Attaching cardiac monitor
- Administering IV pain medication
- Hanging IV fluids and antibiotic

Affective

The student will be able to:

1. Reflect upon personal performance in the care of a patient with thoracic trauma.
2. Describe feelings about working with team members to provide care for a patient with thoracic trauma.
3. Reflect upon feelings in caring for an elderly patient with suspected abuse.
4. Identify areas of performance during the simulation that were appropriate.
5. Identify areas of performance during the simulation that need improvement.
6. Develop self-confidence in the care of the patient with traumatic injuries.

Communication

The student will be able to:

1. Communicate effectively with members of the health-care team while providing care for the patient with traumatic injuries.
2. Apply the principles of Therapeutic Communication while caring for the patient and family with traumatic injuries.
3. Will practice Transparent Thinking (thinking out loud) to facilitate group problem solving.
4. Use Directed Communication (directing a message to specific individual) when delegating tasks.
5. Employ Closed-Loop Communication (acknowledgment of receipt of the message and status) to acknowledge communications from others.

Safety

The student will be able to:

Administer and maintain specific protecting interventions with attention to safety of the client and healthcare professional.

1. Demonstrates a safe environment with attention to hazards to healthcare providers, visitors, and the client. Includes body mechanics, tripping hazards, and equipment issues.
2. Demonstrates attention to national patient safety goals. Includes patient identification standards, effective communication among healthcare providers, and safe medication administration.
3. Demonstrates attention to standard precautions. Includes hand washing, infection control measures, and use of personal protective equipment (PPE) as needed.

Leadership and Management/Delegation

The student will be able to:

1. Identify tasks that can be legally, ethically, and safely delegated to unlicensed assistive personnel (UAP) or licensed practical nurse (LPN) in the care of a patient with traumatic injuries.
2. Prioritize the care of a patient with traumatic injuries.

Legal/Ethical

The students will be able to identify specific situations that require reporting abuse to the authorities.

OVERVIEW OF THE PROBLEM

Blunt Force Trauma

Definition

Blunt trauma occurs as a result of energy forces compressing tissues when the energy is transferred from the blunt object, in this case the assailant's fists, to the victim's body. The force in which the assailant's fists repeatedly make contact with the victim's body causes compression and shearing of tissues and blood vessels and may cause bones to fracture.

Pathophysiology

Trauma is now recognized as a disease process where injury results from exposure to energy. The energy can be in the form of:

- Kinetic (motor vehicle crash [MVC], gunshot wound, fall)
- Chemical, electric, radiation
- Lack of essential energy such as oxygen or heat (drowning, frostbite)

There are two major categories of trauma: blunt and penetrating. *Blunt trauma* is injury without interruption of skin integrity. The extent of the injury may be masked. There is a transfer of energy to the surrounding tissue. In *penetrating trauma*, the energy to body tissue is from a moving object which interrupts skin integrity. Energy to surrounding tissue can also cause deformity.

Risk Factors

Risk factors for trauma include:

- Age
- Gender
- Environmental conditions
- Alcohol and drug use

Elderly patients are especially at risk for trauma-related injuries. Age-related physiological changes and preexistent health problems put them at a greater risk for death from trauma than younger patients.

Assessment

The approach to trauma care requires a systematic, level-headed approach. Trauma care always begins with the primary assessment or survey. This can be remembered by using the mnemonic ABCDE (airway, breathing, circulation/hemorrhage, disability, and exposure/environment). Resuscitation and interventions occur simultaneously. The primary survey is followed by the secondary survey. During the secondary survey all injuries are identified by conducting a thorough head-to-toe assessment, getting a full set of vital signs, keeping the patient warm, and collecting a thorough history.

Thoracic trauma is commonly seen in motor vehicle crashes and falls. Evaluation of the patient's ability to ventilate and oxygenate is essential. Injuries that occur from thoracic trauma include pulmonary contusion, myocardial contusion, fractured ribs, flail chest, pneumothorax (closed, open, and tension), and hemothorax. A focused respiratory and cardiovascular assessment with ongoing monitoring is essential.

Subjective

- Severe, sudden, sharp pain
- Dyspnea
- Anxiety, restlessness, fear, weakness

Objective Data

- Vital signs
- Skin color
- Thorax
  - Asymmetrical expansion
  - Chest wound
  - Crepitus
  - Deviation of trachea, mediastinal shift
- Pneumothorax
- Hemothorax
- Shock
- Hemoptysis
- Distended neck veins

Diagnostic Tests

- Chest x-ray
- Arterial blood gases

Treatment

- Air-occlusive dressing for chest wounds
- Endotracheal intubation
- Oxygen
- Needle decompression
- Insertion of chest tubes

Nursing Management

Goal: restore adequate ventilation and prevent further air escape from pleural cavity.

- Air-occlusive dressing
- Assist with intubation

- Assist with thoracentesis or chest tube insertion
- Monitor vital signs for signs of shock
- Monitor blood gases to detect acid-base imbalance
- Administer pain medications with caution to avoid respiratory depression

Evaluation/Outcome Criteria

- Lung re-expands, stable respiratory status
- Shock and hemorrhage are prevented
- No further damage to surrounding tissues
- Pain is controlled

Elder Abuse/Neglect

The nurse must also be aware of the possibility of abuse in trauma-related injuries. Children and the elderly are at the highest risk. Elderly abuse has gained recognition in recent years and may take many forms. These can include physical, emotional, sexual abuse and exploitation. The National Center on Elder Abuse, which is directed by the US Administration on Aging, provides valuable information on this subject. Their mission is to promote understanding and action on elder abuse, neglect, and exploitation.

Definition

Battering, psychological abuse, sexual assault, or any act or omission by caregiver, family, or legal guardian that results in harm or threatened harm.

Types of Abuse

- Financial
- Neglect
- Psychological
- Physical
- Sexual

Risk Factors

Victim

- Poor health
- Impaired memory
- Impaired thinking

Abuser

- Substance abuse, stressful life events
- Interpersonal problems

Both

- Mental illness
- Hx of family violence
- Financial difficulties
- Dependency
- Shared living space

Assessment

Subjective

- Agitation
- Anger
- Denial
- Fear
- Confusion
- Depression
- Withdrawal
- Stories don't match the pattern of injury

Objective

- Weight loss
- Unexplained injuries
- Poor hygiene or unkempt appearance
- Noncompliance with medical treatment regimen

Financial Matters

- Recent changes in will
- Unusual banking activity
- Missing checks or belongings
- Forced signatures
- Unwillingness to spend money on the elder

Nursing Mangement

Primary Prevention

- Case finding
- Early treatment
- Referral

Secondary Prevention

- Report to law enforcement agency
- Provide hotline information
- Initiate plan for safety of elder

Tertiary Prevention

- Counseling
- Support
- Self-help
- Legal action

Evaluation/Outcome Criteria

- Elder develops trust without fear of future abuse; physical, psychosocial and spiritual well-being is enhanced.

REVIEW QUESTIONS

1. List the steps of the primary and secondary assessment.
   Answer:

2. For each assessment performed in the primary assessment, identify one priority nursing intervention.
   Answer:

3. Identify three factors that place the elderly patient at increased risk for traumatic injury.
   Answer:

4. Describe five critical nursing responsibilities when caring for a patient with a chest drainage system.
Answer:

5. Discuss the physiological changes that are associated with aging which may have an influence on your assessment and intervention with an elderly trauma victim.
Answer:

Related Evidenced-Based Practice Guideline

The Joint Commission National Patient Safety Goals Hospital Program. Retrieved from http://www.jointcommission.org/GeneralPublic/NPSG/10_npsgs.htm

SBAR Technique for Communication: A situational briefing model published by The Institute for Healthcare Improvement was downloaded on December 19, 2008, from http://www.ihi.org/IHI/Topics/PatientSafety/SafetyGeneral/Tools/SBARTechniqueforCommunicationASituationalBriefingModel.htm

National Guidelines Clearing House Elder Abuse http://www.guideline.gov/browse/browsecondition.aspx

National Guidelines Clearing House Trauma http://www.guideline.gov/browse/browsecondition.aspx

Topics to Review Prior to the Simulation

You will be caring for an elderly patient who sustains traumatic injury as a result of abuse by a relative. The patient is brought to the Emergency Department by her neighbor. You are the RN receiving the patient in the trauma unit.

In preparation for this clinical simulation, please complete the following activities prior to attending the simulation:

- Review the physiology and pathophysiology of thoracic trauma.
- Review the risk factors for traumatic injury in the elderly population.
- Review information on elder abuse including prevalence, signs and symptoms, and responsibilities of healthcare professionals.

In addition to your textbook, the following references should assist you in preparing for this assignment:

Elder abuse:
www.helpguide.org (search for elder abuse)
www.ncea.aoa.gov
www.emedicine.com/EMERG/topic160.htm
Merboth, M. (2000). Managing pain: the fifth vital sign. *Nursing Clinics of North America, 35*(2), 375-383.
Trauma:
www.trauma.org
Presumptive antibiotics for chest tube insertion, summary. Retrieved February 2008
Trauma care:
Laskowski-Jones, L. (2006). Responding to trauma: Your priorities in the first hour. *Nursing, 39*, 52-58.
Trauma care of the elderly patient:
Steffen, K. (2003). When your trauma patient is over 65. *Nursing, 33*, 53-56.

SIMULATION

Client Background

Biographical Data

- Age: 72
- Gender: female
- Height: 5 ft 7 in
- Weight: 140 lb

Cultural Considerations

- Language: English
- Ethnicity: Irish
- Nationality: American
- Culture: no significant cultural considerations identified

Demographic

- Marital status: widow
- Educational level: college graduate, doctorate in education
- Religion: Catholic
- Occupation: retired public school superintendent

Current Health Status

Mrs. Martha Scott is a 72-year-old white female who was admitted with traumatic injuries secondary to a physical assault by a family member. Mrs. Scott states that she was beaten by her nephew after she refused to give him money to buy alcohol. She states that her nephew asked her for money to buy beer and cigarettes and became angry when she refused and struck her several times across the face. She left the room to call her sister and he followed behind her yelling that he was sorry. When Mrs. Scott picked up the phone and attempted to dial her sister's number, her nephew snatched the phone from her and punched her in the chest. Mrs. Scott stated that she was able to run out of the house with the nephew following her. When the nephew caught up with her, he continued to punch her in the chest and then pushed her off of the porch.

A neighbor found Mrs. Scott lying on her right side screaming and shivering on the ground in her front yard below her front porch. As the neighbor arrived, she noted Mrs. Scott's nephew driving away.

Mrs. Scott states that her nephew drinks too much and recently lost another job due to his drinking problem. She states that he is a good person, but has trouble controlling his temper, especially after he loses a job.

History

- Psychosocial history
  - Social support: sister living nearby, no children, nephew who sometimes lives with her
- Past health history
  - Medical: osteoarthritis
  - Surgical: bilateral cataracts
- Family history
  - Father died at age 68 of stroke
  - Mother died at age 60 of pneumonia secondary to fractured hip
  - Husband died of cancer at age 60

Admission Sheet

Name:	Martha Scott
Age:	72
Gender:	Female
Marital Status:	Widow
Educational Level:	College graduate, doctorate in education
Religion:	Catholic
Ethnicity:	Irish
Nationality:	American
Language:	English
Occupation:	Retired public school superintendent

Hospital Provider's Orders — **Patient's Name: Martha Scott** — **Allergies: NKDA**

Diagnosis: Right pneumothorax

Date	Time	Order	Signature
2:00 PM	Admission to ER	Vital signs: Continuous cardiac monitoring and SpO_2 monitoring	
		Diet: NPO	
		Activity: Bed rest	
		IV therapy: 1,000 mL of normal saline for infusion	
		Diagnostic tests: CBC Type and screen BMP Stat portable lateral C-spine x-ray, CT head Stat portable chest x-ray UA	
		Oxygen via nasal cannula, titrate to keep O_2 sat >95%	Dr. Thomas
2:20 PM	Chest tube inserted	Chest tube to drainage system Suction 20 cm H_2O	

Continued

Diagnosis: Right pneumothorax—cont'd			
Date	**Time**	**Order**	**Signature**
		Repeat chest x-ray: AP and lateral views	
		Medications: Morphine sulfate 2 mg IV push every 2 hr prn pain Tetanus diptheria toxoid vaccine 0.5 mL IM Lidocaine 1% 10 mL to bedside for chest tube insertion	Dr. Thomas
3:00 PM		Admit to telemetry unit Ancef 1,000 mg IVPB now and q 6 hr	
		Social service consult	
		Clean and dress abrasions	
		Notify attending MD of admission and for futher orders	
			Dr. Thomas

Nursing Report 1:50 PM

Mrs. Scott was brought to the emergency room minutes ago by her neighbor. The neighbor found her screaming and shivering on the ground by her front porch. She has multiple abrasions to the right side of her face, anterior thorax, and right arm. She is alert and oriented to time, place and current events. She is crying but able to answer questions appropriately.

The patient care tech has placed her on a stretcher in trauma room 1.

Student Simulation Prep Assignments

1. Identify items and their purpose in the care of an elderly patient with thoracic trauma.

Item	Purpose
IV with pump	
O_2 nonrebreather mask, cannula	
Pulse ox	
Foley	
Monitor	

2. Identify team members and their specific roles in the care of an elderly patient with thoracic trauma.

Team Member	Role
Primary nurse	
Secondary nurse	
Physician	
Patient care technician	

3. *Relevant Data Exercise:* Fill in the columns below.

Relevant Data from Background and Report	Relevant Data from Other Sources	Data Missing	Sources for Missing Data	Data Requiring Follow-up

4. *Initial Focused Assessment*

After reviewing the client background and nursing report, you are ready to assess your client's current status. Under each category, identify how you would target your assessment and what you would expect to find for the patient with thoracic trauma.

History

Are there any questions you need to ask the patient or family to obtain additional relevant data?

Physical exam

- General appearance:
- Integumentary:
- HEENT:
- Respiratory:
- CV:
- Breasts:
- Abdominal:
- Neuro:
- Musculoskeletal:
- Reproductive:
- Additional:
- Developmental:

What are the nursing implications considering the developmental stage of your patient?

Answer:

5. *Diagnostic Tests*

What diagnostic test results relevant to the patient's current problem are needed to plan care?

Complete the table using Van Leeuwen et al, *Davis's Comprehensive Handbook of Laboratory and Diagnostic Testing with Nursing Implications* 4e, or other diagnostic test reference.

Diagnostic	Significance
Serum glucose 110 mg/dL	
Electrolytes Na 137 mEq/L K 3.7 mEEq/L Cl 109 mEq/L Ca 10.2 mg/dL	

Continued

Diagnostic	Significance
BUN 30 mg /dL Creatinine 1.7 mg/dL	
Hemoglobin 10.3 g/dL Hematocrit 30.9%	

6. Treatment

Identify drugs that are used to treat a patient with thoracic trauma

Complete the table using Deglin et al, *Davis's Drug Guide for Nurses* 12e, or other drug reference.

Medication	Dose, Route, Frequency	Indications	Side Effects	Nursing Implications
Morphine sulfate	2 mg IV q 2 hr prn pain			
Ancef	1,000 mg IV q 6 hr			
Tetanus diphtheria toxoid vaccine	Unimmunized: 2 doses 0.5 mL IM 1–2 mo apart, then a third 6–12 mo later Immunized: booster every 10 years			
Lidocaine 1%	As needed			

7. Nursing Problems/Diagnoses

Identify three priority nursing problems/diagnoses.

Assessment Data	Priority Problem	Intervention	Expected Patient Outcome	Which Interventions Could Be Delegated to Unlicensed Personnel?
1.				
2.				
3.				

References

Chulay, M., & Burns, M. (2005). *AACN essentials of critical care nursing*. New York: McGraw-Hill.

Coughlin, A., & Parchinsky, C. (2006). Go with the flow of chest tube therapy. *Nursing, 36*(3), 36-41.

Deglin, J. H., & Vallerand, A. H. (2009). *Davis's drug guide for nurses* (11th ed.). Philadelphia: F. A. Davis.

Dillon, P. (2007). *Nursing health assessment: A critical thinking and case studies approach* (2nd ed.). Philadelphia: F. A. Davis.

Eastern Association for the Surgery of Trauma (EAST) (2004). *Practice guidelines for pain management in blunt thoracic trauma.* Winston-Salem, NC: Eastern Association for the Surgery of Trauma. Retrieved February, 2008 from the National Guideline Clearinghouse at http://www.guidelines.gov

Erikson, E.H. (1950). *Childhood and society.* New York: Norton

Jacobs, B. (2000). *Trauma nursing core curriculum provider manual* (5th ed.). DesPlaines, IL. Emergency Nursing Association.

Lagerquist, S. (2006). *Davis's NCLEX-RN success*. Philadelphia: F. A. Davis.

Laskowski-Jones, L. (2006). Responding to trauma. *Nursing, 39*(9), 52-58.

Nursing. (*Lippincott's Q&A Certification Review Emergency* (2005). Ambler, PA: Lippincott Williams & Wilkins.

Schumacher, L., & Chernecky, C. (2005). *Critical care and emergency nursing.* St. Louis: Elsevier Saunders.

Sellas, M. (2006). Elder abuse. Retrieved February, 2008 from www.emedicine.com/EMERG/topic160.htm

Steffen, K. (2003). When your trauma patient is over 65. *Nursing, 33*(4), 53-56.

Van Leeuwen, A. M., Poelhuis-Leth, D. J., & Bladh, M. L. (2011). *Davis's comprehensive handbook of laboratory and diagnostic tests with nursing implications.* (4th ed.). Philadelphia: F. A. Davis.

Web sites:

Elder Abuse

www.ncea.aoa.gov

www.helpguide.org

Trauma

www.trauma.org

Presumptive antibiotics for chest tube insertion, summary. Retrieved February, 2008 from http://www.surgicalcriticalcare.net/Guidelines/CT%20antibiotics.pdf

6-2 Syncopal Attack

GERIATRICS

STANDARD FORMS

These templates are included in the Appendix; copy before each use.

LEARNING OUTCOMES

Cognitive

The student will be able to:

1. Identify pertinent history question relevant a patient with syncope.
2. Differentiate the causes of syncope.
3. Correlate the pathophysiology associated with causes of syncope.
4. Identify appropriate diagnostic studies for a patient with syncope.
5. Describe appropriate treatment for syncope.

Psychomotor

The student will be able to:

1. Obtain a pertinent health history from a patient with syncope.
2. Perform appropriate assessment for a patient with syncope.
3. Implement patient safety standards for a patient with syncope.

Affective

The student will be able to:

1. Reflect upon performance in performing an assessment on a patient with syncope.
2. Identify factors that worked well during the simulation of care of a patient.
3. Identify factors that needed improvement during the simulation of care of a patient with syncope.
4. Develop self-confidence in performing an assessment on a patient with syncope.

Communication

The student will be able to:

1. Communicate effectively with the patient while performing an assessment on a patient with syncope.
2. Use SBAR when communication assessment findings.
3. Accurately and succinctly document assessment findings.
4. Will practice Transparent Thinking (thinking out loud) to facilitate group problem solving.
5. Use Directed Communication (directing a message to specific individual) when delegating tasks.
6. Employ Closed-Loop Communication (acknowledgment of receipt of the message and status) to acknowledge communications from others.

Safety

The student will be able to:

Administer and maintain specific protecting interventions with attention to safety of the client and health care professional.

1. Demonstrate a safe environment with attention to hazards to healthcare providers, visitors and the client. Includes body mechanics, tripping hazards, and equipment issues.
2. Demonstrate attention to national patient safety goals. Includes patient identification standards, effective communication among healthcare providers, and safe medication administration.
3. Demonstrate attention to standard precautions. Includes hand washing, infection control measures, and use of personal protective equipment (PPE) as needed.

Leadership and Management/Delegation

The student will be able to:

1. Identify and prioritize patient's needs in care of a patient with syncope.
2. Identify tasks that can be legally, ethically, and safely delegated to unlicensed assistive personnel (UAP) or licensed practical nurse (LPN) in the care of a patient with syncope.

Teaching

The student will be able to:

1. Develop a discharge plan for a patient with syncope.
2. Develop a teaching plan for the patient with syncope.
3. Make appropriate referrals for the patient with syncope.
4. Implement an effective teaching plan for the patient with syncope.
5. Evaluate the discharge and teaching plan for the patient with syncope.

OVERVIEW OF PROBLEM

Syncope

Definition

Temporary loss of consciousness, and a drop in blood pressure resulting in decreased cerebral perfusion and loss of consciousness.

Pathophysiology

Cardiac

- Cardiac arrhythmias
  - Sick sinus syndrome (sinus node dysfunction)
  - Heart block
- Severe aortic stenosis
- Mitral valve prolapse
- Pulmonary hypertension

Vascular

- Vasovagal—the most common
  - Inappropriate bradycardia and vasodilation in response to position change instead of the normal vasoconstriction, tachycardia response
- Orthostatic hypotension
  - Drop in BP with change of position from supine to standing position (+ orthostatic drop with a decrease in BP >20/10 measured 2 min after moving from supine, to sitting, to standing position with increase in pulse 20 bpm and complaints of dizziness, weakness, and loss of consciousness)
  - Decrease in venous return to heart due to venous pooling or inadequate volume leads to decrease in cardiac output and drop in BP
    - Decrease volume such as dehydration, hemorrhage
    - Impaired muscle pump secondary to prolonged bed rest
    - Interference with cardiovascular reflexes; e.g., medications that decrease heart rate or cause vasodilation
    - Disorders of autonomic nervous system
    - Effect of aging on baroreflex function
- Carotid stenosis
  - Narrowing of the carotids with decreased cerebral perfusion
- Carotid sinus hypersensitivity
  - Hypersensitivity of the carotid sinus results in bradycardia and decrease arterial resistance (drop in blood pressure)
  - Usually in older adults with underlying atherosclerotic heart disease
- Cerebrovascular disease
  - Vertebrobasilar insufficiency of midbrain which affects the Reticular Activating System (RAS)
  - TIAs
- Postprandial hypotension
  - Drop in BP 2 hr after eating high-carbohydrate meal
  - More common in older adults
  - Causes: excess insulin, inadequate sympathetic response and baroreceptor function, or vasopeptide-induced vasodilatation
- Valsalva's maneuver
  - Causes decrease decreased venous return, such as when defecating
- Postmicturation syndrome
  - Syncope after emptying a full bladder; Valsalva's maneuver implicated
- Posttussive syncope
  - May occur in patients with chronic bronchitis after severe coughing; results is decreased venous return and increased cerebral vascular resistance

Neurological/Psychiatric

- Anxiety
- Depression
- Panic disorders
- Hysteria
- Seizures

Metabolic

- Hypoglycemia
- Hyperventilation
- Hypoxia

Other

- Prolonged immobility
  - Especially in older adults
  - Venous pooling

Assessment

Subjective

- What were you doing before you passed out?
- How did you feel before you passed out?
- Medications
- Medical history

Objective

- Check for orthostatic drop of BP (supine, sitting, standing)
- Check pulse
- Check carotids for thrills and bruits

Diagnostic Tests

- ECG
- Holter 24-hr monitoring
- Echocardiogram
- Carotid US
- BMP
- CBC

Treatment

- Based on cause

Nursing Management

- Assist with diagnostic procedures
- Assess for symptoms of underlying causes

- Teach patient to recognize warning signs of syncopal episode
- Instruct patient to change position gradually if orthostatic hypertension present
- Maintain adequate hydration
- Administer medications as ordered
  - Review medications and side effects with patient.
- Provide patient teaching regarding cause, prevention, and treatments
  - Instruct patient to avoid wearing tight constricting garments

Evaluation/Outcome Criteria

- Syncopal attacks are prevented
- Injury does not occur
- Underlying cause is identified and treated
- Patient understands cause, prevention, and treatment

REVIEW QUESTIONS

1. What effect does vagal stimulation have on the cardiovascular system?
Answer:

2. What factors would place an older adult at greater risk for developing orthostatic hypotension?
Answer:

3. What effect does the Valsalva's maneuver have on the cardiovascular system?
Answer:

4. In patients with carotid hypersensitivity, what could stimulate a response?
Answer:

5. How do you assess the carotids for bruits?
Answer:

Related Evidence-Based Practice Guidelines

Search http://www.guideline.gov, syncope

The Joint Commission National Patient Safety Goals Hospital Program. Retrieved from http://www.jointcommission.org/GeneralPublic/NPSG/10_npsgs.htm

SBAR Technique for Communication: A situational briefing model published by The Institute for Healthcare Improvement was downloaded on December 19, 2008, from http://www.ihi.org/IHI/Topics/PatientSafety/SafetyGeneral/Tools/SBARTechniqueforCommunicationASituationalBriefingModel.htm

Patient Education for Orthostatic Hypotension

- Review medications and side effects with patient
- Instruct patient to change position slowly
- Avoid wearing tight constricting garments
- Maintain adequate fluid intake

Topics to Review Prior to the Simulation

- Health assessment
- Cardiovascular nursing

SIMULATION

Client Background

Biographical Data

- Age: 84
- Gender: female
- Height: 5 ft 3in
- Weight: 120 lb

Cultural Considerations

- Language: English
- Ethnicity: Irish
- Nationality: American
- Culture: no significant cultural considerations identified

Demographic

- Marital status: married
- Educational level: college
- Religion: Catholic
- Occupation: retired teacher

Current Health Status

- Felt dizzy last night, passed out. Husband prevented fall.

History

- Psychosocial history
  - Social support: family
- Past health history
  - Medical: + HTN, CAD, DJD
  - Surgical: no surgeries
- Family history: + CVD, HTN

Admission Sheet

Name:	Mary Duffy
Age:	84
Gender:	Female
Marital Status:	Married
Educational Level:	College
Religion:	Catholic
Ethnicity:	Irish
Nationality:	American
Language:	English
Occupation:	Retired teacher

Hospital
Provider's Orders

Patient's Name: Mary Duffy
Allergies: NKDA

Diagnosis: Syncope

Date	Time	Order	Signature
		Admit to telemetry	
		Cardiac monitor	
		Vital signs: q 4 hr with neuro check BP supine, sitting, standing	
		Diet: low sodium, cardiac diet	
		Activity: BRP with assistance	
		IV therapy: 1,000 mL NSS over 12 hr	
		TEDS, pneumatic stockings	
		Medications: • Toprol 25 mg po daily • HCTZ 25 mg po daily • Tylenol 650 mg po q 4 hr prn fever or pain • Protonix 40 mg IV push daily	
		Diagnostic studies: • ECG • Echocardiogram • CT scan head done in ER • US carotids • Repeat CBC, BMP in AM • Cardiac enzymes done in ER • Routine UA	
		Treatments: • Oxygen 2 L via NC • Cardiac monitor	Dr. C. Schmidt

Nursing Report

Mary Duffy, an 84-year-old white female, was admitted from the ER during the night with the diagnosis of syncopal attack. Past history of HTN, CAD, DJD. Admitted to telemetry for monitoring and workup. CT head negative. Monitor NSR. Labs: Her H&H was a little low and her BUN was a little elevated, cardiac enzymes negative. INT left hand with 1,000 mL NSS over 12 hr. Was taking Toprol, HCTZ daily, Motrin prn pain. Toprol cut in half, Motrin d/c. Can have Tylenol prn and Protonix daily. Scheduled for diagnostic tests in AM. Patient said she had a "GI bug" the other day with the "runs and couldn't keep anything down." This lasted 24 hr. VS: BP 150/85, negative orthostatic drop, pulse 87 regular, respirations 20, temperature 97.6°F, pulse ox 96% on 2 L O_2 via nasal cannula.

Student Simulation Prep Assignments

1. Identify items and their purpose in the care of a patient with syncope.

Item	Purpose
IV with pump	
O_2 cannula	
Monitor	

2. Identify team members and their specific roles in the care of a patient with syncope.

Team Member	Role
Primary nurse	
Physician	
Secondary nurse	
UAP	

3. Relevant Data Exercise: Fill in the columns below.

Relevant Data from Report	Relevant Data from Other Sources	Data Missing	Sources for Missing Data	Data Requiring Follow-up

4. Initial Focused Assessment

After reviewing the client background and nursing report, you are ready to assess your client's current status. Under each category, identify how you would target your assessment and what you would expect to find for the patient with syncope.

History

Are there any questions you need to ask the patient or family to obtain additional relevant data?

Physical Exam

- General appearance:
- Integumentary:
- HEENT:
- Respiratory:
- CV:
- Breasts:
- Abdominal:
- Neuro:
- Musculoskeletal:
- Reproductive:
- Developmental:

What are the nursing implications considering the developmental stage of your patient?

Answer:

5. Diagnostic Tests

What diagnostic test results relevant to the patient's current problem are needed to plan care?

Complete the table using Van Leeuwen et al, *Davis's Comprehensive Handbook of Laboratory and Diagnostic Testing with Nursing Implications* 4e, or other diagnostic test reference.

Diagnostic Test	Significance to This Patient's Problem
CT scan	
CBC	
BMP • Glucose • Lytes • BUN • Creatinine	
Cardiac enzymes	
UA	
ECG	
US carotids	
Echocardiogram	

6. Treatment

Identify drugs that are used to treat a patient with syncope.

Complete the table using Deglin et al, *Davis's Drug Guide for Nurses* 12e, or other drug reference.

Medication	Dose, Route, Frequency	Indications	Side Effect	Nursing Implications
Toprol	25 mg daily			
HCTZ	25 mg daily			
Motrin (at home)	400 mg q 6 hr prn			
Protonix	40 mg IVP daily			

Medication	Dose, Route, Frequency	Indications	Side Effect	Nursing Implications
Tylenol	2 tabs q 4 hr prn pain or fever			

References

Deglin, J. H., & Vallerand, A. H. (2009). *Davis's drug guide for nurses* (11th ed.). Philadelphia: F. A. Davis.

Dillon, P. (2007). *Nursing health assessment: A critical thinking and case studies approach* (2nd ed.). Philadelphia: F. A. Davis.

Erikson, E.H. (1950). *Childhood and society.* New York: Norton

Goroll, A., & Mulley, A., Jr. (2009). *Primary care medicine* (6th ed.). Philadelphia: Lippincott Williams & Wilkins.

Langerquist, S. (2006). *Davis's NCLEX-RN success* (2nd ed.). Philadelphia: F. A. Davis.

Mattson Porth, C. (2005). *Pathophysiology concepts of altered health states* (7th ed.). Philadelphia: Lippincott Williams & Wilkins.

Van Leeuwen, A. M., Poelhuis-Leth, D. J., & Bladh, M. L. (2011). *Davis's comprehensive handbook of laboratory and diagnostic tests with nursing implications.* (4th ed.). Philadelphia: F. A. Davis.

6-3 Dementia vs Delirium

GERIATRICS

STANDARD FORMS

These templates are included in the Appendix; copy before each use.

LEARNING OUTCOMES

Cognitive

The student will be able to:

1. Describe recognize signs and symptoms of delirium.
2. Differentiate dementia vs delirium.
3. Identify the risk factors for delirium.
4. Identify appropriate intervention for a patient with delirium.

Psychomotor

The student will be able to perform a neurological assessment on a patient with change in mental status.

Affective

The student will be able to:

1. Reflect upon performance in caring for a patient with delirium.
2. Identify what worked well during the scenario.
3. Identify areas that need improvement.
4. Reflect on overall feeling about the scenario.
5. Discuss feelings related to working as a team member.
6. Develop confidence in caring for a patient with delirium.
7. Do self-reflective evaluation.

Communication

The student will be able to:

1. Communicate effectively with healthcare team members.
2. Communicate with a confused patient.
3. Communicate effectively with the family members.
4. Use SBAR when communicating with healthcare team members.
5. Work collaboratively as part of the healthcare team.
6. Accurately and succinctly document assessments, interventions, and evaluations.
7. Practice Transparent Thinking (thinking out loud) to facilitate group problem solving.
8. Use Directed Communication (directing a message to specific individual) when delegating tasks.
9. Employ Closed-Loop Communication (acknowledgment of receipt of the message and status) to acknowledge communications from others.

Safety

The student will be able to:

Administer and maintain specific protecting interventions with attention to safety of the client and healthcare professional.

1. Demonstrate a safe environment with attention to hazards to healthcare providers, visitors, and the client. Includes body mechanics, tripping hazards, and equipment issues.
2. Demonstrate attention to national patient safety goals. Includes patient identification standards, effective communication among healthcare providers, and safe medication administration.
3. Demonstrate attention to standard precautions. Includes hand washing, infection control measures, and use of personal protective equipment (PPE) as needed.

Leadership and Management/Delegation

The student will be able to:

1. Identify tasks that can be legally, ethically, and safely delegated to unlicensed assistive personnel (UAP), licensed practical nurse (LPN), or registered nurse (RN).
2. Identify and prioritize patient's needs in the care of a patient with delirium.

OVERVIEW OF PROBLEM

Delirium

Definition

An acute onset of disturbance in consciousness with decreased ability to focus, sustain, or shift attention; a change in cognition and perceptual disturbances (Source: American Psychiatric Association [2000]. *Diagnostic and statistical manual for mental disorders* [4th ed.]. Washington, DC: APA.)

Pathophysiology

Delirium is characterized by an acute change in mental status with impaired attention, disorganized thinking, or incoherent speech; clouded consciousness; perceptual disturbances; sleep-wake problems; psychomotor agitation; or lethargy and disorientation. This condition is produced by changes in brain chemistry or tissue by metabolic toxins, direct trauma, drug effects, or withdrawal.

Epidemiology

- Incidence during hospitalization: 10–53% (Kuehn, 2010)
- Postoperative incidence: 15–72%
- Onset: usually third day of hospitalization
- Duration: <5 days, symptoms can last 3–6 mo

(Source: Hartford Institute for Geriatric Nursing http://consultgerirn.org)

Outcomes

- Decreased independence, loss of ability for self-determination
- Increased morbidity, such as falls, pressure ulcers, adverse effects from medications, infections, continued cognitive impairment, institutionalization
- Increased mortality; six times more than nondelirious patients
- Increased length of stay, increased acuity, increased cost

Risk Factors

- Increased age
- Increased severity of illness
- Multiple health problems, polypharmacy
- History of dementia, depression, or previous delirium
- Substance or alcohol abuse
- Sleep deprivation
- Immobility
- Sensory impairment

Causes of Delirium

- Acute illness
- Infection (UTI, URI)
- Medications (anticholinergics, sedatives, psychotropics, narcotics, H2 blockers)
- Dehydration and electrolyte imbalance
- Hemodynamic status, hypovolemia
- Environmental challenge (sensory overload or deprivation)
- Pain

Acute Delirium

This condition is seen in postoperative electrolyte disturbance, systemic infection, renal and liver failure, oversedation, and metastatic cancer.

Assessment

- Disorientation to time, especially at night
- Hallucinations, delusions, illusions
- Alterations in mood
- Increased emotional lability
- Agitation
- Lack of cooperation
- Withdrawal
- Sleep disturbance
- Alterations in food intake

Diagnostic Tests

- CBC
- Electrolytes
- Thyroid functions
- Liver enzymes
- Urinalysis
- ECG

Treatment

- Medications
- Low-dose phenothiazines
  - Avoid barbiturates and sedatives that may increase agitation, confusion, and disorientation.

Nursing Management

- Vital signs and pulse oximetry
- Intake and output
- Identify and remove toxic substance
- Treat underlying cause

Goal: Provide therapeutic environment

- Appropriate sensory stimulation
- Reassure and reorient
- Consistent caregivers
- Encourage family members to be at bedside
- Sensory aids
- Minimize relocation
- Simplify environment
- Avoid excessive medication and restraints

Goal: Provide general supportive nursing care

- Comfort measures
- Prevent complications of immobility
- Assist with basic needs
- Communicate clearly
- Reassure and educate family
- Minimize invasive procedures

Evaluation/Outcome Criteria

- Oriented to person, place, and time
- Cooperative
- Decreased agitation

Assessment/Screening Tools for Delirium

Assessment

- Confusion Assessment Method (CAM)
- Cognitive function:
  - Ask:
    - Change in thinking or memory
    - Strange thoughts
- Assess:
  - Alertness, hyperalert, lethargy, stupor, comatose
  - Attention, ability to focus digit span, serial subtraction, spelling backwards, clock drawing test
  - Orientation, may be disoriented to time and place
  - Memory, recent and remote
  - Thinking, logical vs disorganized, rambling
  - Perception, recognition of objects and persons
  - Psychomotor, hypo- or hyperkinetic, unusual or inappropriate

Screening Tools

CAM (The Confusion Assessment Method Instrument)

1. Acute onset: acute change in mental status from baseline?

2A. Inattention difficulty focusing, easily distracted?

2B. If present: does behavior come and go, increase or decrease in severity?

3. Disorganized thinking: incoherent, illogical flow of ideas, switching subject?

4. Altered level of consciousness: alert, hyperalert, and overly sensitive to environmental stimuli, lethargic, coma

5. Disorientation: place time, person

6. Memory impairment: unable to remember events in hospital

7. Perceptual disturbances: hallucinations, illusions or misinterpretation

8A. Psychomotor agitation: restlessness

8B. Psychomotor retardation: sluggishness, staring into space.

9. Altered sleep-wake cycle: excessive daytime sleepiness with insomnia at night

CAM Diagnostic Algorithm

Feature 1: Acute onset or fluctuating course
- Acute change in mental status

Feature 2: Inattention
- Difficulty focusing, easily distracted

Feature 3: Disorganized thinking
- Incoherent, illogical, unpredictable thinking

Feature 4: Altered level of consciousness
- Hyperalert, lethargic, stupor, or coma
  - \+ Diagnosis of delirium if features 1 and 2 and either 3 or 4.

(Source: Inouye, S, van Dyck, C., Alessi, C., Balkin, S., Siegal, A., & Horwitz, R. [1990]. Clarifying confusion: the confusion assessment method. *Annals of Internal Medicine*, *113*(12), 941-948.)

REVIEW QUESTIONS

1. How would you differentiate signs and symptoms of delirium from dementia and depression?

Answer:

Characteristics of Dementia, Delirium, and Depression

Feature	Dementia	Delirium	Depression
Onset			
Prognosis			
Course			
Attention			
Memory			
Perception			
Psychomotor behavior			
Cause			

Source: Dillon, P. (2007). *Health assessment: A critical thinking, case study approach*. Philadelphia: F. A. Davis.

Feature	Dementia	Delirium
Onset		
Prognosis		
Course		
Attention		
Memory		

Feature	Dementia	Delirium
Perception		
Psychomotor behavior		
Cause		

2. Identify five causes of delirium?
   Answer:

3. Why would delirium be considered a medical emergency?
   Answer:

4. What are some possible outcomes of untreated delirium?
   Answer:

5. Identify nursing interventions that would be appropriate for a patient with delirium.
   Answer:

Related Evidence-Based Practice Guideline

Search Delirium and Dementia
National guidelines clearinghouse
http://www.guideline.gov/browse/browsecondition.aspx

Assessing cognitive function. In: Evidence-based geriatric nursing protocols for best practice. Hartford Institute for Geriatric Nursing—Academic Institution. 2003 (revised Jan 2008). 16 pages. NGC:006350

The Joint Commission National Patient Safety Goals Hospital Program. Retrieved from http://www.jointcommission.org/GeneralPublic/NPSG/10_npsgs.htm

SBAR Technique for Communication: A situational briefing model published by The Institute for Healthcare Improvement was downloaded on December 19, 2008, from http://www.ihi.org/IHI/Topics/PatientSafety/SafetyGeneral/Tools/SBARTechniqueforCommunicationASituationalBriefingModel.htm

Topics to Review Prior to the Simulation

- Geriatric assessment
- Mental status assessment
- Differentiation of delirium and dementia

SIMULATION

Client Background

Helen McCloskey, age 85, admitted to the hospital with a fracture of right femur.

Biographical Data

- Age: 85
- Gender: female
- Height: 5 ft
- Weight: 110 lb

Cultural Considerations

- Language: English
- Ethnicity: Irish
- Nationality: American
- Culture: no significant cultural considerations identified

Demographic

- Marital status: single
- Educational level: high school
- Religion: Catholic
- Occupation: retired

Current Health Status

Fractured right hip

History

- Psychosocial history
  - Social support: lives alone
- Past health history: not available

Admission Sheet

Name:	Helen McCloskey
Age:	85
Gender:	Female
Marital Status:	Single
Educational Level:	High school
Religion:	Catholic
Ethnicity:	Irish
Nationality:	American
Language:	English
Occupation:	Retired

Hospital
Provider's Orders

Patient's Name: Helen McCloskey
Allergies: NKDA

Diagnosis: Fracture right hip S/P ORIF right hip

Date	Time	Order	Signature
6/20/07	5:00 PM	Vital Signs: q 4 hr	
		Diet: Clear liquids to regular as tolerated	
		Activity: Bed rest OOB in AM	
		Diagnostic tests: Serum electrolytes CBC in AM	
		PT consult	
		Medications: Lovenox 40 mg sq q 12 hr Colace 100 mg po bid Ancef 1 g q 6 hr x 4 doses Morphine 4 mg IM q 4 hr prn for pain Toprol 50 mg po daily	
		IV Therapy: 1,000 mL 5% D/LR 100 cc/hr	
		Treatments: Remove Foley in AM Pump stockings Oxygen 2 L via NC Incentive spirometry 10 x per hour while awake Chest PT BID	Dr. R. Manning

Nursing REPORT from PACU

Helen McCloskey, a 85-year-old white, single female, admitted with fractured right hip. History of DJD, HTN controlled with Lasix and Toprol. Patient had an ORIF of the right hip, general anesthesia, 500 mL blood loss, 1 U of PRBC in PACU. AAOx3, dressings dry and intact, Hemovac with 100 mL bloody drainage, + pedal pulses, toes warm and movable, +1 edema right foot. IV in left forearm 1,000 mL 5% D/LR at 100 cc/hr, Foley draining 200 mL clear yellow urine, monitor NSR, VS: 134/88, 95, 18, 97.6, pulse ox 94% on 2 L O_2 via NC.

Student Simulation Prep Assignments

1. Identify items and their purpose.

Item	Purpose
IV with pump	
O_2 cannula	
Foley	

2. Identify team members and their specific roles in the care of a patient with delirium.

Team Member	Role
Primary nurse	
Secondary nurse	
Physician	

3. Relevant Data Exercise: Fill in the columns below.

Relevant Data from Report	Relevant Data from Other Sources	Data Missing	Sources for Missing Data	Data Requiring Follow-up

4. Initial Focused Assessment

After reviewing the client background and nursing report, you are ready to assess your client's current status. Under each category, identify how you would target your assessment and what you would expect to find for the patient with delirium.

History

Are there any questions you need to ask the patient or family to obtain additional relevant data?

Physical Exam

- General appearance:
- Integumentary:

- HEENT:
- Respiratory:
- CV:
- Musculoskeletal:
- Neuro:
- Reproductive:
- Additional:
  - Renal:
- Developmental:

What are the nursing implications considering the developmental stage of your patient?

Answer:

5. *Diagnostic Tests*

What diagnostic test results relevant to the patient's current problem are needed to plan care?

Complete the table using Van Leeuwen et al, *Davis's Comprehensive Handbook of Laboratory and Diagnostic Testing with Nursing Implications* 4e, or other diagnostic test reference.

Diagnostic Test	Significance to This Patient's Problem
Serum glucose	
Electrolytes	
BUN and creatinine	
CBC	

6. *Treatment*

Identify drugs that are used to treat a patient with delirium.

Complete the table using Deglin et al, *Davis's Drug Guide for Nurses* 12e, or other drug reference.

Medication	Dose, Route, Frequency	Indications	Side Effect	Nursing Implications
Morphine	4 mg			
Lovenox	40 mg			
Ancef	1 g			

Medication	Dose, Route, Frequency	Indications	Side Effect	Nursing Implications
Toprol	50 mg			
Lasix	20 mg			
Colace	100 mg			

7. Nursing Problems/Diagnoses

Identify three priority nursing problems/diagnoses using NANDA diagnoses.
Complete for each problem identified:

Assessment Data	Priority Problem	Intervention	Expected Patient Outcome	Which Interventions Could Be Delegated to Unlicensed Personnel?
1.				
2.				
3.				

References

American Psychiatric Association (2000). *Diagnostic and statistical manual of mental disorders* (4th ed.). Washington, DC: APA.

Deglin, J. H., & Vallerand, A. H. (2009). *Davis's drug guide for nurses* (11th ed.). Philadelphia: F. A. Davis.

Dillon, P. (2007). *Nursing health assessment: A critical thinking and case studies approach* (2nd ed.). Philadelphia: F. A. Davis.

Erikson, E.H. (1950). *Childhood and society.* New York: Norton

Hartford Institute for Geriatric Nursing http://consultgerirn.org/topics/delirium/want_to_know_moreRetrieved 1/2/08

Inouye, S, van Dyck, C., Alessi, C., Balkin, S., Siegal, A., & Horwitz, R. (1990). Clarifying confusion: The confusion assessment method. *Annals of Internal Medicine*, *113*(12), 941-948.

Kuehn, B. (2010). Delirium often not recognized or treated despite serious long-term consequences. *JAMA, 304* (4), 389-390, 395.

Lagerquist, S. (2006). *Davis's NCLEX-RN success*. Philadelphia: F. A. Davis.

Neitzel, J., Sendelbach, S., & Larson, A. (2007). Delirium in the orthopedic patient. *Orthopedic Nursing, 26*(6), 354-363.

Nursing Standard of Practice Protocol: Delirium: Prevention, Early Recognition, and Treatment.

Tullman, D.F, Mion, L.C., Fletcher, K., & Foreman, M.D. (2008).

Van Leeuwen, A. M., Poelhuis-Leth, D. J., & Bladh, M. L. (2011). *Davis's comprehensive handbook of laboratory and diagnostic tests with nursing implications.* (4th ed.). Philadelphia: F. A. Davis.

Waszynski, C. (2007a). *The confusion assessment method* (CAM). *Try this: best practices in Nursing Care to Older Adults*, Issue Number 17. Retrieved from http://www.hartfordign.org/publications/trythis/issue*13*.pdf.

Waszynski, C. (2007b) How to try this: Detecting delirium. *AJN, American Journal of Nursing, 107*(12), 50-59.

Trauma/Emergency Nursing

7

7-1 Placental Abruption

TRAUMA

STANDARD FORMS

These templates are included in the Appendix; copy before each use.

LEARNING OUTCOMES

Cognitive

The student will be able to:

1. Demonstrate care of the pregnant trauma patient.
2. Identify factors in a patient's current condition that increase risk for placental abruption.
3. Identify symptoms of a possible placental abruption.
4. Identify the appropriate interventions for the patient with placental abruption.
5. Describe signs and symptoms of placental abruption.
6. Identify symptoms of antepartum hemorrhage.
7. Assess maternal and fetus by auscultation of fetal heart rate with a hand-held Doppler, palpating the abdomen, and evaluating vaginal bleeding.
8. Identify the significance of ultrasound assessment in placental abruption.
9. Identify indications of disseminated intravascular coagulation (DIC).
10. Analyze lab values for a pregnant trauma victim.
11. Differentiate the roles of team members in response to a pregnant patient with trauma.

Psychomotor

The student will be able to:

1. Assess fetal status using a hand-held Doppler.
2. Request presence of maternity staff to assess ongoing fetal status.
3. Respond to changes in fetal heart rate.
4. Perform appropriate assessment for a patient with placental abruption.
5. Initiate appropriate interventions for a patient with placental abruption.
6. Work collaboratively as part of the healthcare team in the care of a pregnant patient with trauma.

Affective

The student will be able to:

1. Reflect upon performance in the care of a pregnant patient with trauma to the abdomen.
2. Identify personal feelings in delivering care to a pregnant patient with trauma to the abdomen.
3. Discuss feelings related to working as a member of a team in the care of a pregnant patient with trauma to the abdomen.
4. Identify factors that worked well during the simulation of care of a patient with placental abruption.
5. Identify factors that needed improvement during the simulation of care of a patient with placental abruption.
6. Develop self-confidence as a trauma team member in the care of a patient with placental abruption.

Communication

The student will be able to:

1. Communicate effectively with healthcare team members in care of a patient with placental abruption.
2. Communicate effectively with the patient and family in the care of a patient with fetal compromise.
3. Use SBAR format when communicating with team members in the care of a pregnant patient with trauma.
4. Practice Transparent Thinking (thinking out loud) to facilitate group problem solving.
5. Use Directed Communication (directing a message to specific individual) when delegating tasks.
6. Employ Closed-Loop Communication (acknowledgment of receipt of the message and status) to acknowledge communications from others.

Safety

The student will be able to:

Administer and maintain specific protecting interventions with attention to safety of the client and healthcare professional.

1. Demonstrate a safe environment with attention to hazards to healthcare providers, visitors, and the client. Includes body mechanics, tripping hazards, and equipment issues.
2. Demonstrate attention to national patient safety goals. Includes patient identification standards, effective communication among healthcare providers, and safe medication administration.

3. Demonstrate attention to standard precautions. Includes hand washing, infection control measures, and use of personal protective equipment (PPE) as needed.

Leadership and Management/Delegation

The student will be able to:

1. Identify tasks that can be legally, ethically, and safely delegated to unlicensed assistive personnel (UAP) or licensed practical nurse (LPN) in the care of a pregnant patient with trauma.
2. Identify and prioritize patient's needs in placental abruption.
3. Request presence of OB staff to monitor fetal and maternal status.

OVERVIEW OF THE PROBLEM

Definition

Placental abruption (abruptio placentae) is the premature separation of a normally implanted placenta from the uterine wall.

Pathophysiology

Types of placental abruption:

- Partial: small part of placenta separates from uterine wall
- Complete: total placental separation
- Retroplacental: bleeding is concealed
- Marginal: separation occurs at edges, visible vaginal bleeding

Risk Factors

- Multiple gestation
- Prior abruption
- Thrombophilias
- Advanced maternal age
- Intrauterine infection
- Preeclampsia/eclampsia
- Before birth of second twin
- Traction on umbilical cord
- Rupture of membranes
- High parity
- Chronic renal hypertension
- Oxytocin induction or augmentation of labor
- Cocaine use
- Trauma

Assessment

Subjective

- Sudden onset of severe abdominal pain

Objective

- Rigid abdomen, uterine tenderness
- Presence of frequent contractions, uterine irritability or hypertonus (increased uterine tone), no relaxation between contractions
- Vaginal bleeding or increasing fundal height (assess fundal height compared to gestational age of fetus)
- Port wine–colored amniotic fluid
- Evidence of abnormal fetal heart rate pattern
- Fetal hyperactivity, bradycardia, death
- Sudden, rapid profound shock: may seem out of proportion to visible blood loss
- Signs of DIC

Diagnostic Tests

Medical evaluation will link to suspected etiology; tests are ordered based on differential diagnosis:

- Drug screen, thrombophilias, Kleihauer-Betke (KB)
- Screen for DIC: bleeding time, platelet count, prothrombim time (PT), activated partial thromboplastin time (APTT), fibrinogen, d-dimer
- Ultrasound to evaluate fetus and placenta

Treatment

- Fluid or blood replacement
- C-section

Nursing Management

- Position, supine with right hip elevated
- Left lateral side position
- Give oxygen
- Monitor vital signs, blood loss, fetal heart rate pattern and uterine activity
- I&O
- Control hemorrhage
- Administer crystalloid fluid, blood replacement as ordered
- IV heparin may be ordered to treat DIC: reduce coagulation and fibrinolysis
- Prepare for cesarean birth
- Emotional support

Evaluation/Outcome Criteria

- Successful outcome of pregnancy.
- Birth of viable viable newborn, usually via C-section
- Minimal maternal blood loss
- Assessment findings within normal limits
- Capacity for future childbearing is maintained
- No evidence of further complications such as anemia or DIC

REVIEW QUESTIONS

1. What are primary assessments for a pregnant trauma victim?
   Answer:

2. What is the rationale for tilting a pregnant patient to her side?
   Answer:

3. Is morphine (or fentanyl) appropriate for pain control in a pregnant patient?
   Answer:

4. Blood volume is normally increased by what percentage during pregnancy?
   Answer:

5. A trauma team usually consists of which essential team members?
   Answer:

Related Evidence-Based Practice Guidelines

Deering, S. (2007). Abruptio placentae. Retrieved from Emedicine.com/med/topic6.htm

Emergency Nurses Association. (2007). Emergency nursing core curriculum (6th ed.). Philadelphia: Saunders.

Mandeville, L. K., & Troiano,N H. (1999). AWHONN high-risk & critical care intrapartum nursing (2nd ed.). Philadelphia: Lippincott.

The Joint Commission National Patient Safety Goals Hospital Program. Retrieved from http://www.jointcommission.org/GeneralPublic/NPSG/10_npsgs.htm

SBAR technique for communication: A situational briefing model. The Institute for Healthcare Improvement. Retrieved December 19, 2008, from http://www.ihi.org/IHI/Topics/PatientSafety/SafetyGeneral/Tools/SBARTechniqueforCommunicationASituationalBriefingModel.htm

Topics to Review Prior to the Simulation

- Trauma in pregnancy, DIC
- Diagnostic tests: CBC, DIC panel, ultrasound reports
- Treatment: Splinting of an extremity
- Medications: Morphine sulfate, fentanyl
- Massive transfusion protocol: Cryoprecipitate, platelets, fresh frozen plasma

SIMULATION

Client Background

Biographical Data

- Age: 32
- Gender: female
- Height: 5 ft 4 in
- Weight: 187 lb

Cultural Considerations

- Language: English
- Ethnicity: not known
- Nationality: American
- Culture: No significant cultural considerations identified

Demographic

- Marital status: single
- Educational level: community college graduate
- Religion: none listed
- Occupation: paralegal

Current Health Status

- Pregnant 35 weeks' gestation, single-vehicle MVA about 30 min ago. She is being transported to the hospital emergency department by ambulance. She is complaining of pain in the back of the head, chest, abdomen, and right ankle. The pain is severe in the right ankle. She is 35 weeks' pregnant with her second child.

History

- Psychosocial history
  - Social support: father of baby supportive, living together, currently out of town
- Past health history: not known
  - Previous OB history: delivered vaginally at 41 wk male weight 7 lb 10 oz, labor 14 hr.
- Medical: mild anemia, smokes 1/2 ppd × 10 yr.
  - Surgical: none
- Family history: mother has type 2 diabetes. Father and paternal grandfather have hypertension

Admission Sheet

Name:	Ashley Simmons
Age:	32
Gender:	Female
Marital Status:	Single

Continued

Admission Sheet—cont'd

Educational Level:	Community college graduate
Religion:	Unknown
Ethnicity:	Unknown
Nationality:	American
Language:	English
Occupation:	Paralegal

Hospital
Provider's Orders

Patient's Name: Ashley Simmons
Allergies: NKDA

Diagnosis: IUP 35 wks, single-vehicle MVA

Date	Time	Order	Signature
Today	Stat	Vital signs: Trauma protocol	
		Diet: NPO	
		Activity: Bedrest	
		IV therapy: Normal saline 150 mL/hr	
		Medication: Morphine sulfate 2 mg IVP prn Fentanyl 25 mcg q 1 hr prn	
		Diagnostic studies: Trauma labs: CBC, d-dimer UA, type and screen (T&S), amylase, ETOH, chem screen, PT/PTT, urine tox screen X-ray: C-spine, CXR, right ankle, left clavicle Fetal ultrasound	
		Treatments: Splint right ankle	Dr. Storer

Nursing Report

Report given first (ambulance report to ED): "This is Sweet Home Ambulance. We are about to be en route to Samaritan Lebanon Community Hospital with a 32-year-old female from a single-vehicle motor vehicle crash. Her primary care physician is Dr. Blake. She is complaining of severe pain in the right ankle. It was turned in severely and she would not let us splint it. She also has pain in the back of the head, left chest, and abdomen. She is alert and oriented, 35 weeks' pregnant, no contractions, rupture of membranes, or bleeding. Vital signs are stable, we inserted two IVs in her right arm, O_2 is going at 2 L, and a hard cervical collar is in place. We should be there in about 15 min."

Report from EMT as patient arrives: "This is Ashley Simmons from the motor vehicle crash. She was on her way to work in the attorney's office in Sweet Home. Her right foot was pinned under the foot controls. She was wearing a seat belt and has some discomfort where each strap was located. The air bags deployed and her head must have hit the headrest. We gave her 4 mg morphine sulfate for her ankle pain. Vitals are unchanged. Fetal heart sounds were 140s. Her boyfriend is out of town but she did get in touch with her mother and she will be coming down. Her 2-year-old son is with a babysitter.

Student Simulation Prep Assignments

1. Identify items and their purpose in the care of a patient with trauma during pregnancy.

Item	Purpose
Fetal monitor	
Precipitous delivery pack	
Chux pads	
Splinting material	
Cervical collar	
Doppler ultrasound	
Rapid infuser	

2. Identify team members and their specific roles in the care of a patient with trauma during pregnancy.

Team Member	Role
Emergency department physician	
Nurses	
Respiratory therapy	
Supervisor	
Clergy	
Lab, radiology	
Surgeon, OR staff	

3. Relevant Data Exercise: Fill in the columns below.

Relevant Data from Report	Relevant Data from Other Sources	Data Missing	Sources for Missing Data	Data Requiring Follow-up

4. Initial Focused Assessment

After reviewing the client background and nursing report, you are ready to assess your client's current status. Under each category, identify how you would target your assessment and what you would expect to find for the patient with trauma during pregnancy.

History

Are there any questions you need to ask the patient or family to obtain additional relevant data?

Physical Exam

- General appearance:
- Integumentary:
- HEENT:
- Respiratory:
- CV:
- Breasts:
- Abdominal:

- Neuro:
- Musculoskeletal:
- Reproductive:
- Additional: None
- Developmental:

What are the nursing implications considering the developmental stage of your patient.

Answer:

5. Diagnostic Tests

What diagnostic test results relevant to the patient's current problem are needed to plan care?

Complete the table using Van Leeuwen et al, *Davis's Comprehensive Handbook of Laboratory and Diagnostic Testing with Nursing Implications* 4e, or other diagnostic test reference.

Diagnostic Test	Significance to This Patient's Problem
CBC	
D-dimer	
UA	
T&S	
Amylase	
ETOH	
Chem screen	
PT	
PTT	
Urine toxicology screen	
X-ray: C-spine	
CXR	
Right ankle	
Left clavicle	
Fetal ultrasound	

6. Treatment

Identify drugs that are used to treat a pregnant trauma patient

Complete the table using Deglin et al, *Davis's Drug Guide for Nurses* 12e, or other drug reference.

Medication	Dose, Route, Frequency	Indications	Side Effect	Nursing Implications
Morphine sulfate	2 mg IV q 4 hr prn.			

Medication	Dose, Route, Frequency	Indications	Side Effect	Nursing Implications
Fentanyl	Adjunct to general anesthetic. Adults: For low-dose therapy, 2 mcg/kg IV. For moderate-dose therapy, 2–20 mcg/kg IV; then 25–100 mcg IV prn. For high-dose therapy, 20–50 mcg/kg IV then 25 mcg to ½ initial loading dose IV prn.			

7. Nursing Problems/Diagnoses

Identify three priority nursing problems/diagnoses.

Assessment Data	Priority Problem	Intervention	Expected Patient Outcome	Which Interventions Could Be Delegated to Unlicensed Personnel?
1.				
2.				

Continued

Assessment Data	Priority Problem	Intervention	Expected Patient Outcome	Which Interventions Could Be Delegated to Unlicensed Personnel?
3.				

References

Deering, S. (2007). *Abruptio placentae*. Retrieved from Emedicine.com/med/topic6.htm

Deglin, J. H., & Vallerand, A. H. (2009). *Davis's drug guide for nurses* (11th ed.). Philadelphia: F. A. Davis.

Dillon, P. (2007). *Nursing health assessment: A critical thinking and case studies approach* (2nd ed.). Philadelphia: F. A. Davis.

Emergency Nurses Association. (2007) *Emergency nursing core curriculum.* (6th ed.). Philadelphia: Saunders.

Erikson, E.H. (1950). *Childhood and society.* New York: Norton.

Lagerquist, S. L. (2006). *Davis's NCLEX-RN for success.* Philadelphia: F. A. Davis.

Mandeville, L. K., & Troiano, N H. (1999). *AWHONN high-risk & critical care intrapartum nursing* (2nd ed.) Philadelphia: Lippincott.

Van Leeuwen, A. M., Poelhuis-Leth, D. J., & Bladh, M. L. (2011). *Davis's comprehensive handbook of laboratory and diagnostic tests with nursing implications.* (4th ed.). Philadelphia: F. A. Davis.

7-2 Gunshot Wound

TRAUMA

STANDARD FORMS

These templates are included in the Appendix; copy before each use.

LEARNING OUTCOMES

Cognitive

The student will be able to:

1. Describe the initial process that occurs with assessment of all trauma patients.
2. Identify the signs and symptoms (S/S) of hypoxemia and decreased cardiac output.
3. Identify appropriate intervention for a patient with a GSW.
4. Describe potential secondary injuries that occur from a GSW.

Psychomotor

The student will be able:

1. Perform an assessment on a patient with a GSW.
2. Initiate appropriate interventions, such as start and maintain IV, obtain stat vital signs, and administer appropriate medications.
3. Manage the care of a patient with a chest tube.

Affective

The student will be able to:

1. Reflect upon performance in a simulated simulation of care for a patient with a GSW.
2. Identify what worked well during the simulation.
3. Identify areas that need improvement.
4. Reflect on overall feeling about the scenario.
5. Discuss feelings related to working as a team member.
6. Develop confidence in caring for a patient with a GSW.
7. Perform self-reflective evaluation.

Communication

The student will be able to:

1. Communicate effectively with healthcare team members in the care of a patient with a GSW.
2. Communicate effectively with the patient and family members.
3. Use SBAR format when communicating with healthcare team members.
4. Work collaboratively as part of the healthcare team.
5. Accurately and succinctly document assessments, interventions, and evaluations.
6. Practice Transparent Thinking (thinking out loud) to facilitate group problem solving.
7. Use Directed Communication (directing a message to specific individual) when delegating tasks.
8. Employ Closed-Loop Communication (acknowledgment of receipt of the message and status) to acknowledge communications from others.

Safety

The student will be able to:

Administer and maintain specific protecting interventions with attention to safety of the client and healthcare professional.

1. Demonstrate a safe environment with attention to hazards to healthcare providers, visitors, and the client. Includes body mechanics, tripping hazards, and equipment issues.
2. Demonstrate attention to national patient safety goals. Includes patient identification standards, effective communication among healthcare providers, and safe medication administration.
3. Demonstrate attention to standard precautions. Includes hand washing, infection control measures, and use of personal protective equipment (PPE) as needed.

Leadership and Management/Delegation

The student will be able to:

1. Prioritize interventions in the care of a patient with GSW.
2. Identify interventions that can be delegated to unlicensed assistive personnel (UAP) and secondary nurse in the care of a patient with a GSW.
3. Work collaboratively in performing an assessment with the nurse practitioner and physician.
4. Delegate appropriately to team members.

OVERVIEW OF THE PROBLEM

Definition

Trauma is the number one cause of death in the United States for persons aged 1–44 years. (National Trauma Data Bank, 2009 at www.ntdbdatacenter.com)

Types of trauma:

- MVA 41.3%
- Falls 27.2%
- GSW 5.6%
- Drowning 0.1%

Pathophysiology

Trauma deaths:

- First peak: Major neurological or vascular injury results in death within minutes. Intervention usually not successful.
- Second peak (golden hour): Major injury intracranial hematoma, major thoracic, or abdominal injury. Prompt care during the golden hour increases survival rates.
- Third peak: Occurs days to weeks after trauma; death may occur from sepsis or multiple system failure.

Complications of chest trauma:

- Pneumothorax: Presence of air in the pleural cavity
- Hemothorax: Presence of blood in the pleural cavity.
- Pressure builds in the pleural space, lung on affected side collapses, heart and mediastinum shift toward the unaffected lung.

Risk Factors for Trauma

- Larger societal influences and individual psychosocial factors increase the risk of being a victim of violence.

Assessment

- Primary assessment: ABCDE
  - **A:** Airway; stabilize neck if cervical spine injury suspected; intubation with endotracheal tube may be indicated.
  - **B:** Breathing; may need to ventilate; administer oxygen.
  - **C:** Circulation; is there bleeding? check BP, pulses, pulse ox.
  - **D:** Disability; neurovascular assessment; check for mental status, pupils.
  - **E:** Expose injury; remove clothes, recover patient, and rewarm to avoid hypothermia.
- Secondary assessment: SAMPLE
- Interview
  - **S:** Symptoms
  - **A:** Allergies
  - **M:** Medications
  - **P:** Preexisting conditions
  - **L:** Last ate
  - **E:** Events leading up to injury

Subjective

- Sudden, severe, sharp pain
- Dyspnea
- Anxiety, fear, restlessness, weakness

Objective

- Vital signs, signs of shock
- Pallor or cyanosis
- Asymmetrical chest expansion
- Visible chest wound with rush of air through site
- Crepitus over site
- Distended neck veins
- Hemothorax: Blood in the pleural space. From blunt or penetrating trauma. S/S dependent on extent of bleed:
  - SOB
  - Decreased breath sounds
  - Dullness
  - Decreased chest expansion. Decreased pulse ox, massive bleed can lead to mediastinal shift and tracheal deviation.

Diagnostic Tests

- CXR
- ABGs
- CBC
- T&S
- PT/PTT/INR

Treatment

- Thoracic surgey if indicated
- Endotracheal tube
- Ventilation
- Thoracentesis
- Pain medications
- Fluid and or blood replacement

Nursing Management

Initiate interventions

- Apply air-occlusive dressing over wound (as patient exhales forcefully, Valsalva's maneuver helps expand collapsed lung by creating positive intrapulmonary pressure)
- Maintain chest drainage system
- Monitor amount and color of tube drainage every 15 min with vital signs during initial resusicitation then q 2 hr
- Notify physician if drainage >100 mL/hr
- Chest drainage system should be 1 ft (30 cm) below chest insertion site
- Air bubbles may be in water seal chamber 24–48 hr post-insertion
- Persistent air bubbles in water-seal chamber indicates air leak
- Slight fluctuation (tidaling) in water seal is normal and r/t respirations
- Bubbling in suction chamber is normal
- Ensure tube is kink free
- Fowler's position facilitates drainage
- Have sterile air-occlusive dressing at bedside in case of accidental disconnection or if tube becomes disconnected place tubing end in sterile water or saline

- Clamp the tube only when checking for air leaks; the tube should not be clamped for more than 10 sec, may cause tension pneumothorax, or unless ordered by physician (may order chest tube clamped prior to removal to verify readiness for removal)
- Stripping the tube should be avoided because it affects the intrapulmonary pressure and may damage the lung. The chest tube can be gently squeezed between your fingers and released to facilitate drainage
- Check for air leaks: palpate for crepitus around chest tube insertion site
- Medicate for pain prior to removal
- Assess breath sounds before and after removal
  - Maintain ventilation
  - Monitor VS
  - Control pain (give medications with caution to avoid respiratory depression)
- Prevent infection
- Any trauma creates the potential for shock; hemorrhage most common cause
- Treatment:
  - Insert 2 large-gauge intravenous catheters
  - Fluid resuscitation, administer:
    - Lactated Ringer's
    - Blood products
- Monitor VS
- Monitor blood gases
- Monitor urine output

Evaluation/Outcome Criteria

- Respiratory status stabilizes, lung reexpands
- Shock and hemorrhage are prevented
- No further injury occurs
- Pain and anxiety are controlled
- Chest tube is removed when there is little or no drainage
- Air leak disappears
- Fluctuation stops in water seal

REVIEW QUESTIONS

1. What are the steps in priority order of the assessment that should be used on every trauma patient?
Answer:

2. What are the signs and symptoms of a hemothorax?
Answer:

3. Why is a chest tube inserted in a patient with an open chest wound and decreased lung sounds before waiting for an x-ray to confirm?
Answer:

4. Why is a dose of antibiotics given to the patient with no infectious process?
Answer:

5. What is the most important laboratory sample to obtain on any patient with a traumatic injury?
Answer:

6. What are common associated injuries from a GSW to the chest?
Answer:

7. When setting up the chest tube, how much water is used for the water seal? How much for suction?
Answer:

Related Evidence-Based Practice Guidelines

American College of Surgeons (2009). National Trauma Data Bank 2009: Annual report. Retrieved from http://www.facs.org/trauma/ntdb/docpub.html

The Joint Commission National Patient Safety Goals Hospital Program. Retrieved from http://www.jointcommission.org/GeneralPublic/NPSG/10_npsgs.htm

SBAR technique for communication: A situational briefing model. The Institute for Healthcare Improvement. Retrieved December 19, 2008, from http://www.ihi.org/IHI/Topics/PatientSafety/SafetyGeneral/Tools/SBARTechniqueforCommunicationASituationalBriefing Model.htm

Topics to Review Prior to the Simulation

- Trauma care and assessment
- Chest trauma
- Hemothorax
- Pneumothorax
- Care of chest tubes
- IV therapy
- Medication administration

SIMULATION

Client Background

Biographical Data

- Age: 29
- Gender: male
- Height: 6 ft
- Weight: 195 lb

Cultural Considerations

- Language: English
- Ethnicity: African American
- Nationality: American
- Culture: Potential cultural considerations, important for caregivers to avoid stereotyping and making assumptions in the provision of care to victims of violence

Demographic

- Marital status: unknown
- Educational level: unknown
- Religion: unknown
- Occupation: unknown

Current Health Status

- GSW to back. Bystander called 911 outside after hearing gunshots in Chinese take-out store and witnessing someone falling to ground after noise.

History

- Psychosocial history: unknown
  - Social support: unknown
- Past health history
  - Medical: negative
  - Surgical: unknown
- Family History: unknown

Admission Sheet

Name:	Norman Williams
Age:	29
Gender:	Male
Marital Status:	Unknown
Educational Level:	Unknown
Religion:	Unknown
Ethnicity:	African American
Nationality:	American
Language:	English
Occupation:	Unknown

Hospital Provider's Orders

Patient's Name: Norman Williams
Allergies: NKDA

Diagnosis: Gunshot wound left lower back/hemothorax left lower lobe

Date	Time	Order	Signature
6/20/07	1:15 AM	Vital Signs: q 15 min × 4	
		Diet: NPO	
		Activity: Bed rest	
		Diagnostic studies:	
		STAT CBC, BMP, BUN and creatinine PT/PTT,INR T&S, type and cross 4 units, ABGs	
		Large-bore IV × 2, LR 1 L W/O, LR 1 L at 250/hr, monitor, pulse ox, oxygen NRB or NC PRN	

Diagnosis: Gunshot wound left lower back/hemothorax left lower lobe—cont'd

Date	Time	Order	Signature
		Other: Chest tube to wall suction Medications: Morphine 4 mg IVP Tetanus toxoid 0.5 mL IM	
		Cefazolin 1g IVPB	
		IV therapy: 2 large-bore IVs 1,000 mL LR wide open STAT Followed by 1,000 mL LR to maintain SBP >90	
		Oxygen: NRB or NC to maintain saturation 95%	
		Hold in ED until CXR and results	
		Radiology: CXR and abdominal flat plate	Dr. B. Munez

Nursing Report

Fire Rescue: Arrived to find 29-year-old male with bleeding from back after witness heard two bullets fired. Patient denies any medical history, allergies, or medications. Awakens to verbal stimuli. Vital signs HR 120, BP 96/40, and RR 24.

Student Simulation Prep Assignments

1. Identify items and their purpose in the care of a patient with a GSW.

Item	Purpose
LR bags/IV tubing	
O_2 non-rebreather mask, cannula	
IM syringe	
Chest tube and insertion set	
Pleurovac	
Autotransfuser	

2. Identify team members and their specific roles in the care of a patient with a GSW.

Team Member	Role
Nurse practitioner	
Primary nurse	
Secondary nurse	
Physician	
UAP	
Pastoral care	

Continued

3. *Relevant Data Exercise:* Fill in the columns below.

Relevant Data from Report	Relevant Data from Other Sources	Data Missing	Sources for Missing Data	Data Requiring Follow-up

4. *Initial Focused Assessment*

After reviewing the client background and nursing report, you are ready to assess your client's current status. Under each category, identify how you would target your assessment and what you would expect to find for the patient with gun shot wounds Initial focused assessment should include ABCs.

History

Are there any questions you need to ask the patient or family to obtain additional relevant data?

Physical Examination

- General appearance:
- Integumentary:
- HEENT:
- Respiratory:
- CV:
- Breasts:
- Abdominal:
- Neuro:
- Musculoskeletal:
- Reproductive:
- Additional:
- Renal:
- Developmental:

What are the nursing implications considering the developmental stage of your patient?

Answer:

5. *Diagnostic Tests*

What diagnostic test results relevant to the patient's current problem are needed to plan care?

Complete the table using Van Leeuwen et al, *Davis's Comprehensive Handbook of Laboratory and Diagnostic Testing with Nursing Implications* 4e, or other diagnostic test reference.

Diagnostic Test	Significance to This Patient's Problem
BMP	
BUN and creatinine	
ABGs	
CBC	
PT, PTT, INR	
UA	
T&S and T&C 4 units	
Flat plate abdomen	
Chest x-ray	

6. Treatment

Identify drugs that are used to treat a patient with a GSW.

Complete the table using Deglin et al, *Davis's Drug Guide for Nurses* 12e, or other drug reference.

Medication	Dose, Route, Frequency	Indications	Side Effect	Nursing Implications
Tetanus toxoid	0.5 mL IM			
Morphine	4 mg IV push			
Cefazolin (Ancef)	1 g IVPB			

7. Nursing Problems/Diagnoses

Identify three priority nursing problems/diagnoses.

Complete for each problem identified.

Assessment Data	Priority Problem	Intervention	Expected Patient Outcome	Which Interventions Could Be Delegated to Unlicensed Personnel?
1.				

Continued

Assessment Data	Priority Problem	Intervention	Expected Patient Outcome	Which Interventions Could Be Delegated to Unlicensed Personnel?
2.				
3.				

References

American Heart Association. (2006). *Heartsaver first aid with CPR and AED.* Dallas: APA.

Deglin, J. H., & Vallerand, A. H. (2009). *Davis's drug guide for nurses* (11th ed.). Philadelphia: F. A. Davis.

Dillon, P. (2007). *Nursing health assessment: A critical thinking case studies approach* (2nd ed.). Philadelphia: F. A. Davis.

Erikson, E.H. (1950). *Childhood and society.* New York: Norton.

Lagerquist, S. L. (2006). *Davis's NCLEX-RN for success* (2nd ed.). Philadelphia: F. A. Davis.

Ouimet Perrin, K. (2009). *Understanding the essentials of critical care nursing.* Upper Saddle River, NJ: Pearson Prentice Hall.

Van Leeuwen, A. M., Poelhuis-Leth, D. J., & Bladh, M. L. (2011). *Davis's comprehensive handbook of laboratory and diagnostic tests with nursing implications.* (4th ed.). Philadelphia: F. A. Davis.

7-3 Stroke

EMERGENCY DEPARTMENT, ADULT HEALTH

STANDARD FORMS

These templates are included in the Appendix; copy before each use.

LEARNING OUTCOMES

Cognitive

The student will be able to:

1. Describe signs and symptoms of cerebrovascular ischemia.
2. Correlate signs and symptoms of cerebrovascular ischemia to the pathophysiology of cerebrovascular infarction.
3. Identify factors in a patient's history that increase risk for cerebrovascular disease.
4. Identify factors in a patient's current condition that increase risk for cerebrovascular infarction.
5. Identify the appropriate interventions for the patient with altered cerebral tissue perfusion.
6. Differentiate the roles of team members in response to a patient with acute stroke.

Psychomotor

The student will be able to:

1. Perform appropriate assessment for a patient with altered cerebral tissue perfusion.
2. Initiate appropriate interventions to initiate when responding to a patient with an acute stroke emergency.
3. Work collaboratively as part of the healthcare team in the care of a patient with altered cerebral tissue perfusion.
4. Identify the medication history and accurately calculate medication dosages.
5. Perform a dysphagia assessment using an evidenced-based bedside screening tool.

Affective

The student will be able to:

1. Reflect upon performance in the care of a patient with acute stroke symptoms.
2. Identify personal feelings in delivering care to a patient with acute alteration in neurological status.
3. Discuss feelings related to working as a member of a team in the care of a patient with acute stroke symptoms.
4. Identify factors that worked well during the simulation of care of a patient with acute stroke emergency.
5. Identify factors that needed improvement during the simulation of care of a patient with acute stroke emergency.
6. Develop self-confidence in the care of a patient with altered cerebral tissue perfusion.

Communication

The student will be able to:

1. Communicate effectively with healthcare team members in care of a patient with altered cerebral tissue perfusion.
2. Communicate effectively with the patient and family in the care of a patient with acute stroke.
3. Use SBAR format when communicating with team members in the care of a patient with acute stroke.
4. Practice Transparent Thinking (thinking out loud) to facilitate group problem solving.
5. Use Directed Communication (directing a message to specific individual) when delegating tasks.
6. Employ Closed-Loop Communication (acknowledgment of receipt of the message and status) to acknowledge communications from others.

Safety

The student will be able to:

Administer and maintain specific protecting interventions with attention to safety of the client and healthcare professional.

1. Demonstrate a safe environment with attention to hazards to healthcare providers, visitors, and the client. Includes body mechanics, tripping hazards, and equipment issues.
2. Demonstrate attention to national patient safety goals. Includes patient identification standards, effective communication among healthcare providers, and safe medication administration.
3. Demonstrate attention to standard precautions. Includes hand washing, infection control measures, and use of personal protective equipment (PPE) as needed.

Leadership and Management/Delegation

The student will be able to:

1. Identify tasks that can be legally, ethically, and safely delegated to unlicensed assistive personnel (UAP) or licensed practical nurse (LPN) in the care of a patient with altered cerebral tissue perfusion.
2. Identify and prioritize patient's needs in care of acute stroke emergency.
3. Discuss the necessary teaching related to diagnostic workup of acute stroke.
4. Describe the cultural communication needs of a patient who does not speak English and how patient's ethnicity affects treatment plan.

5. State the nursing priorities for initial evaluation of a stroke patient.
6. Identify legal/ethical considerations if FDA treatment is not offered.
7. Discuss the barriers to providing care if hospital does not have a systematic detailed plan for emergency care in an acute stroke where time is crucial.

OVERVIEW OF THE PROBLEM

DEFINITION

Two problems are discussed: Transient ischemic attack (TIA) and stroke.

- TIA is temporary, complete, or relatively complete cessation of cerebral blood flow to a localized brain area producing symptoms (2–30 min) ranging from weakness and numbness to blindness; an important precursor to stroke.
- Stroke (cerebral vascular accident or brain attack): neurological changes caused by interruption of blood supply to a part of the brain. Two types:
  - Ischemic stroke: commonly due to thrombosis or embolism, more common.
  - Hemorrhagic stroke: rupture of a cerebral vessel, causing a brain bleed, most common after 50 years of age.

Pathophysiology

- Reduced or interrupted blood flow causes interruption of nerve impulses, leading to decreased or absent voluntary movement on one side of the body. Later, autonomous reflex activity leads to spastic and rigid muscles.

Risk Factors

- Hypertension
- Prior TIAs
- Cardiovascular disease
- Oral contraceptives
- Emotional stress
- Family history
- Advancing age
- Diabetes mellitus
- Smoking

Assessment

Subjective

- Weakness
- Difficulty speaking
- Difficulty swallowing
- Nausea/vomiting
- History of TIAs

Objective

- Vitals signs: Blood pressure elevated with thrombosis; widened pulse pressure with hemorrhage; temperature elevated; pulse normal or slow; respirations: tachypnea, altered pattern, deep, sonorous.
- Neurological symptoms vary by type and location of injury: Altered level of consciousness; unequal pupils; visual field blindness; ptosis; hemiplegia; loss of sensation and reflexes; incontinence; aphasia; central and peripheral palsy.

Diagnostic Tests

- CT scan of head: Negative if no hemorrhage, indicates ischemic stroke

Treatment

- Medications
- Ventilation
- IV fluids

Medical and Nursing Management

Goal: Reduce cerebral anoxia.

- Patient airway:
  - Oxygen as ordered
  - Suctioning as needed
  - Turn, cough, deep breathe
- Activity:
  - Bed rest, progressing as tolerated
- Position: Maximize ventilation:
  - Support with pillows
  - Hand rolls, arm slings, etc., as ordered

Goal: Promote cerebral perfusion and maintain function.

- Vitals signs
- Medication:
  - Ischemic stroke: thrombolytic agents within 3 hr of onset, antihypertensives if BP >185 systolic or 105 diastolic, mannitol to decrease ICP, heparin only if at risk for cardiogenic emboli, antiplatelet agents to decrease thrombus formation
  - Hemorrhagic stroke: antihypertensives for systolic >160, never treat with thrombolytics, mannitol to decrease ICP
- Fluids
- ROM exercises
- Skin care

Goal: Provide for emotional relaxation.

- Identify grief reaction
- Encourage expression of feelings

Goal: Client safety.

- Identify sensory deficits
- Use side rails and assists
- Ambulation safety

Goal: Health teaching

- Exercise
- Diet
- Resumption of self-care as tolerated
- Use of supportive devices

Evaluation/Outcome Criteria

- No complications
- Functional independence
- Return of control of body functions

REVIEW QUESTIONS

1. Identify the two types of stroke.
   Answer:

2. Hypoglycemia is ruled out using which of the following:
   A. Point of care testing
   B. Serum lab sample
   C. Urine dip test
   Answer:

3. A noncontrast CT scan shows which of the following :
   A. Blood vessels
   B. Carotid arteries
   C. Intracranial hemorrhage
   D. Blood flow to brain
   Answer:

4. All of the following are signs of a stroke except:
   A. Weakness/numbness face, arm and leg
   B. Severe headache
   C. Abdominal discomfort
   D. Difficulty with speech
   Answer:

5. The medication that may reverse an ischemic stroke given in first 3 hours from symptom onset is:
   A. Heparin
   B. Integrillin
   C. Activase
   D. Plavix
   Answer:

Related Evidence-Based Practice Guidelines

ACLS Training Center. ACLS Suspected Stroke Algorithm. Available at: http://www.acls.net/acls-suspected-stroke-algorithm.htm

Summers, D., Leonard, A., Wentworth, D., Saver, J., Simpson, J., Spilker, J., et al. (2009, May). Stroke. Comprehensive overview of nursing and interdisciplinary care of the acute ischemic stroke patient. A scientific statement from the American Heart Association. doi:10.1161/STROKEAHA.109.192362. Retrieved from http://stroke.ahajournals.org/cgi/reprint/STROKEAHA.109.192362

Pugh, S., Mathiesen, C., Meighan, M., Summers D. (2007). Guide to the care of the patient with ischemic stroke. AANN reference series for clinical practice (2nd ed.). Retrieved from http://stroke. ahajournals.org/cgi/reprint/STROKEAHA.109.192362

Update to the AHA/ASA recommendations for the prevention of stroke in patients with stroke and transient ischemic attack (2008). Retrieved Jan 2011 from :http://stroke.ahajournals.org/cgi/content/full/39/5/1647Guidelines for the early management of adults with ischemic stroke. (2007). Retrieved Jan 2011 from http://stroke.ahajournals.org/cgi/content/full/38/5/1655

The Joint Commission National Patient Safety Goals Hospital Program. Retrieved from http://www.jointcommission.org/GeneralPublic/NPSG/10_npsgs.htm

SBAR Technique for Communication: A situational briefing model. The Institute for Healthcare Improvement. Retrieved December 19, 2008, from http://www.ihi.org/IHI/Topics/PatientSafety/SafetyGeneral/Tools/SBARTechniqueforCommunicationASituationalBriefingModel.htm

Topics to Review Prior to the Simulation

- Neurological Assessment
  - NIH stroke scale available at: http://www.ninds.nih.gov/doctors/NIH_Stroke_Scale.pdf
  - Bedside dysphagia screening
  - Assessment for Bell's palsy
- Fluid and electrolytes for neuro patient
- Oxygenation
- Pharmacology
- Cerebral autoregulation
- Brain physiology

Additional suggested reading:

Mathiesen, C., Tavianini H., Palladino K. (2006). Best practices in stroke rapid response: A case study. *Medical-surgical nursing, 15*(6), 364–369.

SIMULATION

Client Background

Biographical Data

- Age: 24
- Gender: female
- Height: 5 ft 2 in
- Weight: 190 lb

Cultural Considerations

- Language: Spanish
- Ethnicity: Hispanic
- Nationality: Puerto Rican
- Culture: Recently immigrated from Puerto Rico. Extended large Hispanic family arrives and wants information about patient condition. Most do not speak English.

Demographic

- Marital status: single
- Educational level: 12th grade
- Religion: Catholic
- Occupation: cashier at Wal-Mart

Current Health Status

- 24-year-old white Hispanic female with acute-onset right facial droop, right-sided weakness, dysarthia, aphasia onset at 10 AM.

History

- Psychosocial history: single, history of depression
  - Social support: family live in Puerto Rico, patient living with relatives.
- Past health history:
  - Medical: migraines, hypertension, irregular heart rate, obesity, asthma, chronic low back pain, + smoker 1 ppd since age 13.
  - Surgical: no surgeries
- Family history
  - Mother died at age 45 of cerebral aneurysm
  - Father has diabetes, high blood pressure, and has had two heart attacks
  - Four siblings: one deceased of heart disease, sister with diabetes, one brother with asthma, and one brother with high blood pressure and thyroid problems

Admission Sheet

Name:	Maria Lopez
Age:	24
Gender:	Female
Marital Status:	Single
Educational Level:	12th grade, GED
Religion:	Catholic
Ethnicity:	Hispanic
Nationality:	Puerto Rican
Language:	Spanish, English second language
Occupation:	Cashier at local Wal-Mart

Hospital
Provider's Orders

Patient's Name: Maria Lopez
Allergies: Shellfish, sulfa

Diagnosis: Rule out acute stroke

Date	Time	Order	Signature
		Vital signs: q 15 min	
		Diet: NPO pending dysphagia assessment	
		Activity: Bed rest	
		IV therapy: 0.9 NSS at 125 cc/hr	
		Start 2 lines	
		Medications: Activase 0.9 mg/kg. Give 10% bolus over 1–2 min Hang remaining 90 % amount over 1 hr Total dose should not exceed 90 mg Labetalol 10–20 mg IV q 10 min if SBP >185 mm Hg or DBP >105 mm Hg	

Diagnosis: Rule out acute stroke—cont'd

Date	Time	Order	Signature
		Cardene 25 mg/250 NSS titrate to keep SBP <180 mm Hg prn	
		Hold heparin for 24 hr following t-PA infusion	
		Diagnostic studies:	
		Noncontrast CT head r/o bleed stat	
		CBC, Chem 7, MI profile, coagulation profile	
		If on Coumadin, send T&S	
		Urine HCG	
		Treatments:	
		Document vital signs and neuro checks q 15 min for 2 hr, then q 30 min for 6 hr, and finally every hr for 16 hr	
		NIH Stroke Scale on admission and if any neurological worsening	
		Bleeding precautions: Check puncture sites for bleeding or hematomas. Apply pressure to bleeding sites. No intra-arterial puncture, IM injections, or central venous access during t-PA infusion or for 12 hr following infusion	
		Insert Foley catheter before t-PA started	
		Notify physician:	
		Systolic BP >185 or <110	
		Diastolic BP >105 or <60	
		P <50	
		RR >24 or <10	
		Decline in neurological status or worsening of stroke symptoms	
		Monitor for signs of allergic reaction or anaphylaxis	
		If diabetic or blood sugar >120, point of care finger stick blood sugar q 6 hr; if blood sugar >150, follow insulin protocol.	
		Consults:	
		Critical care medicine re: medical management	
		Rehab team: physical therapy, occupational therapy, and speech therapy assess rehab needs	
		Smoking cessation	
		Other orders:	
		Carotid doppler ultrasound	
		CT angio of head and neck	
		Cerebral arteriogram	
		2D echocardiogram	
		MRI/MRA of brain	
		Provide stroke education	
			Dr. Newman

Nursing Report

Patient received from EMS: 24-year-old Hispanic woman sudden onset of right facial droop, right-sided weakness, and difficulty with speech. Visibly upset woman elevated blood pressure, rapid respirations, and pulse oximeter is reading 90%.

Hand off from triage to primary nurse: 24-year-old woman with stroke symptoms: onset <3 hr. BP 174/92, HR 98, RR 24/min on r/a, pulse ox 90%. IV started left antecubital 18-gauge NSS running at KVO. Neuro: right-sided symptoms, difficulty with speech. Primary nurse and ED team (physician + pharmacy + UAP). Begin the workup using ACLS guideline to treat acute ischemic stroke.

Student Simulation Prep Assignments

1. Identify items and their purpose in the care of a patient with acute ischemic stroke.

Item	Purpose
Stroke ACLS algorithm	
TPA checklist	
NIH stroke scale	
IV equipment	
Bedside swallowing assessment	

2. Identify team members and their specific roles in the care of a patient with acute ischemic stroke in an emergency department setting.

Team Member	Role
Triage nurse	
Primary nurse	
Pharmacy	
Unlicensed assistive personnel	
Translator	
Physician	

3. Relevant Data Exercise: Fill in columns below.

Relevant Data from Report	Relevant Data from Other Sources	Data Missing	Sources for Missing Data	Data Requiring Follow-up

4. Initial Focused Assessment

After reviewing the client background and nursing report, you are ready to assess your client's current status. Under each category, identify how you would target your assessment and what you would expect to find for the patient with alteration in cerebral tissue perfusion.

History

Are there any questions you need to ask the patient or family to obtain additional relevant data?

Physical Exam

- General appearance:
- Integumentary:
- HEENT:
- Respiratory:
- CV:
- Breasts:
- Abdominal:
- Neuro:
- Musculoskeletal:
- Reproductive:
- Additional:
- Developmental:

What are the nursing implications considering the developmental stage of your patient?

Answer:

5. Diagnostic Tests

Which diagnostic test results relevant to the patient's current problem are needed to plan care?

Complete the table using Van Leeuwen et al, *Davis's Comprehensive Handbook of Laboratory and Diagnostic Testing with Nursing Implications* 4e, or other diagnostic test reference.

Diagnostic Test	Significance to This Patient's Problem
CBC	
Chem 7	
Coagulation profile	
MI profile	
Pregnancy test	

6. Treatment

Identify drugs that are used to treat a patient with stroke.

Complete the table using Deglin et al, *Davis's Drug Guide for Nurses* 12e, or other drug reference.

Medication	Dose, Route, Frequency	Indications	Side Effect	Nursing Implications
Activase	0.9 mg/kg			
Labetalol	10–20 mg			
Cardene	5 mg/hr may titrate to 15 mg			

7. Nursing Problems/Diagnoses

Identify three priority nursing problems/diagnoses

Assessment Data	Priority Problem	Intervention	Expected Patient Outcome	Which Interventions Could Be Delegated to Unlicensed Personnel?
1.				
2.				
3.				

References

Adams, H., Adams, R., Del Zoppo, G., & Goldstein, L. (2005). ASA scientific statement: Guidelines for the early management of patients with ischemic stroke. *Stroke, 36*, 916–923.

Albers, G. W., Amarenco, P., Easton, J. D., Sacco, R. L., & Teal, P. (2004, September). Antithrombotic and thrombolytic therapy for ischemic stroke: The seventh ACCP conference on antithrombotic and thrombolytic therapy. *Chest, 126*(3 suppl), 483S–512S.

Alberts, M., Hademenos, G., Latchaw, R., Jagoda, A., Marler J., Mayberg, M., et al. (2000). Recommendations for the establishment of primary stroke centers. *JAMA, 283,* 3102–3109.

Comprehensive overview of nursing and interdisciplinary care of the acute ischemic stroke patient: a scientific statement from the American Heart Association. Summers, D., Leonard, A., Wentworth, D., Saver, J. L., Simpson, J., Spilker, J. A., Hock, N., Miller, E., Mitchell, P. H. (2009). American Heart Association Council on Cardiovascular Nursing and the Stroke Council. *Stroke, 40*(8), 2911-44. Epub 2009 May 28.

Deglin, J. H., & Vallerand, A. H. (2009). *Davis's drug guide for nurses* (11th ed.). Philadelphia: F. A. Davis.

Dillon, P. (2007). *Nursing health assessment: A critical thinking and case studies approach* (2nd ed.). Philadelphia: F. A. Davis.

Erikson, E.H. (1950). *Childhood and society.* New York: Norton.

Goldstein, L. B., & Simel, D. L. (2005). Is this patient having a stroke? *JAMA, 293*(19), 2391–2402.

Institute for Clinical Systems Improvement (ICSI). (2005, February). *Diagnosis and initial treatment of ischemic stroke.* Bloomington, MN: ICSI.

Lagerquist, S. L. (2006). *Davis's NCLEX-RN for success.* Philadelphia: F. A. Davis.

Marler, J., Jones, P., & Emr, M. (1997). *Rapid identification and treatment of acute stroke.* Proceedings of a National Symposium of Neurological Institutes of Health. Bethesda, MD: National Institute of Neurological Disorders and Stroke, National Institutes of Health.

Mathiesen, C., Tavianini, H., & Palladino, K. (2006). Best practices in stroke rapid response: A case study. *Medical-surgical nursing, 15*(6), 364–369.

McDaniel, J. (2003). Code gray case studies. *Critical Care Nurse Quarterly, 26*(4), 303–315.

Miller, J., & Elmore, S. (2005). Call a stroke code! *Nursing, 35*(3), 58–63.

Nolan S., Naylor G., & Burn, M. (2003). Code gray: An organized approach to inpatient stroke. *Critical Care Nurse Quarterly, 26*(4), 296–302.

Pugh, S., Mathiesen, C., Meighan, M., & Summers, D. (2007). *Guide to the care of the patient with ischemic stroke. AANN reference series for clinical practice* (2nd ed.). Available at: www.aann.org/pubs/guidelines.html.

Repasky, T. M., & Pfeil, C. (2005). Experienced critical care nurse. Led rapid response teams rescue patients on in-patient units. *Journal of Emergency nursing,* 31, 376–379.

Van Leeuwen, A. M., Poelhuis-Leth, D. J., & Bladh, M. L. (2011). *Davis's comprehensive handbook of laboratory and diagnostic tests with nursing implications.* (4th ed.). Philadelphia: F. A. Davis.

7-4 Adult Asthma

EMERGENCY NURSING/ACUTE CARE

STANDARD FORMS

These templates are included in the Appendix; copy before each use.

LEARNING OUTCOMES

Cognitive

The student will be able to:

1. Identify the signs and symptoms of moderate and severe respiratory distress.
2. Identify appropriate intervention for a patient with an asthma exacerbation.
3. Describe the physiological process that occurs with asthma (inflammation and constriction).
4. Give a concise and thorough report using SBAR format to transfer care to another nurse.

Psychomotor

The student will be able to:

1. Perform an assessment of a patient with respiratory distress.
2. Initiate appropriate interventions, such as start and maintain IV, obtain stat vital signs, and administer appropriate medications.
3. Manage the care of a patient requiring nebulized medications.
4. Demonstrate and educate the patient on the proper technique for utilizing a peak flowmeter.

Affective

The student will be able to:

1. Reflect upon performance in caring for a patient with acute respiratory distress/asthma exacerbation.
2. Identify what worked well during the scenario.
3. Identify areas that need improvement
4. Reflect on overall feeling about the scenario.
5. Discuss feelings related to working as a team member.
6. Develop confidence in caring for a patient with respiratory distress.
7. Perform self-reflective evaluation.

Communication

The student will be able to:

1. Communicate effectively with healthcare team members in the care of a patient with acute respiratory distress/asthma exacerbation.
2. Communicate effectively with the patient and family members.
3. Use SBAR format when communicating with healthcare team members.
4. Work collaboratively as part of the healthcare team.
5. Accurately and succinctly document assessments, interventions, and evaluations.
6. Practice Transparent Thinking (thinking out loud) to facilitate group problem solving.
7. Use Directed Communication (directing a message to specific individual) when delegating tasks.
8. Employ Closed-Loop Communication (acknowledgment of receipt of the message and status) to acknowledge communications from others.

Safety

The student will be able to:

Administer and maintain specific protecting interventions with attention to safety of the client and healthcare professional.

1. Demonstrate a safe environment with attention to hazards to healthcare providers, visitors, and the client. Includes body mechanics, tripping hazards, and equipment issues.
2. Demonstrate attention to national patient safety goals. Includes patient identification standards, effective communication among healthcare providers, and safe medication administration.
3. Demonstrate attention to standard precautions. Includes hand washing, infection control measures, and use of personal protective equipment (PPE) as needed.

Leadership and Management/Delegation

The student will be able to:

1. Identify tasks that can be legally, ethically, and safely delegated to unlicensed assistive personnel (UAP) or licensed practical nurse (LPN) in the care of a patient with acute respiratory distress/asthma exacerbation.
2. Prioritize the care of a patient with acute respiratory distress/asthma exacerbation.

OVERVIEW OF THE PROBLEM

Definition

Asthma, also known as reactive airway disease (RAD), is a complex inflammatory process that can result in airway tissue damage, characterized by airway inflammation and hyperresponsiveness to a variety of stimuli (triggers). Triggers include allergens, cold, dust, smoke, exercise, medications (e.g., ASA), food additives.

Status asthmaticus is a life-threatening asthma attack that does not respond to standard treatment; a medical emergency.

Types of asthma:

- Immunological or allergic asthma.
- Atopic (hypersensitivity state may have hereditary influence); immunoglobulin E usually elevated.
- Nonimmumniological or nonallergic asthma: repeated respiratory infections; usually >35 years.
- Mixed combined immunological and nonimmunological: any age, allergen, or nonspecific stimuli.

Pathophysiology

- Triggers initiate the release of inflammatory mediators, such as histamine, that produce airway obstruction through smooth muscle constriction, microvascular leakage, mucous plugging, swelling, and, for many patients, chronic inflammation.

Risk Factors

- History of allergies, seasonal or environmental
- Recurrent respiratory infection

Assessment

Subjective

- History of URI, allergies, family history of asthma
- Tightness of chest, dyspnea
- Anxiety, restlessness

Objective

- Peak flowmeter levels drops
- Increased respirations
- Expiratory wheezes
- Hyperresonance
- Retraction
- Use of accessory muscles
- Tachycardia, tachypnea
- Dry, hacking, persistent cough
- General appearance: pallor, cyanosis, diaphoresis, barrel chest, distended neck veins, orthopnea
- Thick mucous sputum

Diagnostic Tests

- Forced vital capacity (FVC) decreased
- Forced expiratory volume in 1 second (FEV1) decreased
- Peak expiratory flow rates decreased
- Residual volume increased

Treatment

- Oxygenation and ventilation
- Rescue and maintenance medications
- Antibiotics

Nursing Management

Goal: Promote pulmonary ventilation:

- Position: high Fowler's
- Administer medications as ordered:
  - Rescue medications: Steroids (Medrol, prednisone), beta-adrenergic agonists (Albuterol, metaproterenol)
  - Maintenance medications: Nonsterodial anti-inflammatory drugs; steroids; leukotriene inhibitors/receptor antagonists; theophylline; beta agonists; mast cell stabilizers
- Antibiotics
- Oxygen
- Frequent monitoring for respiratory distress
- Rest

Goal: Facilitate expectoration of secretions

- Humidification
- Fluids
- Monitor for dehydration
- Respiratory therapy

Goal: Health teaching

- Identify triggers
- Importance of peak flow meters
- Management of disease
- Medications

Evaluation/Outcome Criteria

- No complications
- Has fewer attacks
- Takes medications as prescribed
- Avoids infections
- Pulmonary function tests return to normal

REVIEW QUESTIONS

1. Asthma attacks are often triggered by irritants. Name at least three triggers.
   Answer:

2. Steroids are often used to treat patients with asthma attack. What is the rationale for administering steroids?
   Answer:

3. Name at least three side effects associated with steroid use.
   Answer:

4. Differentiate an asthma attack from status asthmaticus.
Answer:

5. A patient with asthma is on Singulair, a leukotriene inhibitor. What is the action of a leukotriene inhibitor?
Answer:

Related Evidence-Based Practice Guidelines

National Heart Lung and Blood Institute Expert Panel Report 3 (EPR3): Guidelines for the Diagnosis and Management of Asthma Available at: http://www.nhlbi.nih.gov/guidelines/asthma/asthgdln.htm

National Guideline Clearinghouse Clinical practice guideline for management of asthma in children and adults. Available at: http://www.guideline.gov/content.aspx?id=15706&search=asthma

The Joint Commission National Patient Safety Goals Hospital Program. Retrieved from http://www.jointcommission.org/GeneralPublic/NPSG/10_npsgs.htm

SBAR technique for communication: A situational briefing model. The Institute for Healthcare Improvement. Retrieved December 19, 2008, from http://www.ihi.org/IHI/Topics/PatientSafety/SafetyGeneral/Tools/SBARTechniqueforCommunicationASituationalBriefingModel.htm

Topics to review prior to the simulation

- Respiratory assessment
- Medication administration, IV, nebulizer

SIMULATION

Client Background

Biographical Data

- Age: 37
- Gender: female
- Height: 5 ft 6 in
- Weight: 130 lb

Cultural Considerations

- Language: English, Spanish
- Ethnicity: Hispanic, born in Puerto Rico
- Nationality: American
- Culture: Assess communication ability in English and Spanish for potential language barrier

Demographic

- Marital status: married
- Educational level: business school at local community college
- Religion: Roman Catholic
- Occupation: office administrator

Current Health Status

- Complaint of shortness of breath for 2 days but it suddenly got worse today and her inhaler wasn't helping
- History: not available

Admission Sheet

Name:	Rachel Rodriguez
Age:	37
Gender:	Female
Marital status:	Married
Educational level:	Business school at local community college
Religion:	Roman Catholic
Ethnicity:	Hispanic, born in Puerto Rico
Nationality:	American
Language:	English, Spanish
Occupation:	Office administrator

Hospital
Provider's Orders

Patient's Name: **Rachel Rodriguez**
Allergies: **NKDA**

Diagnosis: **Respiratory distress/asthma exacerbation**

Date	Time	Order	Signature
6/20/07	8 PM	Vital signs: q 4 hr	
		Diet: NPO	
		Activity: Bed rest	
		Diagnostic tests: Urine HCG	
		Medications: Albuterol 5 mg neb × 3 Atrovent 0.5 mg neb × 1 (power source O_2) Solumedrol 125 mg IV × 1	
		IV therapy: NSS KVO	
		Oxygen: NRB or NC to maintain saturation 95%	
		Radiology: CXR	Dr. B. Hart

Nursing Report

No report. You are the ED nurse and first to see patient.

Student Simulation Prep Assignments

1. Identify items and their purpose in the care of a patient with asthma.

Item	Purpose
LR bags/IV tubing	
O_2 nonrebreather mask, cannula, nebulizer	
Monitor	

2. Identify team members and their specific roles in the care of a patient with asthma.

Team Member	Role
Primary nurse	
Secondary nurse	
Physician	

3. *Relevant Data Exercise:* Fill in columns below.

Relevant Data from Report	Relevant Data from Other Sources	Data Missing	Sources for Missing Data	Data Requiring Follow-up

4. *Initial Focused Assessment*

After reviewing the client background and nursing report, you are ready to assess your client's current status. Under each category, identify how you would target your assessment and what you would expect to find for the patient with asthma.

History

Are there any questions you need to ask the patient or family to obtain additional relevant data?

Physical Exam

- General appearance:
- Integumentary:
- HEENT:
- Respiratory:
- CV:
- Breast:
- Abdominal:
- Neuro:
- Musculoskeletal:
- Reproductive:
- Additional:
  - Renal:
- Developmental:

What are the nursing implications considering the developmental stage of your patient?

Answer:

5. *Diagnostic Tests*

What diagnostic test results relevant to the patient's current problem are needed to plan care?

Complete the table using Van Leeuwen et al, *Davis's Comprehensive Handbook of Laboratory and Diagnostic Testing with Nursing Implications* 4e, or other diagnostic test reference.

Diagnostic Test	Significance to This Patient's Problem
BMP	
BUN and creatinine	
Urine HCG	
CXR	

6. Treatment

Identify drugs that are used to treat a patient with asthma.

Complete the table using Deglin et al, *Davis's Drug Guide for Nurses* 12e, or other drug reference.

Medication	Dose	Action	Side Effect	Nursing Implications
Albuterol	5 mg nebulized			
Atrovent	0.5 mg nebulized			
Solumedrol	125 mg IVP			

7. Nursing Problem/Diagnoses

Identify three priority nursing problems/diagnoses.

Assessment Data	Priority Problem	Intervention	Expected Patient Outcome	Which Interventions Could be Delegated to Unlicensed Personnel?
1.				

Continued

Assessment Data	Priority Problem	Intervention	Expected Patient Outcome	Which Interventions Could be Delegated to Unlicensed Personnel?
2.				
3.				

References

American Heart Association. (2006). *Heartsaver first aid with CPR and AED.* Dallas: AHA.

Deglin, J. H., & Vallerand, A. H. (2009). *Davis's drug guide for nurses* (11th ed.). Philadelphia: F. A. Davis.

Dillon, P. (2007). *Nursing health assessment, a critical thinking case studies approach* (2nd ed.). Philadelphia: F. A. Davis.

Erikson, E.H. (1950). *Childhood and society.* New York: Norton.

Lagerquist, S. L. (2006). *Davis's NCLEX-RN for success* (2nd ed.). Philadelphia: F. A. Davis.

Van Leeuwen, A. M., Poelhuis-Leth, D. J., & Bladh, M. L. (2011). *Davis's comprehensive handbook of laboratory and diagnostic tests with nursing implications.* (4th ed.). Philadelphia: F. A. Davis.

Critical Care Nursing

8

8-1 Shock

CRITICAL CARE

STANDARD FORMS

These templates are included in the Appendix; copy before each use.

LEARNING OUTCOMES

Cognitive

The student will be able to:

1. Identify the patient in shock.
2. Describe the pathophysiology of shock.
3. Differentiate types of shock.
4. Describe appropriate interventions for a patient in shock.

Psychomotor

The student will be able to:

1. Perform an assessment on a patient in shock.
2. Implement appropriate interventions for a patient in shock.
3. Starting and maintaining IV therapy.
4. Administer blood transfusion.
5. Perform nasogastric tube insertion.
6. Perform nasagastric lavage.
7. Administer IV antibiotics.

Affective

The student will be able to:

1. Reflect upon performance in the care of a patient with shock.
2. Identify elements that worked well during the simulation.
3. Identify areas that need improvement.
4. Reflect on overall feeling about the simulation.
5. Discuss feelings related to working as a team member.
6. Develop confidence in caring for a patient with shock.
7. Perform self-reflective evaluation.

Communication

The student will be able to:

1. Communicate effectively with healthcare team members in the care of a patient with shock.
2. Communicate with a confused patient.
3. Communicate effectively with the family members.
4. Use SBAR format when communicating with healthcare team members.
5. Work collaboratively as part of the healthcare team.
6. Accurately and succinctly document assessments, interventions, and evaluations.
7. Practice Transparent Thinking (thinking out loud) to facilitate group problem solving.
8. Use Directed Communication (directing a message to specific individual) when delegating tasks.
9. Employ Closed-Loop Communication (acknowledgment of receipt of the message and status) to acknowledge communications from others.

Safety

The student will be able to:

Administer and maintain specific protecting interventions with attention to safety of the client and healthcare professional.

1. Demonstrate a safe environment with attention to hazards to healthcare providers, visitors, and the client. Includes body mechanics, tripping hazards, and equipment issues.
2. Demonstrate attention to national patient safety goals. Includes patient identification standards, effective communication among healthcare providers, and safe medication administration.
3. Demonstrate attention to standard precautions. Includes hand washing, infection control measures, and use of personal protective equipment (PPE) as needed.

Leadership and Management/Delegation

The student will be able to:

1. Identify and prioritize patient's needs in care of a patient with shock.
2. Identify tasks that can be legally, ethically, and safely delegated to unlicensed assistive personnel (UAP) or licensed practical nurse (LPN) in the care of a patient with shock.

OVERVIEW OF THE PROBLEM

Definition

Shock is severe deficit of nutrients, oxygen, and electrolytes to body tissue with subsequent increase in cellular wastes resulting from cardiac failure, insufficient blood volume, or increased vascular bed size.

Pathophysiology

Major types of shock:.

- Hypovolemic: Decreased blood volume (hemorrhage or plasma loss from intestinal obstruction, burns, physical trauma, or dehydration) leads to decreased venous return, and cardiac output which leads to decreased tissue perfusion.
- Cardiogenic: Pump failure (MI) leads to decreased cardiac output, pulmonary congestion, hypoxia, and inadequate circulation. Associated with high mortality rates.
- Distributive: Massive vasodilation leading to decreased venous return and tissue hypoxia.
- Neurogenic: Massive vasodilation from reduced vasomotor, vasoconstrictor tone (spinal shock, head injuries, anesthesia, pain) and interruption of sympathetic nervous system; blood volume is normal but inadequate leading to decreased venous return and tissue hypoxia.
- Vasogenic: Massive vasodilation from histamine release leading to venous stasis and decreased venous return (anaphylactic, septic endotoxic—severe reaction to foreign protein such as insect bites, drugs, toxic substance, aerobic, gram-negative organisms).

	Hypovolemic	Cardiogenic	Distributive: Vasogenic	
			Anaphylactic	Septic
CVP	<5 cm H_2O	>15 cm H_2O		Possible >15 cm H_2O
Skin	Cool, clammy	Cool, clammy, mottled	Urticaria	Warm, flushed
Neuro	Dizziness, syncope, orthostasis	Syncope	Anxious	Restless
Vital signs	Decrease in BP Increase in HR Increase in RR	Dysrhythmias, tachycardia/ bradycardia orthopnea	Increase in HR Increase in RR Decrease in BP	Increase in HR Increase in RR Widening pulse pressure Bounding pulses
Additional assessment findings		NVD (neck vein distention) Crackles	Hives Wheezes Edema	Peripheral edema
				Cold shock phase: Decrease in BP Skin cool, clammy, pallor or cyanosis Petechiae, ecchymosis, bleeding

Assessment

Subjective

- Anxious, restless
- Dizziness, fainting
- Thirst, nausea

Objective

- Vital signs:
  - Blood pressure: hypotension, postural hypotension, systolic <70 mm late in shock
  - Pulse: tachycardia, thready, irregular or could be slow d/t conduction problem in cardiogenic shock
  - Respirations: increased depth and rate, wheezing with anaphylaxsis
  - Temperature: decreased, elevated with septic shock
- Skin:
  - Pale, mottled, cool, clammy, warm in septic shock
  - Urticaria with anaphylactic shock
- Level of consciousness: alert to decreased
- CVP:
  - Hypovolemia <5 cm H_2O
  - Cardiogenic, and possibly septic >15 cm H_2O
- Swanz-Gantz catheter: elevated pulmonary capillary wedge pressure
- Urine output: decreased <30 mL/hr

Diagnostic Tests

Tests used will vary according to type of shock (Laboratory studies [CBC, electrolytes]—not useful in the immediate [8-12 hr] acute phase of hemorrhage.)

- CBC count with differential
- Urinalysis
- Electrolytes
- BUN
- Creatinine
- Glucose
- Urine cultures
- Blood cultures
- Arterial blood gas
- Serum lactate if metabolic acidosis is present
- Sputum Gram stain and culture in suspected pneumonia

The following if hepatic insufficiency or abdominal condition suspected:

- Serum bilirubin
- Alkaline phosphatase
- Aspartate aminotransferase (AST), alanine aminotransferase (ALT)
- Prothrombin time (PT)/activated partial thromboplastin time (aPTT)/INR (International Normalized Ratio)
- Amylase, lipase

The following if disseminated intravascular coagulation (DIC) suspected:

- PT, aPTT, fibrin split products, D-dimer assay, fibrinogen level, and platelet count
- Peripheral blood smear for signs of erythrocyte changes

Others:

- Imaging studies to identify source of bleeding
- Esophagogastroduodenoscopy for upper acute GI bleeding
- Lumbar puncture
- ECG
- Chest x-ray
- Ultrasonography/echocardiography
- Cardiac enzymes

Treatment

- Treat underlying cause
- Fluid replacement (except cardiogenic)
- Mechanical support
- Medications, according to cause:
  - Vasopressors (cardiogenic, neurogenic, septic)
  - Antiarrythmics (cardiogenic)
  - Cardiac glycosides (cardiogenic)
  - Adrenocorticoids (anaphylactic)
  - Vasodilators (cardiogenic)
  - Antihistamines (anaphylactic)

Nursing Management

- Position: Foot of bed elevated 20 degrees with head slightly elevated. Head elevated with breathing problems or head injuries in the absence of spinal injuries.
- Fluids: Hypovolemia: replace fluids, blood, or plasma expanders.
- Vital signs: CVP, arterial line, PA catheter (pulmonary artery catheter); Foley catheter with uriometer; cardiac monitor.
- Administer medications as ordered and monitor response.
- Initiate and maintain mechanical support: Maintain blood pressure and respirations.

Evaluation/Outcome Criteria

- Vital signs stable within normal limits
- Alert, oriented
- Urine output >30 mL/hr

REVIEW QUESTIONS

1. Hypotension and tachycardia are common signs for all types of shock. How would you differentiate signs and symptoms of cardiogenic shock from hemorrhagic shock?
   Answer:

2. How would you explain the signs of crackles and neck vein distention associated with cardiogenic shock?
   Answer:

3. What is the rationale for administering antihistamines and steroids to patients with anaphylactic shock?
   Answer:

4. What are some possible outcomes of untreated shock?
   Answer:

5. Identify nursing interventions that would be appropriate for a patient in cardiogenic shock.
   Answer:

Related Evidence-Based Practice Guidelines

American Heart Association

Advanced Cardiovascular Life Support Provider Manual

The Joint Commission National Patient Safety Goals Hospital Program. Retrieved from http://www.jointcommission.org/GeneralPublic/NPSG/10_npsgs.htm

National Guideline Clearinghouse

Guidelines on the management of massive blood loss. 2006 Dec. NGC:006194 British Committee for Standards in Haematology -Professional Association. http://www.guideline.gov/content.aspx?id=12231&search=shock

National Guideline Clearinghouse

Surviving sepsis campaign: international guidelines for management of severe sepsis and septic shock: 2008. 2004 (revised 2008 Jan). NGC:006316 Society of Critical Care Medicine - Professional Association. http://www.guideline.gov/content.aspx?id=12231&search=shock

SBAR technique for communication: A situational briefing model. The Institute for Healthcare Improvement. Retrieved December 19, 2008, from http://www.ihi.org/IHI/Topics/PatientSafety/SafetyGeneral/Tools/SBARTechniqueforCommunicationASituationalBriefingModel.htm

Topics to Review Prior to the Simulation

- Peptic ulcer disease (PUD)
- Shock

SIMULATION

Client Background

Biographical Data

- Age: 63
- Gender: male
- Height: 5 ft 11 in
- Weight: 235 lb

Cultural Considerations

- Language: English
- Ethnicity: English heritage
- Nationality: American
- Culture: no significant cultural considerations identified

Demographic

- Marital status: married
- Educational level: college
- Religion: Protestant
- Occupation: accountant

Current Health Status

- Gastric ulcer

History

- Not available
- Psychosocial history
  - Social support
- Past health history
  - Medical
  - Surgical
- Family history

Admission Sheet

Name:	Harold Dunbrow
Age:	63
Gender:	Male
Marital Status:	Married
Educational Level:	College
Religion:	Protestant
Ethnicity:	English heritage
Nationality:	American
Language:	English
Occupation:	Accountant

Hospital
Provider's Orders

Patient's Name: Harold Dunbrow
Allergies: NKDA

Diagnosis: PUD r/o GI bleed

Date	Time	Order	Signature
6/20/07	2 PM	Vital signs: q 4 hr.	
		Diet: Clear liquids	
		Activity: Bed rest	
		IV therapy: 1,000 mL 5% D/LR 100 cc/hr	

Diagnosis: PUD r/o GI bleed—cont'd

Date	Time	Order	Signature
		Medications: Dilaudid 1 mg q 4 hr prn Pepcid 20 mg IV q 12 hr	
		Diagnostic studies: CBC, serum electrolytes UA ECG	
		Treatments: Pump stockings Oxygen 2 L via nasal cannula	
		Schedule endoscopy in AM	Dr. S. Knack

Nursing Report

Mr. Dubrow, age 63, was seen by his family physician for stomach pain and fatigue. After being seen by his physician, Mr. Dunbrow is admitted to the hospital for further workup for PUD. He has been diagnosed with a gastric ulcer. On admission he tells you he doesn't feel so well, "My stomach hurts." He is very tired, been feeling dizzy, and a little SOB. VS: BP 130/90, P 97 bpm, RR 24, pulse ox 94% on RA.

Student Simulation Prep Assignments

1. Identify items and their purpose in the care of a patient with shock.

Item	Purpose
IV with pump	
O_2 cannula	
NG tube and suction	
Foley with urometer	
Blood transfusion filter	

2. Identify team members and their specific roles in the care of a patient with shock.

Team Member	Role
Primary nurse	
Secondary nurse	
Physician	

3. *Relevant Data Exercise*

Fill in the columns below.

Relevant Data from Report	Relevant Data from Other Sources	Data Missing	Sources for Missing Data	Data Requiring Follow-Up

4. *Initial Focused Assessment*

After reviewing the client background and nursing report, you are ready to assess your client's current status. Under each category, identify how you would target your assessment and what you would expect to find for the patient with shock.

History

Are there any questions you need to ask the patient or family to obtain additional relevant data?

Physical Exam

- General appearance:
- Integumentary:
- HEENT:
- Respiratory:
- CV:
- Breasts: No findings
- Abdomen:
- Musculoskeletal:
- Neuro:
- Renal:
- Reproductive:
- Additional:
- Developmental:

Because of the age of your client, are there any developmental issues you need to address?

Answer:

5. *Diagnostic Tests*

What diagnostic test results relevant to the patient's current problem are needed to plan care?

Complete the table using Van Leeuwen et al, *Davis's Comprehensive Handbook of Laboratory and Diagnostic Testing with Nursing Implications* 4e, or other diagnostic test reference.

Diagnostic Test	Significance to This Patient's Problem
ECG	
Electrolytes	
BUN and creatinine	
CBC	
Type and cross (T&C)	
Coagulation studies	
Chest x-ray	
Urinalysis	

6. Treatment

Identify drugs that are used to treat a patient with shock.

Complete the table using Deglin et al, *Davis's Drug Guide for Nurses* 12e, or other drug reference.

Medication	Dose, Route, Frequency	Indications	Side Effect	Nursing Implications
Dilaudid	1 mg IV q 4 hr			
Pepcid	20 mg			
Rocephin	1 g			
Unasyn	1.5 g			
Benadryl	50 mg			
Tylenol	650 mg			

7. Nursing Problems/Diagnoses

Identify three priority nursing problems/diagnoses.

Complete for each problem identified.

Assessment Data	Priority Problem	Intervention	Expected Patient Outcome	Which Intervention Could Be Delegated to Unlicensed Personnel?
1.				

Continued

Assessment Data	Priority Problem	Intervention	Expected Patient Outcome	Which Intervention Could Be Delegated to Unlicensed Personnel?
2.				
3.				

References

Deglin, J. H., & Vallerand, A. H. (2009). *Davis's drug guide for nurses* (11th ed.). Philadelphia: F. A. Davis.

Dellinger, R. P., Levy, M. M., Carlet, J. M., Bion, J., Parker, M. M., Jaeschke, R., et al.. (2008). Surviving sepsis campaign: International guidelines for management of severe sepsis and septic shock: 2008. *Intensive Care Medicine, 34,* 17–60. doi: 10.1007/s00134-007-0934-2.

Dillon, P. (2007). *Nursing health assessment: A critical thinking and case studies approach* (2nd ed.). Philadelphia: F. A. Davis.

Erikson, E.H. (1950). *Childhood and society.* New York: Norton.

Lagerquist, S. L. (2006). *Davis's NCLEX-RN for success* (2nd ed.). Philadelphia: F. A. Davis.

Surviving Sepsis Campaign (2008, December). *Surviving sepsis.*. Retrieved from http://www.survivingsepsis.org

Van Leeuwen, A. M., Poelhuis-Leth, D. J., & Bladh, M. L. (2011). *Davis's comprehensive handbook of laboratory and diagnostic tests with nursing implications.* (4th ed.). Philadelphia: F. A. Davis.

8-2 Acute Respiratory Distress Syndrome (ARDS)

CRITICAL CARE/HIGH ACUITY MEDICAL-SURGICAL

STANDARD FORMS

These templates are included in the Appendix; copy before each use.

LEARNING OUTCOMES

Cognitive

The student will be able to:

1. Describe signs and symptoms of ARDS.
2. Correlate signs and symptoms of ARDS to the pathphysiology of ARDS.
3. Identify factors in a patient's history that increase risk for ARDS.
4. Explain factors in a patient's current condition that increase risk for ARDS.
5. Relate appropriate interventions for the patient with ARDS.
6. Differentiate the roles of team members in response to a patient with ARDS.

Psychomotor

The student will be able to:

1. Demonstrate appropriate assessment for a patient with ARDS.
2. Initiate appropriate interventions (respiratory assessment, gather appropriate assessment data and notify physician, prioritize physician orders, demonstrate appropriate collection of specimens, accurately calculate and administer medications) for a patient with ARDS.
3. Work collaboratively as part of the healthcare team in the care of a patient with ARDS.

Affective

The student will be able to:

1. Reflect upon performance in the care of a patient with ARDS.
2. Identify personal feelings in delivering care to a patient with ARDS.
3. Discuss feelings related to working as a member of a team in the care of a patient with ARDS.
4. Identify factors that worked well during the simulation of care of a patient with ARDS.
5. Identify factors that needed improvement during the simulation of care of a patient with ARDS.
6. Develop self-confidence in the care of a patient with ARDS.

Communication

The student will be able to:

1. Communicate effectively with healthcare team members in the care of a patient with ARDS.
2. Communicate effectively with the patient and family in the care of a patient with ARDS.
3. Utilize effective cross-cultural communication techniques with a client and family of Vietnamese descent.
4. Model family responses to hospitalization for the client with ARDS (family member).
5. Use SBAR format when communicating with team members in the care of a patient with ARDS.
6. Practice Transparent Thinking (thinking out loud) to facilitate group problem solving.
7. Use Directed Communication (directing a message to specific individual) when delegating tasks.
8. Employ Closed-Loop Communication (acknowledgment of receipt of the message and status) to acknowledge communications from others.

Safety

The student will be able to:

Administer and maintain specific protecting interventions with attention to safety of the client and healthcare professional.

1. Demonstrate a safe environment with attention to hazards to healthcare providers, visitors, and the client. Includes body mechanics, tripping hazards, and equipment issues.
2. Demonstrate attention to national patient safety goals. Includes patient identification standards, effective communication among healthcare providers, and safe medication administration.
3. Demonstrate attention to standard precautions. Includes hand washing, infection control measures, and use of personal protective equipment (PPE) as needed.

Leadership and Management/Delegation

The student will be able to:

1. Identify and prioritize patient's needs in care of a patient with ARDS.
2. Identify tasks that can be legally, ethically, and safely delegated to unlicensed assistive personnel (UAP) or licensed practical nurse (LPN) in the care of a patient with ARDS.

OVERVIEW OF THE PROBLEM

Definition

ARDS is characterized by noncardiogenic pulmonary infiltrations resulting in stiff wet lungs and refractory hypoxemia in an adult who was previously healthy. Acute hypoxemic respiratory failure occurs without hypercapnia.

Pathophysiology

- Damage to alveolar capillary membrane
- Increased vascular permeability creating noncardiac pulmonary edema and impaired gas exchange
- Decreased surfactant production
- Atelectasis
- Severe hypoxia refractory to decreased FiO_2
- Possible death

Risk Factors

Primary

- Shock, multiple trauma
- Infections
- Aspiration, inhalation of chemical toxins
- Drug overdose
- Disseminated intravascular coagulation (DIC)
- Emboli, especially fat emboli

Secondary

- Overaggressive fluid administration
- Oxygen toxicity

Assessment

Subjective

- Restlessness, anxiety
- History of risk factors
- Severe dyspnea

Objective

- Cyanosis
- Tachycardia
- Hypotension
- Hypoxemia, acidosis
- Crackles
- X-ray: bilateral patchy infiltrates
- Death if untreated

Diagnostic Tests

- ABG
- Chest x-ray
- CBC
- Metabolic panel

Treatment

- Oxygen
- Antibiotics
- Sedation/analgesics
- Bronchodilators
- Low molecular weight heparin (DVT prophylaxis)
- Steroids
- Diuretics

Nursing Management

Goal: Assist in respirations.

- Intensive care unit
- Mechanical ventilation
- Positive end expiratory pressure (PEEP)
- Oxygen
- Monitor blood gases
- Suctioning
- Cough and deep breathe
- Rotation therapy and/or prone position

Goal: Prevent complications

- Monitor for and prevent gastrointestinal bleeding
- Monitor for and correct acidosis
- Monitor for dysrhythmias
- Decrease anxiety, conserve energy, calm atmosphere, comfort, and emotional support
- Hemodynamic monitoring (central venous and pulmonary artery pressures)
- Maintain fluid balance
- Accurate I&O: Assess for bleeding tendencies (potential for disseminated intravascular coagulation)
- Protect from infection (aseptic technique, DVT prophylaxis)
- Maintain nutrition
- Skin care

Goal: Health teaching.

- Procedures
- Follow-up care
- Risk factors

Evaluation/Outcome Criteria

- Alert and oriented
- Skin warm to touch
- Respiratory rate and other assessments within normal limits
- Urine output >30 mL/hr

REVIEW QUESTIONS

1. Describe the pathophysiology of ARDS.
   Answer:

2. Identify five potential causes of ARDS.
   Answer:

3. Describe the progression sequence of ARDS (onset/exudative phase, progression/fibroproliferative phase, resolution) with associated clinical manifestations, and laboratory/diagnostic findings of each phase.
   Answer: Complete the table on page 339.

Phase	Clinical Manifestations	Laboratory/Diagnostic Findings
Onset/ Exudative		
Progression/ Fibroproliferative		
Resolution		

4. List five anticipated medical/pharmacological interventions for the client with ARDS and give rationales for each.
Answer:

Intervention	Rationale
1.	
2.	
3.	
4.	
5.	

Related Evidence-Based Practice Guidelines

CDC

Guidelines for preventing healthcare associated pneumonia (2003). Retrieved from http://www.cdc.gov/mmwr/preview/mmwrhtml/rr5303a1.htm

The Joint Commission National Patient Safety Goals Hospital Program. Retrieved from http://www.jointcommission.org/GeneralPublic/NPSG/10_npsgs.htm

AARC Clinical Practice Guideline

Nasotracheal suctioning 2004 revision & update. Retrieved from http://www.aarc.org/daz/rcjournal/rcjournal/x.RCJOURNAL.COM%2002.21.07/contents/09.04/09.04.1080.asp
National Guideline Clearing House
Practice management guideline for pulmonary contusion/flail chest (2006). Retrieved from http://www.guideline.gov/content.aspx?id=10167
Surviving sepsis campaign guidelines for management of severe sepsis and septic shock (2004). Retrieved from http://www.guideline.gov/content.aspx?id=12231
SBAR technique for communication: A situational briefing model. The Institute for Healthcare Improvement. Retrieved December 19, 2008, from http://www.ihi.org/IHI/Topics/PatientSafety/SafetyGeneral/Tools/SBARTechniqueforCommunicationASituationalBriefingModel.htm

Topics to Review Prior to the Simulation

- Acute medical-surgical nursing, ARDS.
- Mechanical ventilation (SIMV, PEEP).
- Arterial blood gas interpretation.
- Trauma, pulmonary contusion.
- Antibiotic administration.
- Sputum specimen collection.
- IV sedation administration (lorazepam [Ativan], morphine IV).

The Richmond Agitation and Sedation Scale: The RASS http://www.icudelirium.org/docs/CAM_ICU_worksheet.pdf

SIMULATION

Client Background

Biographical Data

- Age: 55
- Gender: male
- Height: 5 ft 5 in
- Weight: 141 lb

Cultural Considerations

- Language: English and Vietnamese
- Ethnicity: Vietnamese
- Nationality: American
- Culture: Vietnamese

Demographic

- Marital status: married
- Educational level: 6th grade
- Religion: Buddhist
- Occupation: shrimper

Current Health Status

- Acute respiratory failure

History

- Psychosocial history
  - Social support: family
- Past health history: not available
  - Medical
  - Surgical
- Family History: not available

Admission Sheet

Name:	Ty Nguyen
Age:	55
Gender:	Male
Marital Status:	Married
Educational Level:	6th grade
Religion:	Buddhist
Ethnicity:	Vietnamese
Nationality:	American
Language:	Primarily Vietnamese, minimal English
Occupation:	Shrimper, owner of boat

Hospital
Provider's Orders

Patient's Name: Ty Nguyen
Allergies: NKDA

Diagnosis: Acute respiratory failure

Date	Time	Order	Signature
		Vital signs: q hr	
		Diet: NPO	
		Activity: Bed rest	
		IV therapy: 0.9% NS at KVO	
		Medications: Diagnostic studies: CBC and BMP in AM, ABG's at 8 AM	
		Treatments: Respiratory therapy assessment Vent settings: TV 550 Assist control 10, FiO_2 55% Call if O_2 saturation <90%	
			Dr. Know

Nursing Report

Mr. Nguyen was shrimping 3 days ago. Upon arriving at the dock, he was trying to untangle his shrimp nets that were 25 feet off the ground. When his leg got caught in a net, it caused him to fall 25 feet, landing on his chest. He was able to get up, refused emergency medical attention, and went home. Today he presented to the emergency department with shortness of breath, pulse oximetry 89% on RA, and sinus tachycardia with frequent PVCs. Mr. Nguyen has a 60 pack/yr smoking history. His only additional history includes a laceration of his leg which required 20 stitches in 1988.

Mr. Nguyen's oxygen saturation continued to drop to 82% on 100% NRBM. He was intubated in the emergency department. Etomidate 20 mg IV and Anectine 100 mg IV were given prior to intubation 30 min ago. Mr. Nguyen currently has a 7.5 cm ETT at 22 cm at teeth, right side of mouth. Vent settings are TV 550, assist control 10, FiO_2 55%. ABGs were done prior to transfer to ICU (15 min ago). A chest x-ray was also done after intubation. BMP and CBC results are pending. Mr. Nguyen's daughter is at the bedside.

Student Simulation Prep Assignments

1. Identify items and their purpose in the care of a patient with mechanical ventilation and ARDS.

Item	Purpose
Oropharyngeal or nasopharyngeal airway	
Manual resuscitation bag and face mask with 100% oxygen	
Magic slate, magnetic board with plastic letters, pictures, alphabet boards, flash cards	

Continued

Item	Purpose
Yankauer suction catheter	
Wall mount or gomco suction unit	
In-line suction catheter	
Oral care swabs, toothbrush, mouth rinse, mouth moisturizer, and pharyngeal suction catheter	
Pulse oximetry	

2. Identify team members and specific roles in the care of a patient with mechanical ventilation and ARDS.

Team Member	Role
Staff nurse	
Practitioner/physician	
Respiratory therapist	
Registered dietitian	
Physical therapist	
Pharmacist	

3. *Relevant Data Exercise:* Fill in columns below.

Relevant Data from Report	Relevant Data from Other Sources	Data Missing	Sources for Missing Data	Data Requiring Follow-Up

4. *Initial Focused Assessment*

After reviewing the client background and nursing report, you are ready to assess your client's current status. Under each category, identify how you would target your assessment, and what you would expect to find for the patient with ARDS.

History

Are there any questions you need to ask the patient or family to obtain additional relevant data?

Physical Exam

- General appearance:
- Integumentary:
- HEENT:
- Respiratory:
- CV:
- Breasts:
- Abdominal:
- Neuro:

- Musculoskeletal:
- Renal:
- Reproductive:
- Additional:
- Developmental:

What are the nursing implications considering the developmental stage of your patient?

Answer:

5. Diagnostic Tests

What diagnostic test results relevant to the patient's current problem are needed to plan care?

Complete the table using Van Leeuwen et al, *Davis's Comprehensive Handbook of Laboratory and Diagnostic Testing with Nursing Implications* 4e, or other diagnostic test reference.

Diagnostic Test	Significance to This Patient's Problem
ABGs: pH PCO_2 PaO_2 HCO_3 SaO_2	
Chest x-ray	
Hgb	
Hct	
BUN	
Creatinine	

6. Treatment

Identify drugs that are used to treat a patient with ARDS.

Complete the table using Deglin et al, *Davis's Drug Guide for Nurses* 12e, or other drug reference.

Medication	Dose Route, Frequency	Indications	Side Effect	Nursing Implications
Furosemide (Lasix)	IV (acute pulmonary edema) 40 mg, after 1 hr may give additional 80 mg			

Medication	Dose Route, Frequency	Indications	Side Effect	Nursing Implications
Albuterol (Proventil)	3 mL unit dose (1 mg/mL, 2 mg/mL, 5 mg/mL)			
Ipratropium (Atrovent)	0.02% in single-dose vials containing 500 mcg			
Methylprednisolone (Solumedrol)	10–40 mg IV			

Continued

Medication	Dose Route, Frequency	Indications	Side Effect	Nursing Implications
Morphine	4–10 mg q 3–4 hr			
Lorazepam (Ativan)	Not to exceed 2 mg IV (do not exceed 8 mg/12 hr)			

Medication	Dose Route, Frequency	Indications	Side Effect	Nursing Implications
Imipenem/ cilastatin sodium (Primaxin)	250 mg–1 g q 6–8 hr IV			

7. Nursing Problems/Diagnoses

Identify three priority nursing problems/diagnoses.

Assessment Data	Priority Problem	Intervention	Expected Patient Outcome	Which Interventions Could Be Delegated to Unlicensed Personnel?
1.				

Continued

Assessment Data	Priority Problem	Intervention	Expected Patient Outcome	Which Interventions Could Be Delegated to Unlicensed Personnel?
2.				
3.				

References

Deglin, J. H., & Vallerand, A. H. (2009). *Davis's drug guide for nurses* (11th ed.). Philadelphia: F. A. Davis.

Dillon, P. (2007). *Nursing health assessment: A critical thinking and case studies approach* (2nd ed.). Philadelphia: F. A. Davis.

Erikson, E.H. (1950). *Childhood and society.* New York: Norton.

Guidelines for preventing healthcare associated pneumonia (2003). Retrieved January 4, 2008, from http://www.guideline.gov/summary/summary.aspx?doc id=4872&nbr =003506&string=pulmonary+AND+trauma

Lagerquist, S. L., McMillin, J. L., Nelson, R. M., & Snider, K. E. (2006). *Davis's NCLEX-RN for success* (2nd ed.). Philadelphia: F. A. Davis.

Nasotracheal suctioning (2004 revision and update). Retrieved January 4, 2008 from http://www.guideline.gov/summary/summary.aspx?doc_id=6514&nbr=004083&string=sputum+AND+collection

Practice management guideline for pulmonary contusion/flail chest (2006). Retrieved January 4, 2008, from http://www.guideline.gov/summary/summary.aspx?doc_id=10167&nbr=005352&string=mechanical+AND+ventilation

Richmond Agitation Sedation Scale (RASS). Retrieved January 27, 2008, from http://www.icudelirium.org/delirium/training-pages/RASS.pdf.

The Richmond Agitation-Sedation Scale: Validity and reliability in adult intensive care unit patients. *American Journal of Respiratory and Critical Care Medicine, 166*, 1338–1344.

Sessler, C. N., Gosnell, M., Grap, M. J., Brophy, G. T., O'Neal, P. V., Keane, K. A., et al. (2002). *Surviving sepsis campaign guidelines for management of severe sepsis and septic shock.* (2004). Retrieved January 4, 2008, from http://www.guideline.gov/summary/ summary.aspx?doc_id=4911&nbr = 003508&string=sedation

Urden, L. D., Stacy, K. M., & Lough, M. E. (2006). *Thelan's critical care nursing: Diagnosis and management* (5th ed). St. Louis: Mosby.

Van Leeuwen, A. M., Poelhuis-Leth, D. J., & Bladh, M. L. (2011). *Davis's comprehensive handbook of laboratory and diagnostic tests with nursing implications.* (4th ed.). Philadelphia: F. A. Davis.

8-3 Hyperglycemic Hyperosmolar Nonketosis (HHNK)

CRITICAL CARE

STANDARD FORMS

These templates are included in the Appendix; copy before each use.

LEARNING OUTCOMES

Cognitive

The student will be able to:

1. Describe signs and symptoms of HHNK.
2. Correlate signs and symptoms to the pathophysiology of HHNK.
3. Identify factors in a patient's history that increase risk for HHNK.
4. Identify factors in a patient's current condition that increase risk for hypovolemic shock.
5. Differentiate between the clinical signs of diabetic ketoacidosis and HHNK.
6. Identify the appropriate interventions for the patient with HHNK.
7. Differentiate the roles of team members in response to a patient with HHNK.
8. Correctly calculate medication dosages.
9. Interpret significance of diagnostic test results.
10. Identify potential clinical sequelae related to HHNK.

Psychomotor

The student will be able to:

1. Perform appropriate assessment for a patient with HHNK.
2. Initiate appropriate interventions for a patient with HHNK.
3. Initiate ECG monitoring.
4. Initiate and monitor IV medications and solutions.
5. Insert a Foley catheter using sterile technique.
6. Institute seizure precautions.
7. Work collaboratively as part of the healthcare team in the care of a patient with HHNK.

Affective

The student will be able to:

1. Reflect upon performance in the care of a patient with HHNK.
2. Identify personal feelings in delivering care to a patient with HHNK.
3. Discuss feelings related to working as a member of a team in the care of a patient with HHNK.
4. Identify factors that worked well during the simulation of care of a patient with HHNK.
5. Identify factors that needed improvement during the simulation of care of a patient with HHNK.
6. Develop self-confidence in the care of a patient with HHNK.

Communication

The student will be able to:

1. Communicate effectively with healthcare team members in the care of a patient with HHNK.
2. Communicate effectively with the patient and family in the care of a patient with HHNK.
3. Use SBAR format when communicating with team members in the care of a patient with HHNK.
4. Document assessments, interventions, and evaluations.
5. Practice Transparent Thinking (thinking out loud) to facilitate group problem solving.
6. Use Directed Communication (directing a message tospecific individual) when delegating tasks.
7. Employ Closed-Loop Communication (acknowledgment of receipt of the message and status) to acknowledge communications from others.

Safety

The student will be able to:

Administer and maintain specific protecting interventions with attention to safety of the client and healthcare professional.

1. Demonstrate a safe environment with attention to hazards to healthcare providers, visitors, and the client. Includes body mechanics, tripping hazards, and equipment issues.
2. Demonstrate attention to national patient safety goals. Includes patient identification standards, effective communication among healthcare providers, and safe medication administration.
3. Demonstrate attention to standard precautions. Includes hand washing, infection control measures, and use of personal protective equipment (PPE) as needed.

Leadership and Management/Delegation

The student will be able to:

1. Identify and prioritize patient's needs in care of a patient with HHNK
2. Identify tasks that can be legally, ethically, and safely delegated to unlicensed assistive personnel (UAP) or licensed practical nurse (LPN) in the care of a patient with HHNK.

OVERVIEW OF THE PROBLEM

Definition

Hyperglycemic hyperosmolar nonketosis (HHNK) is characterized by profound hyperglycemia and dehydration without ketosis or ketoacidosis. It is seen in non–insulin-dependent diabetics, usually precipitated by infection or illness. It is a critical condition that may lead to impaired consciousness and seizures, with a mortality rate greater than 50%.

Pathophysiology

Hyperglycemia >1,000 mL/dL causes osmotic diuresis, depletion of extracellular fluid, and hyperosmolarity. The patient is unable to replace fluid volume with oral intake.

Risk Factors

- Advanced age
- Non–insulin-dependent diabetes
- Infections
- Renal failure
- Shock
- Hemorrhage
- Medications: diuretics, glucocorticoids
- Tube feedings

Assessment

Subjective

- Confusion
- Lethargy

Objective

- Nystagmus
- Dehydration
- Aphasia
- Nuchal rigidity
- Hyperreflexia

Diagnostic Tests

- Blood glucose >1,000 mg/dL
- Serum Na and Cl normal to elevated
- BUN >60 mg/dL
- Arterial pH slightly decreased

Treatment

- Regular insulin
- Treat the precipitating condition

Nursing Management

Goal: Promote fluid and electrolyte balance.

- IV fluid and electrolyte replacement
- Rate of infusion determined by assessment
- Monitor I&O
- Treat precipitating condition

Goal: Prevent complications.

- Administer regular insulin
- Monitor for complications

Evaluation/Outcome Criteria

- Blood sugar returns to normal level
- Client is alert and oriented
- Primary medical problem is resolved
- Client recognizes and reports signs of imbalance

REVIEW QUESTIONS

1. What are the similarities and differences between HHNK and DKA? Include physical assessment findings and diagnostic laboratory data.
   Answer: Complete the table on pages 350 and 351.

Parameter	DKA	HHNK
Serum glucose		
Serum osmolality		
Serum bicarbonate		
Arterial blood pH		
Serum ketones		
Urine ketones		
Serum sodium		
BUN		
Diabetes mellitus		
Onset		
Clinical Presentation		

Clinical Presentation	DKA	HHNK

2. What risk factors may precipitate an episode of HHNK in a vulnerable patient?
Answer:

3. Describe two potential clinical sequelae (include precipitating factors) associated with HHNK.
Answer:

Clinical Sequelae	Precipitating Factors

4. Explain why 0.9% sodium chloride may be used as opposed to D5W or 0.45% sodium chloride as fluid replacement in the treatment of HHNK.
Answer:

5. Why is the blood pH normal or slightly acidotic (7.3 or greater) in the patient experiencing HHNK?
Answer:

Related Evidence-Based Practice Guidelines

American Diabetic Association
Position Statement: Hyperglycemic Crises in Diabetes, retrieved from: http://care.diabetesjournals.org/content/27/suppl_1/s94.full.pdf+html
SBAR technique for communication: A situational briefing model. The Institute for Healthcare Improvement. Retrieved December 19, 2008, from http://www.ihi.org/IHI/Topics/PatientSafety/SafetyGeneral/Tools/SBARTechniqueforCommunicationASituationalBriefingModel.htm
The Joint Commission National Patient Safety Goals Hospital Program. Retrieved from http://www.jointcommisssion.org/GeneralPublic/NPSG/10_npsgs.htm

Topics to Review Prior to the Simulation

- Pathophysiology of HHNK and diabetic ketoacidosis (DKA) giving careful consideration to the differences and similarities between these two disease entities.
- Vulnerable patient population and risk factors for developing HHNK.
- Expected signs and symptoms of the patient experiencing HHNK.
- Typical diagnostic findings (lab results) related to HHNK.
- Nursing and collaborative interventions that are used to treat the patient with HHNK.
- Pharmacological interventions for a patient with HHNK.

SIMULATION

Client Background

Biographical Data

- Age: 78
- Gender: male
- Height: 5 ft 11 in (71 in)
- Weight: 224 lb (101.8 kg)

Cultural Considerations

- Language: English
- Ethnicity: English/Irish
- Nationality: American
- Culture: He lives in an upscale, retirement community with Maggie, his wife of 58 yr. He and his wife are active members of the Congregational Church and residential community.

Demographic

- Marital status: married
- Educational level: masters degree
- Religion: Congregational Church
- Occupation: retired mechanical engineer

Current Health Status

- Jeremy is lethargic and weak upon admission to the ICU and his wife states he has been "terribly sick for 1 to 2 days." He has complaints of nausea, vomiting, and frequent diarrhea. His wife states he has been unable to "keep anything down, not even water," for the last 36 hr but he was reluctant to come to the hospital.

History

- Psychosocial history: does not drink alcohol or smoke cigarettes
  - Social support: wife, three grown children live nearby
- Past Health History:
  - Medical: osteoarthritis, hyperlipidemia, hypertension, gastroesophageal reflux disease (GERD), and a right total hip replacement in 1999. He has recently been diagnosed with diabetes mellitus type 2.
  - Surgical: total hips in 1999
- Family history: none significant

Admission Sheet

Name:	Jeremy Slade
Age:	78
Gender:	Male
Marital Status:	Married
Educational Level:	Masters degree
Religion:	Protestant
Ethnicity:	Irish/English
Nationality:	American
Language:	English
Occupation:	Retired mechanical engineer

The following orders accompany the patient to the ICU.

Hospital
Provider's Orders

Patient's Name: Jeremy Slade
Allergies: Morphine sulfate

Diagnosis: Severe dehydration

Date	Time	Order	Signature
	1400	Admit to ICU	
		Vital signs: q 1 hr; call for a HR >120 bpm, SBP <90 mm Hg	
		Strict intake and output q 1 hr; call for a UO <30 mL/hr	

Diagnosis: Severe dehydration—cont'd

Date	Time	Order	Signature
		Diet: NPO	
		Activity: Bed rest	
		IV therapy: 0.9% NSS at 250 mL/hr	
		Medications: Protonix 40 mg po daily Lopressor 50 mg po daily; hold for HR <55 bpm and/or SBP <100 mm Hg Hydrochlorothiazide 12.5 mg po daily Zestril 5 mg po daily Glyburide 2.5 mg po daily Lovenox 40 mg SQ q 12 hr	
		Titrate oxygen to keep SpO_2 ≥92% prn	
		Diagnostic studies: Complete metabolic profile (CMP) and CBC q AM	
			Dr. Fisher

Nursing Report

From the ED nurse: Mr. Slade came into the ED via ambulance in the company of his wife. She is the historian since he is profoundly lethargic and difficult to arouse. His wife states he has been sick with nausea, vomiting, and diarrhea for about 2 days, and he is unable to keep solid foods or liquids down. His wife also states he has been "peeing all the time" and has been unable to "get to the bathroom" since he has become "weak and dizzy." He has not had an episode of diarrhea in 24 hr. He had been complaining of nausea and thirst. She called an ambulance when she could not wake him up this morning.

He has recently been diagnosed with type 2 diabetes. His medications include Nexium, Lopressor, Glyburide, and Zestril. She is not sure of the dosages.

Vital signs 30 minutes ago were T 36.8°C, HR 122, sinus rhythm without ectopy, RR 28 and shallow, BP 90/62 supine. Chest x-ray and ECG were unremarkable.

Complete chemistry panel and CBC are pending. Urine dipstick was negative for ketones. ABG results: pH 7.34, PO_2 90, PCO_2 34 and HCO_3^- 24.

He has an 18-gauge peripheral IV in the left antecubital fossa with 0.9% NaCl infusing at 150 mL/hr. Patient was incontinent of urine while in the ED.

Between the time the patient leaves the ED and is delivered to you in the ICU, the laboratory calls for a critical serum glucose level of 1,050 mg/dL and the other lab results have arrived on the unit. The hospital intensivist wrote the admission orders while the patient was in the ED.

Student Simulation Prep Assignments

1. Identify items and their purpose in the care of a patient with HHNK.

Item	Purpose
IV tubing	
IV solutions	
Infusion pump and pole	
Cardiac monitor	

Continued

Item	Purpose
Pulse oximeter	
Gloves	
Stethoscope	
Regular insulin	
Syringes	

2. *Identify team members and their specific roles in the care of a patient with HHNK.*

Team Member	Role
Nurse	
Clinical leader	
Physician	
Significant other	

3. *Relevant Data Exercise:* Fill in the columns below.

Relevant Data from Report	Relevant Data from Other Sources	Data Missing	Sources for Missing Data	Data Requiring Follow-Up

4. *Initial Focused Assessment*

After reviewing the client background and nursing report, you are ready to assess your client's current status. Under each category, identify how you would target your assessment, and what you would expect to find for the patient with HHNK.

History

Are there any questions you need to ask the patient or family to obtain additional relevant data?

Physical Exam

- General appearance:
- HEENT:
- Respiratory:
- CV:
- Breasts:
- Abdominal:
- Neuro:
- Musculoskeletal:
- Reproductive:
- Genitourinary:
- Additional:
- Developmental:

What are the nursing implications considering the developmental stage of your patient?

Answer:

5. Diagnostic Tests

What diagnostic test results relevant to the patient's current problem are needed to plan care?

Complete the table using Van Leeuwen et al, *Davis's Comprehensive Handbook of Laboratory and Diagnostic Testing with Nursing Implications* 4e, or other diagnostic test reference.

Diagnostic Test	Significance to This Patient's Problem
Serum glucose (typically >800 mg/dL)	
Serum osmolality	
Serum bicarbonate	
Arterial blood pH	
BUN	
Serum potassium >6.5	
Serum potassium <3	
Urine ketones	
Serum sodium	

6. Treatment

Identify drugs that are used to treat a patient with HHNK.

Complete the table using Deglin et al, *Davis's Drug Guide for Nurses* 12e, or other drug reference.

Medication	Dose Route, Frequency	Indications	Side Effect	Nursing Implications
0.9% NSS	15–20 mL/kg/hr (ADA, 2004)			
0.45% NSS	15–20 mL/kg/hr (ADA, 2004)			
D5W with 0.45% NSS	Variable rate (Gahart, 2006)			
Regular insulin	Bolus: 0.15 units/kg (ADA, 2004) Infusion: 0.1–0.2 units/kg/hr (ADA, 2004)			

Continued

Medication	Dose Route, Frequency	Indications	Side Effect	Nursing Implications
KCl	If initial serum K+ is <3.3, hold insulin and give 40 mEq K+ until K+ ≥3.3 (ADA, 2004) If initial serum K+ is ≥5 mEq/L, do not give K+ (ADA, 2004) If initial K+ is ≥3.3 but <5, give 20–30 mEq K+ in each L of IV fluid to keep serum K+ at 4–5 mEq/L (ADA, 2004)			

7. Nursing Problems/Diagnoses

Identify three priority nursing problems/diagnoses.

Assessment Data	Priority Problem	Intervention	Expected Patient Outcome	Which Intervention Could be Delegated to Unlicensed Personnel?
1.				

Assessment Data	Priority Problem	Intervention	Expected Patient Outcome	Which Intervention Could be Delegated to Unlicensed Personnel?
2.				
3.				

References

American Diabetes Association (2004). Hyperglycemic crises in diabetes. *Diabetes Care, 27,* S94–S101. Retrieved June 29, 2007, from http://care.diabetesjournals.org/cgi/reprint/27/suppl_1/S94

Brenner, Z. R. (2005). Endocrine alterations. In M. L. Sole, D. G. Klein, & M. J. Moseley (Eds.). *Introduction to critical care nursing* (4th ed.). St. Louis: Elsevier Saunders.

Cheever, K. H., Dooling, E., Hagler, D., Keuth, J., Pool, D., Stillwell, S. B, et al. (2006). In S. B. Stillwell (Ed.), *Critical care nursing reference* (4th ed.). St. Louis: Mosby.

Deglin, J. H., & Vallerand, A. H. (2009). *Davis's drug guide for nurses* (11th ed.). Philadelphia: F. A. Davis.

Dillon, P. (2007). *Nursing health assessment: A critical thinking and case studies approach* (2nd ed.). Philadelphia: F. A. Davis.

Erikson, E.H. (1950). *Childhood and society.* New York: Norton.

Gahart, B. L. (2006). *Intravenous medications* (22nd ed.). St. Louis: Mosby.

Lagerquist, S. L. (2006). *Davis's NCLEX-RN for success* (2nd ed.). Philadelphia: F. A. Davis.

Litwack, K. (2006). *Core curriculum for critical care nurses* (6th ed.). St. Louis: Elsevier Saunders.

Van Leeuwen, A. M., Poelhuis-Leth, D. J., & Bladh, M. L. (2011). *Davis's comprehensive handbook of laboratory and diagnostic tests with nursing implications.* (4th ed.). Philadelphia: F. A. Davis.

8-4 Diabetic Ketoacidosis (DKA)

CRITICAL CARE

STANDARD FORMS

These templates are included in the Appendix; copy before each use.

LEARNING OUTCOMES

Cognitive

The student will be able to:

1. Describe signs and symptoms of DKA.
2. Differentiate diabetes mellitus type 1 and type 2.
3. Correlate the signs and symptoms of DKA to the pathophysiology.
4. Identify the signs and symptoms of hyperglycemia and hypoglycemia.
5. Identify appropriate intervention for a patient with DKA.

Psychomotor

The student will be able:

1. Perform an assessment on a patient with DKA.
2. Initiate appropriate interventions, such as start and maintain IV, insert Foley catheter, place patient on monitor.

Affective

The student will be able to:

1. Reflect upon performance in a simulated situation and care of a patient with DKA.
2. Identify areas that worked well during the scenario.
3. Identify areas that need improvement.
4. Reflect on overall feeling about the scenario.
5. Discuss feelings related to working as a team member.
6. Develops confidence in caring for a patient with DKA.
7. Perform self-reflective evaluation.

Communication

The student will be able to:

1. Communicate effectively with healthcare team members in the care of a patient with DKA.
2. Communicate effectively with the patient and family members.
3. Use SBAR format when communicating with healthcare team members.
4. Work collaboratively as part of the healthcare team.
5. Accurately and succinctly document assessments, interventions, and evaluations.
6. Practice Transparent Thinking (thinking out loud) to facilitate group problem solving.
7. Use Directed Communication (directing a message to specific individual) when delegating tasks.
8. Employ Closed-Loop Communication (acknowledgment of receipt of the message and status) to acknowledge communications from others.

Safety

The student will be able to:

Administer and maintain specific protecting interventions with attention to safety of the client and healthcare professional.

1. Demonstrate a safe environment with attention to hazards to healthcare providers, visitors, and the client. Includes body mechanics, tripping hazards, and equipment issues.
2. Demonstrate attention to national patient safety goals. Includes patient identification standards, effective communication among healthcare providers, and safe medication administration.
3. Demonstrate attention to standard precautions. Includes hand washing, infection control measures, and use of personal protective equipment (PPE) as needed.

Leadership and Management/Delegation

The student will be able to:

1. Identify and prioritize patient's needs in care of a patient with DKA.
2. Identify those interventions that can be delegated to unlicensed assistive personnel (UAP) or licensed practical nurse (LPN).

OVERVIEW OF THE PROBLEM

Definition

Diabetic ketoacidosis (DKA) is a major metabolic complication occurring when there is insufficient insulin for metabolism of carbohydrates, fats, and proteins. It is seen most often in patients who are insulin dependent, and can be precipitated by stressors such as infection, trauma, and major illness that increase insulin needs.

Pathophysiology

In DKA, circulating glucose cannot be used due to a lack of insulin, which "turns on" ketogenic pathways. The supply of ketones exceeds peripheral demand, and ketosis results.

Risk Factors

- Insufficient insulin or oral hypoglycemics
- Noncompliance with dietary regimen
- Major illness/infection
- Steroid therapy
- Trauma/surgery
- Elevated blood sugar >200 mg/dL

Assessment

Assessment	Subjective	Objective
Behavior	Irritable, confused	
Visual		Soft, sunken eyeballs
Skin		Decreased turgor, flushed face, pruritus vulvae
Vital signs		Tachycardia, thready pulse, Kussmaul's respirations, hypotension, hypovolemic shock
Gastrointestinal	Increased thirst and hunger, abdominal pain, nausea	Vomiting, diarrhea, dry mucous membranes, lips and tongue red and parched, fruity breath (acetone)
Neurological	Headache, irritability, confusion, lethargy	
Muskuloskeletal	Fatigue, malaise, weakness	Decreased muscle tone and strength
Renal		Polyuria
Blood sugar		>300 mg/dL

Treatment

- Regular insulin
- Fluid replacement
- Bicarbonate and electrolyte replacement

Nursing Management

Goal: Promote normal balance of intake and insulin.

- Administer regular insulin as ordered and monitor response
- IV saline as ordered
- Bicarbonate and electrolyte replacement
- Potassium replacement once therapy begins and urine output is adequate

Goal: Provide health teaching

- Diet, desired and side effects of insulin or hypoglycemic therapy, importance of recognizing signs of imbalance

Evaluation/Outcome Criteria

- Follows prescribed diet
- Takes medication as ordered
- Avoids serious complication

REVIEW QUESTIONS

1. How would you differentiate signs and symptoms of hyperglycemia from those of hypoglycemia?
   Answer:

2. What physical findings would result from hyperosmolar diuresis?
   Answer:

3. How does the body attempt to compensate for metabolic acidosis?
   Answer:

4. DKA is a medical emergency; why is it a life-threatening crisis?
   Answer:

5. Regular insulin is used to treat DKA. Explain the rationale of using regular insulin rather than NPH insulin.
   Answer:

Related Evidenced-Based Practice Guidelines

The Joint Commission National Patient Safety Goals Hospital Program. Retrieved from http://www.jointcommission.org/GeneralPublic/NPSG/10_npsgs.htm

SBAR technique for communication: A situational briefing model. The Institute for Healthcare Improvement. Retrieved December 19, 2008, from http://www.ihi.org/IHI/Topics/PatientSafety/SafetyGeneral/Tools/SBARTechniqueforCommunicationASituationalBriefingModel.htm

National Guidline Clearinghouse: Search Type 1 diabetes

Type 1 diabetes. In: Prevention, detection and treatment of diabetes in adults. 4th edition.

Type 1 diabetes practice guidelines. In: Mazze RS, Strock E, Simonson GD, Bergenstal RM. Prevention, detection and treatment of diabetes in adults. 4th ed. Minneapolis (MN): International Diabetes Center; 2007. p. Various. http://www.guideline.gov/content.aspx?id=14722&search=diabetic+ketoacidosis

Topics to Review Prior to the Simulation

- Diabetes mellitus type 1 and type 2 in pathophysiology text or medical-surgical text.
- Pathophysiology of DKA.
- Appropriate interventions for a patient with DKA.
- Appropriate pharmacological interventions for a patient with DKA.

SIMULATION

Client Background

Biographical Data

- Age: 24
- Gender: female
- Height: 5 ft 8 in
- Weight: 160 lb

Cultural Considerations

- Language: English
- Ethnicity: Irish
- Nationality: American
- Culture: No cultural considerations identified

Demographic

- Marital status: single
- Educational level: college
- Religion: Catholic
- Occupation: accountant

Current Health Status

- Diabetes mellitus type 1, found unconscious after flu illness

History

- Psychosocial history
  - Social support: family
- Past health history
  - Medical: diabetes mellitus type 1 since 3 years of age
  - Surgical: unknown
- Family History: unknown, adopted

Admission Sheet

Name:	Shannon O'Reilly
Age:	24
Gender:	Female
Marital Status:	Single
Educational Level:	College
Religion:	Catholic
Ethnicity:	Irish
Nationality:	American
Language:	English
Occupation:	Accountant

Hospital
Provider's Orders

Patient's Name: **Shannon O'Reilly**
Allergies: **NKDA**

Diagnosis: **DKA**

Date	Time	Order	Signature
6/20/07	3:10 PM	Vital signs: q 15 min	
		Diet: NPO	
		Activity: Bed rest	
		Diagnostic studies: Serum electrolytes, glucose BUN, creatinine, ABGs	
		Medications: IV regular insulin drip at 0.1 units/kg/hr	
		IV therapy: 1,000 mL NSS to maintain systolic BP >100	
		Treatments: Accu-Checks q hr Insert Foley, hourly output Oxygen via NR mask	Dr. L. Fisher
6/20/07	3:15 PM	K rider 40 mEq in 100 mL over 4 hr Repeat ABGs in 1 hr. Repeat	Dr. L. Fisher
6/20/07	5 PM	Change IV to 5% D/½ NSS	
		Admit to ICU	
		Maintain insulin drip Accu-Checks q hr	
		Repeat BUN, creatinine, electrolytes, glucose, ABGs	Dr. L. Fisher

Nursing Report

Mother states she went to work this morning and her daughter was asleep. When mother called home later in the morning daughter didn't answer the phone and she rushed home to check on her. She found her unconscious lying on the sofa. She has had the flu for the past couple days with vomiting and loss of appetite. She was diagnosed with diabetes mellitus type 1 at 3 years of age. Her mother said since her daughter wasn't eating, she hasn't taken her insulin.

Medications she was taking:

10 units Humulin Regular, 20 units of Humilin NPH before breakfast.

10 units Humulin NPH at bed time.

IV line inserted in the field. NSS hanging wide open.

Student Simulation Prep Assignments

1. Identify items and their purpose in the care of a patient with DKA.

Item	Purpose
IV with pump	
O_2 nonrebreather mask, cannula	
Accu-Check	
Foley	
Monitor	

2. Identify team members and their specific roles in the care of the patient with DKA.

Team Member	Role
Primary nurse	
Secondary nurse	
Physician	

3. Relevant Data Assignment: Fill in columns below.

Relevant Data from Report	Relevant Data from Other Sources	Data Missing	Sources for Missing Data	Data Requiring Follow-Up

4. Initial Focused Assessment

After reviewing the client background and nursing report, you are ready to assess your client's current status. Under each category, identify how you would target your assessment and what you would expect to find for the patient with DKA.

History

Are there any questions you need to ask the patient or family to obtain additional relevant data?

Physical Exam

- General appearance:
- Integumentary:
- HEENT:
- Respiratory:
- CV:
- Breasts:
- Abdominal/GI:
- Neuro:

- Musculoskeletal:
- Reproductive:
- Additional
  - Renal:
- Developmental:

What are the nursing implications considering the developmental stage of your patient?

Answer:

5. Diagnostic Tests

What diagnostic test results relevant to the patient's current problem are needed to plan care?

Complete the table using Van Leeuwen et al, *Davis's Comprehensive Handbook of Laboratory and Diagnostic Testing with Nursing Implications* 4e, or other diagnostic test reference.

Diagnostic Test	Significance to This Patient's Problem
Serum glucose	
Electrolytes	
BUN and creatinine	
ABGs	

6. Treatment

Identify drugs that are used to treat a patient with DKA?

Complete the table using Deglin et al, *Davis's Drug Guide for Nurses* 12e, or other drug reference.

Medication	Dose Route, Frequency	Indications	Side Effect	Nursing Implications
Regular insulin	IV regular insulin drip at 0.1 unit/kg/hr			
Potassium	IV not to exceed 10 mEq/hr			

7. Nursing Problems/Diagnoses

Identify three priority nursing problems/diagnoses.

Assessment Data	Priority Problem	Intervention	Expected Patient Outcome	Which Intervention Could Be Delegated to Unlicensed Personnel?
1.				
2.				
3.				

References

Deglin, J. H., & Vallerand, A. H. (2000). *Davis's drug guide for nurses* (11th ed.). Philadelphia: F. A. Davis.

Dillon, P. (2007). *Nursing health assessment: A critical thinking and case studies approach* (2nd ed.). Philadelphia: F. A. Davis.

Erikson, E.H. (1950). *Childhood and society.* New York: Norton.

Lagerquist, S. L.(2006). *Davis's NCLEX-RN for success* (2006). Philadelphia: F. A. Davis.

Van Leeuwen, A. M., Poelhuis-Leth, D. J., & Bladh, M. L. (2011). *Davis's comprehensive handbook of laboratory and diagnostic tests with nursing implications.* (4th ed.). Philadelphia: F. A. Davis.

Psychiatric/Mental Health Nursing

9

9-1 Narcotic Overdose/Bipolar Disorder

BEHAVIORAL HEALTH

STANDARD FORMS

These templates are included in the Appendix; copy before each use.

LEARNING OUTCOMES

Cognitive

The student will be able to:

1. Describe signs and symptoms of a narcotic overdose.
2. Correlate signs and symptoms of a narcotic overdose to the pathophysiology of the human body.
3. Identify factors in a patient's history that increase risk for a narcotic overdose.
4. Identify factors in a patient's current condition that increase risk for a narcotic overdose.
5. Identify the appropriate interventions for the patient in a narcotic overdose.
6. Differentiate the roles of team members in response to a patient in a narcotic overdose.

Psychomotor

The student will be able to:

1. Perform appropriate assessment (neurological assessment) for a patient in a narcotic overdose.
2. Initiate appropriate interventions including recognizing the signs and symptoms of the overdose, maintaining an airway, initiating emergency actions (naloxone hydrochloride [Narcan]), and completing the appropriate documentation.
3. Work collaboratively as part of the healthcare team in the care of a patient in a narcotic overdose.

Affective

The student will be able to:

1. Reflect upon performance in the care of a patient in a narcotic overdose.
2. Identify own feelings in delivering care to a patient in a narcotic overdose.
3. Discuss feelings related to working as a member of a team in the care of a patient in a narcotic overdose.
4. Identify factors that worked well during the simulation of care of a patient in a narcotic overdose.
5. Identify factors that needed improvement during the simulation of care of a patient in a narcotic overdose.
6. Develop self-confidence in the care of a patient in a narcotic overdose.

Communication

The student will be able to:

1. Communicate effectively with healthcare team members in care of a patient in a narcotic overdose.
2. Communicate effectively with the patient and family in the care of a patient in a narcotic overdose.
3. Use SBAR when communication with team members in the care of a patient in a narcotic overdose.
4. Will practice Transparent Thinking (thinking out loud) to facilitate group problem solving.
5. Use Directed Communication (directing a message to specific individual) when delegating tasks.
6. Employ Closed-Loop Communication (acknowledgment of receipt of the message and status) to acknowledge communications from others.

Safety

The student will be able to:

Administer and maintain specific protecting interventions with attention to safety of the client and health care professional.

1. Demonstrate a safe environment with attention to hazards to healthcare providers, visitors, and the client. Includes body mechanics, tripping hazards, and equipment issues.
2. Demonstrate attention to national patient safety goals. Includes patient identification standards, effective communication among healthcare providers, and safe medication administration.
3. Demonstrates attention to standard precautions. Includes hand washing, infection control measures, and use of personal protective equipment (PPE) as needed.

Leadership and Management/Delegation

The student will be able to:

1. Identify and prioritize patient's needs in care of a patient with a narcotic overdose.
2. Identify tasks that can be legally, ethically, and safely delegated to unlicensed assistive personnel (UAP) or licensed practical nurse (LPN) in the care of a patient in a narcotic overdose.
3. Direct second nurse to assist with care of the patient in a narcotic overdose.

OVERVIEW OF PROBLEM

Substance Abuse

Narcotics

Definition

Substance abuse is a pattern of pathological use characterized by daily need of the substance for functioning, inability to stop use, and repeated medical complications from use.

Pathophysiology

Opium and its derivatives (morphine, heroin, codeine, and meperidine [Demerol]) can be abused by "snorting," "skin popping," or "mainlining," which may lead to complications such as abscesses and hepatitis. Narcotics abusers may exhibit decreased pain response, respiratory depression, apathy, detachment from reality, impaired judgment, loss of sexual activity, and pinpoint pupils. Narcotics are CNS depressants, causing sedation, euphoria, pain relief, impaired intellectual functioning, and impaired coordination.

Risk Factors

- Complex psychosocial and environmental factors influence abuse and addiction.

Assessment

Subjective

- Person feels it is impossible to get along without drug
- Disrupted relationships and family dynamics
- Low self-esteem
- Anger
- Denial
- Rationalization
- Social isolation
- Rigid coping pattern
- Poorly defined values and mores
  - Long-term effects include constipation, loss of appetite and weight, temporary impotence, habituation, and addiction with painful withdrawal symptoms.
- Withdrawal
  - Symptoms begin within 12 hr of last dose, peak in 24–36 hr, subside in 72 hr, and disappear in 5–6 days

Objective

- Pupil dilation
- Muscle twitches, tremors, aches and pains
- Gooseflesh (piloerection)
- Lacrimation, rhinorrhea, sneezing, yawning
- Diaphoresis, chills
- Fever
- Vomiting, abdominal pain
- Dehydration
- Rapid weight loss
- Sleep disturbance
- Overdose
  - Signs and symptoms of narcotic/opioid overdose include euphoria, arousable somnolence, nausea, pinpoint pupils, hypoxia, respiratory arrest, coma, and seizures.

Diagnostic Tests

- Blood toxicology

Treatment

- Airway management
- Naloxone
- Charcoal or bowel irrigation if indicated

Nursing Management

Goal: maintain safety and optimum level of physical comfort.

- Supportive physical care
- Vital signs
- Nutrition
- Hydration
- Seizure precautions

Goal: assist with medical treatment, offer support, and reality orientation to reduce anxiety.

- Detoxification: give medications as ordered
- Withdrawal: monitor symptoms and report concerns immediately

Evaluation/Outcome Criteria

- No complications
- Replaces addictive lifestyle with self-reliant plan formulated to maintain substance-free life

REVIEW QUESTIONS

1. What are the physical signs and symptoms of a narcotic overdose?
   Answer:

2. What are the nursing interventions for a patient suffering from a severe narcotic (opioid) overdose?
   Answer:

3. What are the signs and symptoms of narcotic withdrawal?
   Answer:

4. What are the treatments for withdrawal symptoms?
   Answer:

5. What are the five components of a neurological examination?
   Answer:

Related Evidence-Based Practice Guidelines

The Joint Commission National Patient Safety Goals Hospital Program. Retrieved from http://www.jointcommission.org/GeneralPublic/NPSG/10_npsgs.htm

SBAR Technique for Communication: A situational briefing model published by The Institute for Healthcare Improvement was downloaded on December 19, 2008, from http://www.ihi.org/IHI/Topics/PatientSafety/SafetyGeneral/Tools/SBARTechniqueforCommunicationASituationalBriefingModel.htm

The National Guideline Clearinghouse

Substance Abuse and Mental Health Services Administration (U.S.)—Federal Government Agency (U.S.) (2006). Detoxification and substance abuse treatment: Physical detoxification services for withdrawal from specific substances. In: Center for Substance Abuse Treatment (CSAT). Detoxification and substance abuse treatment. Rockville (MD): Substance Abuse and Mental Health Services Administration (SAMHSA); 2006 Jan 18. p. 41-111. (Treatment improvement protocol (TIP); no. 45). Retrieved from http://www .guideline.gov/content.aspx?id=9118

Bipolar Disorder

Definition

Bipolar disorders fall under the heading of mood disorders and are characterized by mood swings alternating from depression to elation, with periods of relative normality between episodes.

Pathophysiology

There is increasing evidence that the etiology involves a biochemical disturbance.

Concepts and Principles

- Manic and depressive episodes are related to hostility, guilt, and anxiety from the struggle between unconscious impulses and the moral conscience.
- During the manic phase, the person projects hostile feelings onto others.
- During the depressive phase, hostility is directed at the self.
- Both phases serve the objective of gaining attention, approval, and emotional support, either biochemically, unconsciously, or both.

Topics to Review Prior to the Simulation

- Drug overdose
- Neurological assessment (Glasgow Coma Scale)
- Bipolar disorder

SIMULATION

Client Background

Biographical Data

- Age: 36
- Gender: male
- Height: 6 ft
- Weight: 165 lb

Cultural Considerations

- Language: English
- Ethnicity: English
- Nationality: Canadian
- Culture: no significant cultural considerations identified

Demographic

- Marital status: single
- Educational level: grade 10
- Religion: not known
- Occupation: unemployed

Current Health Status

- History of bipolar disorder and heroin addiction

History

- Psychosocial history
  - Social support: none
- Past health history
  - Medical: two previous overdoses
  - Surgical: not known
- Family history: father died of alcohol addiction

Admission Sheet

Name:	Mr. Brown
Age:	36
Gender:	Male
Marital Status:	Single
Educational Level:	Grade 10
Religion:	Unknown
Ethnicity:	English
Nationality:	Canadian
Language:	English
Occupation:	Unemployed

Hospital
Provider's Orders

Patient's Name: Mr. Brown
Allergies: NKDA

Diagnosis: bipolar disorder

Date	Time	Order	Signature
		Vital signs with neuro check q 15 min x 2 hr then routine Continuous pulse oximetry monitoring	
		Diet as tolerated	
		Activity: Activity as tolerated	
		IV therapy: Initiate in an emergency and follow overdose protocol	
		Medications: Lithium 300 mg po tid Narcan 0.4 mg IV. Repeat in 1 min if RR <10 Monitor for 2 hr following Narcan administration	
		Diagnostic studies: CBC, BMP, UDS, CXR r/o aspiration, acetaminophen level, salicylate level, ECG, cardiac monitoring	
		Treatments: Psychiatric support	
		1:1 observation, suicide risk	Dr. Bennett

Nursing Report

You are working on a psychiatric inpatient unit. One of your assigned patients has returned from a day pass. You are suddenly called to the dining room to find the patient lying on his back and talking incoherently. He is inappropriate in his responses and his breathing is shallow and labored.

Student Simulation Prep Assignments

1. Identify items and their purpose in the care of a patient in a narcotic overdose.

Item	Purpose
Oxygen via mask and nasal cannula	
BP cuff, thermometer, stethoscope, O_2 saturation machine	
IV equipment	
Airway/Ambu bag	

2. Identify team members and their specific roles in the care of a patient in a narcotic overdose.

Team Member	Role
Primary nurse	
Second nurse	
Psychiatrist	
Respiratory therapy	
Attending physician	

3. Relevant Data Exercise: Fill in the columns below.

Relevant Data from Report	Relevant Data from Other Sources	Data Missing	Sources for Missing Data	Data Requiring Follow-Up

4. Initial Focused Assessment

After reviewing the client background and nursing report, you are ready to assess your client's current status. Under each category, identify how you would target your assessment and what you would expect to find for the patient in a narcotic overdose.

History

Are there any questions you need to ask the patient or family to obtain additional relevant data?

Physical Exam

- General appearance:
- Integumentary:
- HEENT:
- Respiratory:
- CV:
- Breasts:
- Abdominal:
- Neuro:
- Musculoskeletal:
- Reproductive:
- Additional:
- Developmental:

What are the nursing implications considering the developmental stage of your patient?

Answer:

5. Diagnostic Tests

What diagnostic test results relevant to the patient's current problem are needed to plan care?

Complete the table using Van Leeuwen et al, *Davis's Comprehensive Handbook of Laboratory and Diagnostic Testing with Nursing Implications* 4e, or other diagnostic test reference.

Diagnostic Test	Significance to This Patient's Problem
CBC	
Chemistry profile including electrolytes, BUN, creatinine	
ECG	
Drug screen on blood, urine, and gastric analysis as appropriate	
Chest x-ray	
Blood gases	
Liver function tests	

6. Treatment

Identify drugs that are used to treat a patient in a narcotic overdose.

Complete the table using Deglin et al, *Davis's Drug Guide for Nurses* 12e, or other drug reference.

Medication	Dose, Route, Frequency	Indications	Side Effect	Nursing Implications
Lithium	300 mg po tid			

Medication	Dose, Route, Frequency	Indications	Side Effect	Nursing Implications
Naloxone hydrochloride	0.4–2.0 mg q 2–3 mins until respiratory function is restored			

7. Nursing Problems/Diagnoses

Identify three priority nursing problems/diagnoses.

Assessment Data	Priority Problem	Intervention	Expected Patient Outcome	Which Interventions Could Be Delegated to Unlicensed Personnel?
1.				
2.				

Continued

Assessment Data	Priority Problem	Intervention	Expected Patient Outcome	Which Interventions Could Be Delegated to Unlicensed Personnel?
3.				

References

Deglin, J. H., & Vallerand, A. H. (2009). *Davis's drug guide for nurses* (11th ed.). Philadelphia: F. A. Davis.

Dillon, P. (2007). *Nursing health assessment: A critical thinking and case studies approach* (2nd ed.). Philadelphia: F. A. Davis.

Erikson, E.H. (1950). *Childhood and society.* New York: Norton.

Ignatavicius, D., Winkelman, C., Workman, M.L., & Hausman, K. (2010). *Clinical companion for medical-surgical nursing: Critical thinking for collaborative care* (6th ed.). St. Louis: Saunders.

Kee, J. L., Hayes, E. R., & McCuistion L. E. (2009). *Pharmacology: A nursing process approach* (6th ed.). St. Louis: Saunders Elsevier

Lagerquist, S. (2006). *Davis's NCLEX-RN success*. Philadelphia: F. A. Davis.

Potter, P. (2007). *Basic nursing: Essentials for practice* (6th ed.). St. Louis: Mosby.

Van Leeuwen, A. M., Poelhuis-Leth, D.J., & Bladh, M.L. (2011). *Davis's comprehensive handbook of laboratory and diagnostic tests with nursing implications.* (4th ed.). Philadelphia: F.A. Davis.

Varcarolis, E., & Halter, M. (2009) *Foundations of psychiatric mental health nursing: A clinical approach.* St. Louis: Saunders Elsevier.

9-2 Paranoid Schizophrenia

PSYCHIATRIC/MENTAL HEALTH NURSING

STANDARD FORMS

These templates are included in the Appendix; copy before each use.

LEARNING OUTCOMES

Cognitive

The student will be able to:

1. Describe signs and symptoms of schizophrenia.
2. Identify the elements of a mental status assessment.
3. Identify the medications commonly used to treat psychotic disorders with perceptual disturbances.
4. Describe the expected results of medications used for schizophrenia and the possible side effects.
5. Identify the appropriate therapeutic communication interventions for a client with paranoid delusions.
6. Describe the means of ascertaining medication adherence/compliance history.
7. Interpret diagnostic tests.

Psychomotor

The student will be able to:

1. Complete a focused assessment for a client exhibiting psychotic symptoms.
2. Intervene appropriately with a client who is delusional and paranoid.
3. Intervene appropriately with family members.
4. Administer prescribed medications in a safe manner.
5. Implement suicide precautions.

Affective

The student will be able to:

1. Identify one's own feelings in caring for a client with delusions and auditory hallucinations and how these feelings could impact nursing care.
2. Demonstrate self-confidence in the care of a patient with delusions and paranoia.
3. Discuss factors that worked well during the simulation of care of a client with paranoid schizophrenia.
4. Discuss factors that needed improvement during the simulation of care of a client with paranoid schizophrenia.

Communication

The student will be able to:

1. Intervene therapeutically with clients who are demonstrating the following symptoms:
   - Auditory hallucinations
   - Suicidal ideations/thoughts
   - Escalating behaviors
2. Using SBAR, communicate effectively with the following people in the care of a patient with a psychotic disorder.
   - Physician
   - Nursing team members
   - Social worker
   - Security
3. Communicate effectively with the patient and family during a psychiatric crisis.
4. Evaluate and document measures used to treat a patient experiencing delusions and increasing agitation.
5. Will practice Transparent Thinking (thinking out loud) to facilitate group problem solving
6. Use Directed Communication (directing a message to specific individual) when delegating tasks
7. Employ Closed-Loop Communication (acknowledgment of receipt of the message and status) to acknowledge communications from others.

Safety

The student will be able to:

Administer and maintain specific protecting interventions with attention to safety of the client and health care professional.

1. Demonstrate a safe environment with attention to hazards to healthcare providers, visitors, and the client. Includes body mechanics, tripping hazards, and equipment issues.
2. Demonstrate attention to national patient safety goals. Includes patient identification standards, effective communication among healthcare providers, and safe medication administration.
3. Demonstrates attention to standard precautions. Includes hand washing, infection control measures, and use of personal protective equipment (PPE) as needed.

Leadership/Delegation

The student will be able to:

1. Differentiate the roles of team members in response to a family member who expresses concern for a psychiatric client.
2. Appropriately assign roles to staff members when a client exhibits escalating behavior.

Legal/Ethical

The student will be able to discriminate the amount of information members of the hospital team need to know in order to assist in the care of a client with a psychotic disorder.

OVERVIEW OF PROBLEM

Definition

Schizophrenia is a group of interrelated symptoms with a number of common features involving disorders of mood, thought content, feelings, perception, and behavior. The onset is usually between ages 15 and 27.

Pathophysiology

The etiology of schizophrenia is thought to be related to genetics and neurochemical imbalances of dopamine and serotonin. It is not clear whether structural differences in the brains of schizophrenics are a result or a cause of the disease.

Risk Factors

It is possible to develop schizophrenia with no identified risks. The following categories have been identified as factors that may increase risk for developing schizophrenia:

- Family history
- Brain abnormalities
- Environmental factors
- Complications during fetal development or birth
- Early parental loss
- Socioeconomic and cultural factors

Assessment

"Positive" symptoms reflect an excess or distortion of normal function, and are associated with normal brain structure on CT scans, and usually respond well to treatment.

- Delusions
- Hallucinations
- Disorganized thought or speech
- Disorganized behavior

"Negative" symptoms (known as the 4 As) reflect a loss of normal function and structural brain abnormalities, and respond poorly to treatment.

- Associative looseness: impairment of logical thought processes
- Affect: exaggerated, apathetic, flat, inappropriate, or inconsistent
- Ambivalence: simultaneous conflicting feelings or attitudes
- Autism: withdrawal from the external world, preoccupation with fantasies, and idiosyncratic thoughts

  Prodromal or residual symptoms:
  - Social isolation
  - Role impairment
  - Peculiar behavior
  - Impaired personal hygiene
  - Blunt or inappropriate affect
  - Speech alterations
  - Bizarre thinking
  - Unusual perceptual experiences

The *paranoid type of schizophrenia* consists of disturbed perceptions leading to disturbance in thought content of persecutory, grandiose, or hostile nature; projection is a key mechanism, with religion a common preoccupation.

Diagnostic Tests

- Drug screen
- CT, MRI, PET, EEG may be ordered to examine structure and function of the brain

Treatment

- Antipsychotic and antiparkinsonian medications
- Isolation and seclusion if required to maintain safety
- Mileu therapy

Nursing Management of Hallucinatory Behavior

- Provide a structured environment
- Use real objects to keep or stimulate interest
- Protect against injury resulting from hallucinations
- Increase social interaction gradually
- Ask person to describe the hallucinatory experience
- Respond to anything real; focus on feelings
- Distract to something real during hallucinations
- Avoid direct confrontation; do not argue
- Ask one question at a time
- Use clear unambiguous language
- Encourage consensual validation; point out that experience is not shared by you
- Assist family to understand client needs

Evaluation/Outcome Criteria

- Growing self-awareness
- Small positive behavioral change
- Evidence of beginning trust
- Initiates conversation
- Participates in activities
- Decreases amount of time spent alone
- Demonstrates appropriate behavior in public
- Makes positive statements

REVIEW QUESTIONS

1. What are therapeutic communication strategies to use with a patient who is demonstrating paranoid delusions and auditory hallucinations?
   Answer:

2. Name the components of a mental status assessment.
   Answer:

3. What classification of drugs is commonly used to treat schizophrenia?
   Answer:

4. Describe the side effects for which the nurse would monitor when a client is taking antipsychotic mediations? How would the nurse intervene?
Answer:

5. What are appropriate nursing interventions when a patient's behavior indicates agitation?
Answer:

Related Evidence-Based Practice Guidelines

Veterans Administration, Department of Defense. Management of persons with psychoses. Washington (DC):

Department of Veteran Affairs; 2004 May. Various p. Available at:

http://www.ngc.gov/summary/summary.aspx?doc_id=5632&nbr=003794&string=schizophrenia. Best Practice Evidenced-based Guideline: The assessment and management of people at risk of suicide: New Zealand Guidelines Group (NZGG).Available at: http://www.nzgg.org.nz/guidelines/0005/acf50e.pdf

Violence: the short-term management of disturbed/violent behaviour in psychiatric in-patient settings and emergency departments: National Collaborating Centre for Nursing and Supportive Care. London (UK): National Institute for Clinical Excellence (NICE); Feb 2005. 292 p.

The Joint Commission National Patient Safety Goals Hospital Program. Retrieved from http://www.jointcommission.org/GeneralPublic/NPSG/10_npsgs.htm

SBAR Technique for Communication: A situational briefing model published by The Institute for Healthcare Improvement was downloaded on December 19, 2008, from http://www.ihi.org/IHI/Topics/PatientSafety/SafetyGeneral/Tools/SBARTechniqueforCommunicationASituationalBriefingModel.htm

Topics to Review Prior to the Simulation

- Communication
  - Therapeutic communication
  - Interdisciplinary communication
  - Documentation
  - Patient confidentiality
- Psychopharmacology
- Mental status assessment
- Schizophrenia
- Acute care of the psychiatric client
  - Risk factors that may predispose a client with paranoid schizophrenia to experience thought disorders
  - Pertinent assessment(s) the nurse would perform in caring for a hospitalized client with a psychiatric disorder
  - Expected response to therapeutic interventions
  - Treatments for a client who is experiencing auditory hallucinations and paranoia

SIMULATION

Client Background

Biographical Data

- Age: 59
- Gender: male
- Height: 5 ft 9 in
- Weight: 165 lb

Cultural Considerations

- Language: English
- Ethnicity: German
- Nationality: American
- Culture: urban

Demographic

- Marital status: separated from wife and four children for past 3 years
- Educational level: completed 11th grade
- Religion: Baptist
- Occupation: unemployed

Current Health Status

- Diagnosed with paranoid schizophrenia at age 20; prior to hospitalization, attempted to jump in front of a commuter train, stating the voices told him to "jump off rooftops" and "to jump in front of trains."

History

- Psychosocial history: separated 3 years; sees his children about once/month when they come to visit their grandmother; incarcerated 5 years for manslaughter (released 10 years ago); admitted to abusing alcohol and drugs at the time of the crime
  - Social support: currently lives with 75-year-old mother; no other friends
- Past health history
  - Medical: diagnosed HIV positive 3 years ago—asymptomatic; states he does not know how he contracted the disease; hypertension; NKDA
  - Current medications: Atenolol 50 mg po q AM; Spironolactone 100 mg po q AM; Olanzapine 20 mg po q AM

- Surgical: none
- Psychiatric: medical records indicate that he has been in and out of psychiatric hospitals for the past 20 years due to psychotic episodes; first heard voices at the age of 19 while serving in the first Gulf War; subsequently received a medical discharge.
- Family history: unremarkable; 75-year-old mother is in good health except for minor hearing loss

Admission Sheet

Name:	Peter Snyder
Age:	59
Gender:	Male
Marital Status:	Separated
Educational Level:	Completed 11th grade
Religion:	Baptist
Ethnicity:	German
Nationality:	American
Language:	English
Occupation:	Unemployed

Hospital
Provider's Orders

Patient's Name: **Peter Snyder**
Allergies: **NKDA**

Diagnosis: **Paranoid schizophrenia, HTN, HIV**

Date	Time	Order	Signature
dd/mm/yy		Vital signs: q day	
		Weight on admission then q other day	
		Special precautions: Suicide precautions q 15 min	
		Privileges: Routine visits allowed, family members only	
		Diet: 2 g sodium	
		Activity: Up ad lib	
		Medications: Atenolol 50 mg po q AM	
		Tylenol 650 mg po q 4 hr prn for headache/pain Haldol 5 mg IM q 4 hr prn for severe psychotic agitation	
		Diagnostic studies: CBC with diff, ECG, urine toxicology screen, blood alcohol level	
			Albert Nicholson, MD

Nursing Report

Mr. Snyder, a 59-year-old male, was admitted 24-hr ago with a history of paranoid schizophrenia. Prior to admission, patient states he heard voices telling him to "jump off the rooftops" and "jump in front of trains." He states he has not been taking his medications "because they make me tired and I can't have sex." On admission, he was accompanied by his 75-year-old mother with whom he lives since his separation from his wife 3 years ago.

Shift report from night nurse:

Mr. Snyder, a 59-year-old male patient of Dr. Nicholson, threatened another male client when he arrived on the unit last evening, stating the other client accused him of being a homosexual. Mr. Snyder accused the other client of touching him inappropriately. Mr. Snyder was responsive to directions to accompany staff to his assigned room and there were no further incidents before bedtime. He slept poorly last night—said "the voices get worse at night." He awoke early this morning and came to the day room just outside the nurses' station. He was observed glancing around the room mumbling to himself. He admits to hearing voices. He became increasingly more agitated, threatening to hurt other patients, who he said were plotting to kill him. He did not respond to directions to accompany staff back to his room because he was afraid someone was waiting to hurt him. An hour ago, he agreed to an IM injection of Haldol 5 mg for his increasing agitation and "to quiet the voices." He slept for 30 min. He is currently awake and resting in his room.

Urine drug screen is negative; no evidence of alcohol on BAL. CBC WNG except WNL 11,000 mm^3.

Student Simulation Prep Assignments

1. Identify items and their purpose in the care of a patient with paranoid schizophrenia.

Item	Purpose
B/P cuff, thermometer, stethoscope	
Syringe, needle, alcohol wipes, gloves	
Telephone	

2. Identify team members and specific roles in the care of a patient with paranoid schizophrenia.

Team Member	Role
Primary nurse	
Secondary nurse	
Social worker	
Physician	

3. Relevant Data Exercise: Fill in columns below.

Relevant Data from Report	Relevant Data from Other Sources	Data Missing	Sources for Missing Data	Data Requiring Follow-Up

Continued

Relevant Data from Report	Relevant Data from Other Sources	Data Missing	Sources for Missing Data	Data Requiring Follow-Up

4. Initial Focused Assessment

After reviewing the client background and nursing report, you are ready to assess your client's current status. Under each category, identify how you would target your assessment, and what you would expect to find for the patient with paranoid schizophrenia?

History

Are there any questions you need to ask the patient or family to obtain additional relevant data?

Answer:

Physical Exam—WNL

Additional

Mental status assessment:

- Appearance:
  - Posture:
  - Body movement:
  - Dress:
  - Grooming and hygiene:
- Behavior
  - Level of consciousness:
  - Facial expression:
  - Speech:
- Mood and affect:
- Cognition

- Orientation:
- Attention span:
- Recent memory:
- Remote memory:
- New learning:
- Judgment:
- Thought processes:

- Developmental:

What are the nursing implications considering the developmental stage of your patient?

Answer:

5. Diagnostic tests

What diagnostic test results relevant to the patient's current problem are needed to plan care?

Complete the table using Van Leeuwen et al, *Davis's Comprehensive Handbook of Laboratory and Diagnostic Testing with Nursing Implications* 4e, or other diagnostic test reference.

Diagnostic Test	Significance to This Patient's Problem
Complete blood count with differential: WBC Neutrophils Eospinophils Basophils Lymphocytes Monocytes RBC Hemoglobin Hematocrit Platelets	
Urine toxicology screen	
Blood alcohol level	

6. Treatment

Identify drugs that are used to treat a patient with paranoid Schizophrenia.

Complete the table using Deglin et al, *Davis's Drug Guide for Nurses* 12e, or other drug reference.

Medication	Dose, Route, Frequency	Indication	Side Effect	Nursing Implications
Atenolol	50 mg po q AM			

Continued

Medication	Dose, Route, Frequency	Indication	Side Effect	Nursing Implications
Spirinolactone	100 mg po q AM			
Aripiprazole	15 mg po q AM			
Tylenol	650 mg po q 4 rh prn for headache/pain			

Medication	Dose, Route, Frequency	Indication	Side Effect	Nursing Implications
Haloperidol	5 mg IM q 4 hr prn for severe psychotic agitation			

7. Nursing problems/diagnoses.

Assessment Data	Priority Problem	Intervention	Expected Patient Outcome	Which Interventions Could Be Delegated to Unlicensed Personnel?
1.				

Continued

Assessment Data	Priority Problem	Intervention	Expected Patient Outcome	Which Interventions Could Be Delegated to Unlicensed Personnel?
2.				
3.				

References

Deglin, J. H., & Vallerand, A. H. (2009). *Davis's drug guide for nurses* (11th ed.). Philadelphia: F. A. Davis.

Dillon, P. (2007). *Nursing health assessment: A critical thinking and case studies approach* (2nd ed.). Philadelphia: F. A. Davis.

Erikson, E.H. (1950). *Childhood and society.* New York: Norton.

Lagerquist, S. (2006). *Davis's NCLEX-RN success*. Philadelphia: F. A. Davis.

Swearingen, P. (2007). *All-in-one care planning resource.* St. Louis: Mosby Elsevier.

Van Leeuwen, A. M., Poelhuis-Leth, D. J., & Bladh, M. L. (2011). *Davis's comprehensive handbook of laboratory and diagnostic tests with nursing implications.* (4th ed.). Philadelphia: F.A. Davis.

Varcarolis, E. (2006). *The schizophrenias*. In E. M. Varcarolis, V. B. Carson, N. Shoemaker, *Foundations of psychiatric mental health nursing: A clinical Approach*. St. Louis: Saunders Elsevier.

Varcarolis, E., & Halter, M. (2009) *Foundations of psychiatric mental health nursing: A clinical Approach.* St. Louis: Saunders Elsevier.

Wilson, B. A., Shannon, M. T., & Stang, C. L. (Eds.). *Nurse's drug guide 2006* (pp. 9-11, 119-120, 131-133, 792-794, 1494-1496). Upper Saddle River, NJ: Pearson Prentice Hall.

9-3 Lithium Overdose with Renal Failure

MENTAL HEALTH

STANDARD FORMS

These templates are included in the Appendix; copy before each use.

LEARNING OUTCOMES

Cognitive

The student will be able:

1. Identify factors in a client's past medical history that increase risk for lithium overdose.
2. Describe signs and symptoms of lithium overdose.
3. Describe the pathophysiology of lithium overdose/toxicity.
4. Correlate signs and symptoms to the pathophysiology of lithium overdose.
5. Identify appropriate interventions for the client with lithium overdose.
6. Differentiate the roles of team members in response to an overdose emergency.
7. Correctly calculate medication dosages.
8. Interpret significance of diagnostic test results.
9. Describe the importance of maintaining asepsis and standard precautions.

Psychomotor

The student will be able to:

1. Perform appropriate assessment for a client with lithium overdose.
2. Initiate appropriate interventions for a client with lithium overdose.
3. Work collaboratively as part of the healthcare team in the care of a client with lithium overdose.
4. Monitor IV therapy.
5. Apply sterile gloves.
6. Draw up and administer IV medications.
7. Insert Foley catheter using sterile technique.
8. Maintain standard precautions.

Affective

The student will be able to:

1. Reflect thoughtfully upon performance of self and others in a simulated overdose emergency situation.
2. Identify own feelings in a simulated overdose emergency situation.
3. Discuss feelings related to working as a member of a team.
4. Identify factors that worked well during the scenario.
5. Identify factors that needed improvement during the scenario.
6. Develop self-confidence in the care of a client during a simulated overdose emergency.

Communication

The student will be able:

1. Communicate effectively with team members in a simulated overdose emergency.
2. Communicate effectively with the client and family in a simulated overdose emergency.
3. Document assessments, interventions, and evaluations.
4. Maintain HIPAA compliance with respect to client care modalities.
5. Will practice Transparent Thinking (thinking out loud) to facilitate group problem solving.
6. Use Directed Communication (directing a message to specific individual) when delegating tasks.
7. Employ Closed-Loop Communication (acknowledgment of receipt of the message and status) to acknowledge communications from others.

Safety

The student will be able to:

Administer and maintain specific protecting interventions with attention to safety of the client and health care professional.

1. Demonstrate a safe environment with attention to hazards to health care providers, visitors, and the client. Includes body mechanics, tripping hazards, and equipment issues.
2. Demonstrates attention to national patient safety goals. Includes patient identification standards, effective communication among healthcare providers, and safe medication administration.
3. Demonstrates attention to standard precautions. Includes hand washing, infection control measures, and use of personal protective equipment (PPE) as needed.

Leadership and Management/Delegation

The student will be able to:

1. Identify and prioritize patient's needs in a simulated drug toxicity emergency situation.
2. Identify tasks that can be legally, ethically, and safely delegated to unlicensed assistive personnel (UAP) or licensed practical nurse (LPN) in a simulated drug toxicity emergency situation.

Legal/Ethical

The student will be able to:

Identify aspects of HIPAA compliance and state law with regard to protocols and social services evaluation in mental health nursing care.

OVERVIEW OF THE PROBLEM

Definition

Lithium therapy is used to treat an acute manic attack and for the prevention of recurrence of cyclic manic-depressive episodes of bipolar disorders. It affects transport and uptake of neurotransmitters and intracellular enzymes as well as alters membrane permeability.

Dosage

- Therapeutic level: 0.8–1.6 mEq/L (may take several weeks to achieve (4–8 weeks)
- Maintenance dose: 300–1200 mg/day
- Toxic level : >2.0 mEq/L, blood sample drawn in acute phase 10–14 hr after last dose taken

Assessment

Side Effects

Monitoring of therapy is critical since common side effects can be realized ranging from acute to long-term effects. Pronounced neurological and gastrointestinal side effects can occur ranging from twitching, blurred vision, to coma as well as diarrhea, vomiting, and seizures. During the initial management of therapy, the client may experience side effects that can significantly affect compliance with therapy.

Levels 1.6–2.0 mEq:

- Blurred vision
- Tinnitus
- Tremors
- Nausea and vomiting
- Diarrhea
- Polyuria
- Polydipsia
- Ataxia

Levels >2.0 mEq/L:

- Motor weakness
- Headache
- Edema
- Lethargy

Levels >2.5 mEq/L:

- Severe toxicity
- Arrhythmias
- MI
- Cardiovascular collapse
- Oliguria/anuria
- Neurological symptoms: twitching, marked drowsiness, slurred speech, dysathria, atheotosis movements, convulsions, delirium, stupor, coma

Diagnostic Tests

- Baseline labs are indicated with initiation of therapy: CBC, thyroid profile, chemistry, and ECG in order to confirm "normal" functioning of body systems.

Precautions

- Potential for toxicity is increased in the presence of low sodium levels (low-salt diets) and certain uses of concurrent medications that may affect the lithium therapeutic level such as thiazide diuretics, ibuprofen, tetracyclines, and metronidazole.
- Use cautiously in patients with abnormal electrolytes (sweating, dehydration, postoperative), with thyroid problems, heart failure, or impaired renal function.
- Use is contraindicated during pregnancy and/or lactation.

Nursing Management

Goal: anticipate and check for signs and symptoms of toxicity.

- Reduce GI symptoms—take with meals
- Check for edema, daily wt, I&O
- Monitor blood levels and signs of toxicity
- Monitor results of diagnostic tests-thyroid and kidney function
- Withhold drug and notify MD of elevated drug levels (1.5 mEq/L)
- Monitor vital signs
- Assess for fever, diarrhea, prolonged vomiting, and report immediately

Goal: report complications immediately.

- Fever, diarrhea, prolonged vomitting

Goal: monitor effects (therapeutic and toxic) through blood samples.

Blood samples taken:

- 10–14 hr after last dose
- Every 2–3 days until therapeutic level reached
- Once a week while hospitalized
- Every 2–3 mo to maintain therapeutic levels

Goal: health teaching.

- Advise client of delayed effect
- Encourage adequate fluid intake, oral hygiene
- Report polyuria and polydipsia
- Diet: avoid caffeine, fad diets, diet pills, self-prescribed low-sodium diet, alcohol, antacids, high-sodium foods (which increase lithium excretion and reduce drug effect). Use sugarless candy
- Caution against driving and operating machinery if mental alertness is impaired
- Warn against altering or omitting doses

Evaluation/Outcome Criteria

- Changed facial affect
- Improved posture
- Able to concentrate
- Sleep patterns and mood stabilized
- Resumption of self care
- No signs of toxicity

REVIEW QUESTIONS

1. Define the concept of drug overdosage and/or toxicity.
   Answer:

2. Define lithium overdose.
Answer:

3. Describe three potential risk factors for lithium toxicity.
Answer: Fill in the table.

Risk Factor	Assessment Data	Precipitating Factors	Treatment

4. List at least two potential consequences or sequelae of lithium toxicity.
Answer:

Related Evidence-Based Practice Guidelines

National Guideline Clearinghouse, Bipolar disorder. The management of bipolar disorder in adults, children and adolescents, in primary and secondary care. National Collaborating Centre for Mental Health. Bipolar disorder: the management of bipolar disorder in adults, children, and adolescents, in primary and secondary care. Leicester (UK): British Psychological Society, Royal College of Psychiatrists; 2006. 592 p. Available at:http://www.guideline.gov/content.aspx?id=10949&search=bipolar+disorder

Bipolar affective disorder. A national clinical guideline. Scottish Intercollegiate Guidelines Network - National Government Agency [Non-U.S.]. 2005 May. 41 pages. NGC:004338

Available at: http://www.sign.ac.uk/pdf/sign82.pdf

The Joint Commission National Patient Safety Goals Hospital Program. Retrieved from http://www.jointcommission.org/GeneralPublic/NPSG/10_npsgs.htm

SBAR Technique for Communication: A situational briefing model published by The Institute for Healthcare Improvement was downloaded on December 19, 2008, from http://www.ihi.org/IHI/Topics/PatientSafety/SafetyGeneral/Tools/SBARTechniqueforCommunicationASituationalBriefingModel.htm

Topics to Review Prior to the Simulation

- State statutes for psychiatric commitment
- Lithium toxicity
- Risk factors for lithium overdose
- Nursing interventions for lithium overdose
- Pharmacological and other medical interventions for a client with lithium overdose

SIMULATION

Client Background

Hector Martinez, a 31-year-old math instructor, found in a hospital parking lot in a "confused" state. Agitated upon interaction but lethargic when left alone. States he has "not eaten in several hours." Suspected drug overdose as client found with bottle of lithium tablets in his possession. Client brought to the emergency room for triage. Preliminary background assessment information reveals that the individual has been treated for bipolar disorder in the past (onset 3 years ago) but cannot adequately provide detailed information related to prescription and/or dosage of medication. Client also has a history of non–insulin-dependent diabetes recently diagnosed within the past 3 months for which he has been following dietary modifications. Bottle found with client lithium carbonate: 450-mg tablets, 1 tablet by mouth in the morning and one in the evening, dispense 60 tablets. The vial has 45 tablets in it, and the prescription date is within 2 days of when the prescription was filled.

Biographical Data

- Age: 31
- Gender: male
- Height: 5 ft 8 in
- Weight: 141 lb

Cultural Considerations

- Language(s): Spanish, English
- Ethnicity: Hispanic
- Nationality: American
- Culture: Hispanic/American middle class

Demographic

- Marital status: married
- Educational level: master's degree
- Religion: does not attend church; not sure if he believes in any "God"
- Occupation: math instructor

Current Health Status

- Lithium overdose

History

- Psychosocial history: bipolar disorder
    - Social support: wife; other family members stay away from Hector; no children, but wife wants to "start a family" soon
    - Denies alcohol and/or street drug use
    - Denies smoking
    - Heavy coffee drinker—"the real stuff"
    - Stressed about finances and worried about "obtaining tenure" track position at work
- Past health history
    - Medical: recently diagnosed with diabetes type 2, insomnia, underweight
    - Surgical: fractured radius right arm repaired
- Family history: father alcohol abuse, mother hypertension, sister depression, brother healthy

Admission Sheet

Name:	Hector Martinez
Age:	31
Gender:	Male
Marital Status:	Married
Educational Level:	College educated
Religion:	Denies any religious affiliation
Ethnicity:	Hispanic
Nationality:	American
Language:	Spanish, English
Occupation:	Math instructor

Hospital
Provider's Orders

Client's Name: Hector Martinez
Allergies: NKA

Diagnosis: Suspected Lithium Drug Overdose

Date	Time	Order	Signature
xx/xx/xxxx	0830	Admit to telemetry floor Vital signs: q 15 min along with Neuro Flow sheet documentation. Contact physician immediately if there are any changes in presentation.	
		Diet: NPO @ present until evaluated by physician	
		Activity: maintain bed rest 1:1 observation	
		IV therapy: Normal saline @ 50 mL/hr	
		Medications: Dilantin 15 mg/kg IV loading dose followed by 100 mg q 8 hr	
		Bi-Pap 15/5 60% oxygen	
		Blood sugar qid AC Regular insulin: sliding scale subcutaneous administration: BG 70–150: give 0 units BG 151–200: give 2 units BG 201–250: give 4 units BG 251–300: give 6 units BG 301–350: give 8 units BG <70 or >350: notify on-call physician	
		Contact MD for additional orders	
		Diagnostic studies: Stat CBC, CMP, thyroid panel, renal panel. Obtain results from lithium level drawn in ER stat	Dr. House

Nursing Report on Admission to Telemetry Floor

Vital signs: 102/56, pulse 60 and regular, respirations 9 and shallow, temperature 98.8°F, bowel sounds slightly hyperactive. IV of normal saline infusing @ 50 mL/hr in his right forearm. Bilateral wrist restraints applied. Level of consciousness: Rouses easily with slurred speech but remains lethargic unless stimulated by touch or verbal interaction. He has a urinary catheter in place—inserted in ER. Minimal urine output obtained; slightly concentrated urine in bottom of bag with no sediment noted.

Pending lab results: CBC, CMP, thyroid, renal panel and lithium level. Accu-Check result: 250 mg/dL in ER. Sliding scale protocol initiated with client receiving 4 units regular insulin given in ER via subcutaneous route in left upper arm.

Student Simulation Prep Assignments

1. Identify items and their purpose in the care of a patient with lithium overdose.

Item	Purpose
IV access	
Wrist restraints	
Oxygen and supplies	
VS equipment	
Suction equipment	

2. Identify team members and specific roles in the care of a patient with lithium overdose.

Team member	Role
Physician	
Consulting physician	
Primary nurse	
UAP	
Supervisor	

3. Relevant Data Exercise: Fill in the columns below.

Relevant Data from Report	Relevant Data from Other Sources	Data Missing	Sources for Missing Data	Data Requiring Follow-Up

4. Initial Focused Assessment

After reviewing the client background and nursing report, you are ready to assess your client's current status. Under each category, identify how you would target your assessment, and what you would expect to find for the patient with a lithium overdose.

History

Are there any questions you need to ask the patient or family to obtain additional relevant data?

Answer:

Physical Exam

- General appearance:
- Integumentary:
- HEENT:
- Respiratory:
- CV:
- Breasts:
- Abdominal:
- Musculoskeletal:
- Neuro:
- Reproductive:
- Additional:
- Developmental:

What are the nursing implication considering the developmental stage of your patient?

Answer:

5. Diagnostic tests

What diagnostic test results relevant to the patient's current problem are needed to plan care?

Complete the table using Van Leeuwen et al, *Davis's Comprehensive Handbook of Laboratory and Diagnostic Testing with Nursing Implications* 4e, or other diagnostic test reference.

Diagnostic Test	Significance to This Client's Problem
CBC	
CMP	
Thyroid panel	
Renal panel	
Lithium level	
Blood sugar	
Troponin	
Magnesium	
Calcium	

6. Treatment

Identify drugs that are commonly used to treat a client with bipolar disorder.

Complete the table using Deglin et al, *Davis's Drug Guide for Nurses* 12e, or other drug reference.

Medication	Dose, Route, Frequency	Indications	Side Effect	Nursing Implications
Lithium	Usual maintenance dose 300–400 mg 3 times daily			

Medication	Dose, Route, Frequency	Indications	Side Effect	Nursing Implications
Phenytoin	15 mg/kg IV loading dose followed by 100 mg q 8 hr			

7. Nursing Problems/Diagnoses

Identify three priority nursing problems/diagnoses for the client with lithium overdose.

Assessment Data	Priority Problem	Interventions	Expected Patient Outcome	Which Interventions Could Be Delegated to Unlicensed Personnel?
1.				

Continued

Assessment Data	Priority Problem	Interventions	Expected Patient Outcome	Which Interventions Could Be Delegated to Unlicensed Personnel?
2.				
3.				

References

Deglin, J. H., & Vallerand, A. H. (2009). *Davis's drug guide for nurses* (11th ed.). Philadelphia: F. A. Davis.

Dillon, P. (2007). *Nursing health assessment: A critical thinking and case studies approach* (2nd ed.). Philadelphia: F. A. Davis.

Erikson, E.H. (1950). *Childhood and society.* New York: Norton.

Gorman, L. M., & Sultan, D. F. (2008). *Psychosocial nursing for general patient care* (3rd ed.). Philadelphia: F. A. Davis.

Lederer, E., & Dacso, C. C. (2009). Lithium nephropathy. Retrieved from http://emedicine.medscape.com/article/242772-overview

Lee, D. C., & Gupta, A. (2010). Toxicity, lithium. Retrieved from http://www.emedicine.com/EMERG/topic301.htm

Psych Education Organization. (2007). Lithium risks: Thyroid, kidney and weight gain problems (2007). Retrieved from http://www.psycheducation.org/depression/meds/LithiumRisks.htm

Van Leeuwen, A. M., Poelhuis-Leth, D. J., & Bladh, M. L. (2011). *Davis's comprehensive handbook of laboratory and diagnostic tests with nursing implications.* (4th ed.). Philadelphia: F. A. Davis.

Additional Informative Sites:

Dialysis and Depression http://www.hopkinsmedicine.org/gec/studies/dialysis_depression.html

Lithium Warnings and Precautions http://bipolar-disorder.emedtv.com/lithium/lithium-warnings-and-precautions.html

Progressive Renal Failure Caused by Lithium Nephropathy (2002). http://www.ncbi.nlm.nih.gov/pubmed/12148451

Community Health Nursing

10

10-1 Wound Care in Home Setting

COMMUNITY

STANDARD FORMS

These templates are included in the Appendix; copy before each use.

LEARNING OUTCOMES

Cognitive

The student will be able to:

1. Describe signs and symptoms of an infected pressure ulcer.
2. Correlate signs and symptoms of infection to the pathophysiology of the inflammatory response.
3. Identify factors in a client's history that increase the risk for wound infection and pressure ulcers.
4. Identify factors in a client's current condition that increase the risk for wound infection and pressure ulcers.
5. Identify the appropriate interventions for the client with an infected pressure ulcer.

Psychomotor

The student will be able to:

1. Perform appropriate assessment for a client with an infected pressure ulcer including staging of the wound.
2. Initiate appropriate interventions including cleansing, swabbing, measuring, and dressing a wound for a client with venous insufficiency.
3. Use the Braden Scale to complete a pressure ulcer risk assessment.

Affective

The student will be able to:

1. Reflect upon performance in the care of a client with an infected pressure ulcer.
2. Identify own feelings in delivering care to a client with an infected pressure ulcer.
3. Identify factors that worked well during the simulation of care of a client with an infected pressure ulcer .
4. Identify factors that needed improvement during the simulation of care of a client with an infected pressure ulcer.
5. Develop self-confidence in the care of a client with pressure ulcers.

Communication

The student will be able to:

1. Communicate effectively with the client, family, and physician in the care of a patient with a pressure ulcer.
2. Use SBAR when communication with team members in the care of a client with a pressure ulcer.
3. Apply the principles of Therapeutic Communication while caring for the patient and family with a pressure ulcer.
4. Practice Transparent Thinking (thinking out loud) to facilitate group problem solving.
5. Use Directed Communication (directing a message to specific individual) when delegating tasks.
6. Employ Closed-Loop Communication (acknowledgment of receipt of the message and status) to acknowledge communications from others.

Safety

The student will be able to:

Administer and maintain specific protecting interventions with attention to safety of the client and health care professional.

1. Incorporate 2011 Joint Commission Home Care National Patient Safety Goals.
   - Identify patient correctly
   - Prevent infection
   - Reconcile patient medications
   - Prevent falls
   - Identify patient safety risks in the home setting
2. Demonstrate attention to standard precautions. Includes hand washing, infection control measures, and use of personal protective equipment (PPE) as needed.

Leadership and Management/Delegation

The student will be able to:

- Identify and prioritize patient's needs in care of a patient with an ankle ulcer in the home setting.

Teaching and Learning

The student will be able to:

1. Teach the client about the importance of protein, vitamins, and minerals in wound healing.
2. Discuss resources for obtaining high-protein food.

OVERVIEW OF PROBLEM

Skin Breakdown

- Assess presence of risk factors
  - Immobility
  - Inadequate nutrition
  - Lack of position changes
- Subjective data
  - Pain
  - Fatigue
  - Inability to turn without assistance
- Objective data
  - Interruption of skin integrity, especially over ears, occiput, heels, sacrum, scrotum, elbows, trochanter, ischium, scapula
  - Immobilization
  - Malnutrition
- Prevention
  - Change position q 1–2 hr
  - Out of bed when possible
  - Protect from infection
  - Increase intake of protein, carbohydrates, and fluids
- Assess for/reduce contributing factors
  - Incontinence
  - Stationary position
  - Malnutrition
  - Obesity
  - Sensory deficits
  - Emotional disturbances
  - Paralysis
- Promote healing
  - Wash gently, pat dry
  - Clean, dry wrinkle-free linen
  - Massage skin with alcohol-free lotion
  - Protect skin with barriers
  - Avoid donuts or rings

Evaluation/Outcome Criteria

- No skin breakdown.

Pressure Ulcer Stages

- Stage 1: Nonblanchable erythema (redness) of intact skin.
- Stage 2: Partial-thickness skin loss involving epidermis, dermis, or both (e.g., abrasion, blister, or shallow crater).
- Stage 3. Full-thickness skin loss involving damage to or necrosis of subcutaneous tissue that may extend down to but not through underlying fascia (deep crater with or without undermining).
- Stage 4: Full-thickness skin loss with extensive destruction, tissue necrosis, or damage to muscle, bone, or supporting structures (e.g., tendon or joint capsule). *Unstageable:* You cannot see the base of these wounds so they are considered unstageable.
- Deep tissue injury: A pressure-related injury that appears as a bruise over intact skin or a blood-filled blister from pressure or shear.

Wound assessment should include:

- Length, width, depth of wound
- Description of wound bed
- Drainage, amount and type, odor
- Type of wound
- Condition of the periwound
- Undermining or tunneling
- Pain
- Treatment
- Patients with PVD also assess pulses, edema, color, temperature, sensation; measure leg circumferences.

REVIEW QUESTIONS

1. What are the risk factors for impaired wound healing in this scenario?
   Answer:
2. What is peripheral vascular disease (PVD)?
   Answer:
3. What are the treatments for PVD?
   Answer:
4. Describe the four stages of pressure ulcers.
   Answer:
5. What diet suggestions could you make to this client?
   Answer:

Related Evidence-Based Practice Guidelines

The National Guideline Clearinghouse Practice Guidelines: http:www.guideline.gov

Risk assessment & prevention of pressure ulcers and Guideline for management of wounds in patients with lower-extremity neuropathic disease.

Wound, Ostomy, and Continence Nurses Society: http://www.wocn.org/

2011 Home Care National Patient Safety Goals

http://www.jointcommission.org/assets/1/6/2011_OME_NPSG_EASY.pdfSBAR Technique for Communication: A situational briefing model published by The Institute for Healthcare Improvement was downloaded on December 19, 2008, from http://www.ihi.org/IHI/Topics/PatientSafety/SafetyGeneral/Tools/SBARTechniqueforCommunicationASituationalBriefingModel.htm

Topics to Review Prior to the Simulation

- Diabetes
- Peripheral vascular disease (PVD)
- Hypertension
- Obesity
- Aging
- Infection and inflammatory response
- Wound management
- Nutrition to promote healing
- Sterile technique
- Medical asepsis

SIMULATION

Client Background

Biographical Data

- Age: 79
- Gender: male
- Height: 5 ft 10 in
- Weight: 265 lb

Cultural Considerations

- Language: English
- Ethnicity: unknown
- Nationality: Canadian
- Culture: no significant cultural considerations identified

Demographic

- Marital status: married
- Education level: grade 10
- Religion: Anglican
- Occupation: retired mill worker

Current Health Status

- Type 2 diabetic, obese, HTN, PAD, and has an infected pressure ulcer on his ankle

History

- Psychosocial history
  - Social support: three adult children, two grandchildren
- Past health history
  - Medical: myocardial infarction 10 years ago
  - Surgical: appendectomy 15 years ago
- Family history: father had HTN and died of a heart attack at age 64

Admission Sheet

Name:	Robert Smith
Age:	79
Gender:	Male
Marital Status:	Married
Educational Level:	Grade 10
Religion:	Anglican
Ethnicity:	Unknown
Nationality:	Canadian
Language:	English
Occupation:	Retired mill worker

Hospital
Provider's Orders

Patient's Name: **Robert Smith**
Allergies: **Penicillin**

Diagnosis:

Date	Time	Order	Signature
05/21/07	1000	Vital signs: once daily (as per home care visit)	
		Diet: 1,800 calories diabetic diet	
		Activity: activity as tolerated	
		Medications: Metformin 500 mg po daily Metoprolol 150 mg po daily Lisinopril 10 mg po daily Lasix 20 mg po daily	
		Diagnostic studies: Client gets his glucose tested at the lab once a month. Uses an Accu-Chek monitor at home prn	
		Treatments: Change ankle dressing with Aquacel Ag daily and bilateral Tubigrip	
			Dr Adams

Nursing Report

You arrive at 1000 at the client's home. His wife answers the door and the client is sitting in a recliner with his legs elevated. He reports to you that his legs have been "more puffy" and that his heel wound is draining more than yesterday.

Student Simulation Prep Assignments

1. Identify items and their purpose in the care of a client with an infected ankle ulcer.

Item	Purpose
Sterile dressing kit	
Stethoscope and BP cuff	
Apron	
Goggles	
Normal saline	

2. Identify team members and their specific roles in the care of a client with an infected ankle ulcer.

Team Member	Role
Primary nurse	
Physician	
Family member	

3. *Relevant Data Exercise:* Fill in the columns below.

Relevant Data from Report	Relevant Data from Other Sources	Data Missing	Sources for Missing Data	Data Requiring Follow-Up

4. *Initial Focused Assessment*

After reviewing the client background and nursing report, you are ready to assess your client's current status. Under each category, identify how you would target your assessment and what you would expect to find for the client with an infected pressure ulcer on his ankle.

History

Are there any questions you need to ask the patient in family to obtain relevant data

Physical Exam

- General appearance:
- Integumentary:
- HEENT:
- Respiratory:
- CV:
- Breasts:
- Abdominal:
- Neuro:
- Musculoskeletal:
- Reproductive:
- Additional:
- Developmental

What are the nursing implications considering the developmental stage of your patient?

Answer:

5. *Diagnostic Tests*

What diagnostic test results relevant to the patient's current problem are needed to plan care?

Complete the table using Van Leeuwen et al, *Davis's Comprehensive Handbook of Laboratory and Diagnostic Testing with Nursing Implications* 4e, or other diagnostic test reference.

Diagnostic Test	Significance to This Patient's Problem
Doppler ultrasound (detect PVD)	
Ankle-arm (ankle-brachial) index	
Venography or phlebography	
Wound C&S	
Serum pre-albumin level	

6. *Treatment*

Identify drugs that are used to treat a patient with an infected ankle ulcer.

Complete the table using Deglin et al, *Davis's Drug Guide for Nurses* 12e, or other drug reference.

Medication	Dose, Route, Frequency	Indications	Side Effect	Nursing Implications
Metformin 500 mg daily	500 mg daily			
Metoprolol	150 mg po OD			
Lisinopril	10 mg OD			
Lasix	20 mg OD			

7. *Nursing Problems/Diagnoses*

Identify three priority nursing problems/diagnoses.

Assessment Data	Priority Problem	Intervention	Expected Patient Outcome	Which Intervention Could Be Delegated to Unlicensed Personnel?
1.				

Assessment Data	Priority Problem	Intervention	Expected Patient Outcome	Which Intervention Could Be Delegated to Unlicensed Personnel?
2.				
3.				

References

Deglin, J. H., & Vallerand, A. H. (2009). *Davis's drug guide for nurses* (11th ed.). Philadelphia: F. A. Davis.

Dillon, P. (2007). *Nursing health assessment: A critical thinking and case studies approach* (2nd ed.). Philadelphia: F. A. Davis.

Erikson, E.H. (1950). *Childhood and society.* New York: Norton.

Grodner, M., Long, S., & Wackingshaw, B. (2007). *Foundations and clinical applications of nutrition: A nursing approach* (4th ed.). St. Louis: Mosby.

Ignatavicius, D., Winkelman, C., Workman, M. L., & Hausman, K. (2010). *Clinical companion for medical-surgical nursing: Critical thinking for collaborative care* (6th ed.). St. Louis: Saunders.

Lagerquist, S. (2006). *Davis's NCLEX-RN success*. Philadelphia: F. A. Davis.

The National Guideline Clearinghouse Practice Guidelines. Retrieved on July, 8, 2008 from http:www.guideline.gov

Potter, P. (2007). *Basic nursing: Essentials for practice* (6th ed.). St. Louis: Mosby.

Rothrock, J. C. (2006). *Alexander's care of the patient in surgery* (13th ed.). St. Louis: Mosby.

Van Leeuwen, A. M., Poelhuis-Leth, D. J., & Bladh, M. L. (2011). *Davis's comprehensive handbook of laboratory and diagnostic tests with nursing implications.* (4th ed.). Philadelphia: F. A. Davis.

Wound, Ostomy, and Continence Nurses Society. Retrieved on July, 8, 2008 from http://www.wocn.org/

10-2 Unresponsive Patient at Home

COMMUNITY HEALTH NURSING: HOME HEALTH CARE

STANDARD FORMS

These templates are included in the Appendix; copy before each use.

LEARNING OUTCOMES

Cognitive

The student will be able to:

1. Describe signs and symptoms of carbon monoxide poisoning.
2. Differentiate between signs and symptoms of carbon monoxide poisoning and diabetic ketoacidosis/coma.
3. Identify the appropriate interventions for an unresponsive patient in the home setting/the patient with carbon monoxide poisoning.
4. Differentiate the roles of team members in response to an unresponsive patient in the home setting/a patient with carbon monoxide poisoning.
5. List three nursing diagnoses r/t carbon monoxide poisoning.
6. Determine environmental safety hazards for an older adult related to carbon monoxide poisoning.

Psychomotor

The student will be able to:

1. Perform neurological assessment for an unresponsive patient in the home setting.
2. Perform a blood glucose test.
3. Perform a pulse oximetry.
4. Perform an environmental assessment.
5. Draw blood specimens.
6. Initiate appropriate interventions for an unresponsive patient in the home setting d/t a patient with carbon monoxide poisoning:
   - Survey the scene for hazards to the nurse.
   - Immediate assessment of the patient.
     - Assess the patient's ABCs.
   - Call emergency personnel.
     - Communicate history and findings to emergency personnel.
   - Call the home care agency nurse supervisor to report situation and consult on other interventions.
   - Remove patient from the site.
     - Perform a proper one-person transfer from a chair or bed to a blanket to move patient to safety.
7. Work collaboratively as part of the healthcare team for an unresponsive patient in the home setting.

Affective

The student will be able to:

1. Reflect upon performance in the care of an unresponsive patient in the home setting (a patient with carbon monoxide poisoning).
2. Identify personal feelings in delivering care to an unresponsive patient in the home setting.
3. Discuss feelings related to working as a home care nurse team member in the assessment and care of an unresponsive patient in the home setting.
4. Identify factors that worked well during the simulation.
5. Identify factors that needed improvement during the simulation.
6. Develop self-confidence in the care of an unresponsive patient in the home-setting patient (with carbon monoxide poisoning).

Communication

The student will be able to:

1. Communicate effectively with healthcare team members in care of an unresponsive patient in the home setting with carbon monoxide poisoning.
2. Communicate effectively with emergency care personnel in the care of an unresponsive patient in the home with carbon monoxide poisoning.
3. Will practice Transparent Thinking (thinking out loud) to facilitate group problem solving.
4. Use Directed Communication (directing a message to specific individual) when delegating tasks.
5. Employ Closed-Loop Communication (acknowledgment of receipt of the message and status) to acknowledge communications from others.

Safety

The student will be able to:

Administer and maintain specific protecting interventions with attention to safety of the client and healthcare professional.

1. Demonstrate a safe environment with attention to hazards to healthcare providers, visitors, and the client. Includes body mechanics, tripping hazards, and equipment issues.
2. Demonstrate attention to national patient safety goals. Includes patient identification standards, effective

communication among healthcare providers, and safe medication administration.
3. Demonstrates attention to standard precautions. Includes hand washing, infection control measures, and use of personal protective equipment (PPE) as needed.

Leadership and Management/Delegation

The student will be able to:

- Identify and prioritize patient's needs in care of an unresponsive patient in the home setting due to carbon monoxide poisoning.

OVERVIEW OF PROBLEM

Recognizing carbon monoxide (CO) poisoning in a patient in the home care setting requires an awareness of the environmental hazards in a home setting, especially during colder weather or in patients in colder climates, and those who work or live in enclosed areas or homes with older heating systems or alternate methods of heating their environments. It is also important to have knowledge of high-risk behaviors in your patients and their families. Community health nurses can be the first line of defense in assessing for this invisible hazard as they provide nursing care to those in the community.

Carbon Monoxide (CO)

- A poisonous gas resulting from the inefficient and incomplete combustion of organic fuels.
- Colorless, tasteless and odorless, it cannot be detected by the senses.
- CO is distributed widely because of imperfect combustion and oxidation and is found, for example, in the exhaust gas from the internal combustion engines in most motor-powered vehicles, and in sewers, cellars, and mines.

Carbon Monoxide Poisoning

- Toxicity that results from inhalation of small amounts of CO over a long period or from large amounts inhaled for a short time.
- In the United States, where exposure to car exhaust, smoke, and other sources of combustion is common (especially during the winter months), CO poisoning is one of the most frequent, and potentially deadliest intoxications.
- CO poisoning is the third leading cause of unintentional poisoning death in the United States (see CDC.gov).
- Males are at higher risk, especially those in ages ranging 25–44 years of age.
- The elderly are more vulnerable to the effects of CO poisoning, as are those with chronic illnesses. Further, the elderly over the age of 75 are at greater risk for adverse neurological outcomes (see CDC.gov).

Pathophysiology

CO poisoning results from the avid chemical combination of the gas with hemoglobin, forming carboxyhemoglobin (COHb), a long-lasting substance that inhibits the binding of oxygen to hemoglobin and prevents oxygenation of tissues.

Risk Factors

- Heavy cigarette smoking, burning materials containing carbon such as through wood stoves, portable kerosene or propane heaters within the home, fireplaces, and charcoal briquettes burnt within the home for heat
- Improperly maintained oil and gas furnaces and poorly ventilated homes
- Poorly ventilated cars during snowstorms while idling in deep or drifting snow
- Working with chemical fumes without proper personal protective equipment (PPE)
- During power outages, usually 2–3 days after the outage occurs, poisonings occur d/t alternate heating source usage
- When outdoor portable generators are used too close to a living space
- Immigrants and minorities are at higher risk (see CDC.gov)
- Newer homes d/t tight construction and increased levels of insulation causing less ventilation of potential hazardous fumes in the home

Assessment

Subjective

- Symptoms of CO poisoning vary with the level of the exposure and concentration of COHb in the bloodstream
- At levels less than 10% patients may be symptom free or only complain of a headache
  - Heavy cigarette smoking may produce levels as high as 7–9%
  - COHb levels of 30% may produce mild neurological impairment (dizziness, fatigue, nausea, difficulty concentrating)
- Chest pain can occur more frequently in patients with preexisting coronary artery disease

Objective

Physical findings

- COHb levels of 50% may cause seizures or coma
- COHb levels above 70% will likely cause death
- Other signs can be hypotension and life-threatening arrhythmias
- Vital signs associated with carbon monoxide poisoning:
  - BP assess for hypotension
  - Pulse: assess for tachycardia and arrhythmias
  - Respirations: assess for change in pattern
    - Early CO exposure may demonstrate an increased heart and respiratory rate as the body tries to compensate for hypoxia

  - Temperature: nonspecific; however, if patient is trying to stay warm with the use of portable heaters, consider temperatures based on the environment you find the patient in at the time of assessment
- Respiratory assessment may demonstrate pulmonary edema from the increased myocardial workload to compensate for cellular hypoxia by increasing heart and respiratory rates
- Neurological exam:
  - Monitor any changes in mental status, LOC
  - Use Glasgow Coma Scale: generally, the lower the score, the worse the prognosis
  - Pupils: test reaction, speed, and equality
  - Monitor for signs and symptoms of seizures
  - Assess reflexes: hypertonia/hypotonia

Diagnostic Tests

- Pulse oximetry: results are usually falsely elevated measures of hemoglobin saturation with oxygen because pulse oximetry cannot distinguish between carboxyhemoglobin (COHb) and oxyhemoglobin.
- Perform a blood glucose using the patient's home monitor to determine if an abnormally high or low BS is present. This can help exclude other causes of altered mental status when the diagnosis of CO poisoning is inconclusive.
  - You can use a drop of blood from the venipuncture needle, the venipuncture site, or withdraw a minute sample from the Vacutainer to use to check a blood sugar.
- Draw a COHb level into a heparinized tube to prevent clotting. This sample must be kept in an ice slush or surrounded by ice cubes in baggies for transport to the lab.
  - The emergency transporters can bring the specimen to the hospital for evaluation.
- Draw blood samples for clotting analysis and for a basal metabolic panel (BMP), CBC, and liver function tests (LFTs) to assist with determining the patient's status at the time of the assessment.
- Blood gases would be ideal to have available; however, the barriers to maintaining their integrity for analysis would be difficult to achieve in the home setting.

Treatment

- The affected person(s) should be removed immediately from exposure to CO and taken to a safe place.
- Protect yourself from becoming a victim in the environment.
- Notify the emergency system, 911, for transport to the ED.
  - The Fire Department may be called to decontaminate the environment.
- Ventilate the environment and attempt to determine the source. Search for secondary victims in the home. Keep pets in mind as victims as they are also affected by CO and their survival may be very important to the individual/family.
- Notify the patient's physician and or the ED physician of your assessment findings and await any advice.
- If oxygen is available in the home, administer oxygen. A tight-fitting mask with 100% oxygen is given in optimal situations; a nonrebreather mask is also a method to help disassociate the CO from the hemoglobin (Smith, 2006).
  - The hospital will administer oxygen under pressure (hyperbaric) if possible.
- Artificial respiration should be used if indicated.
- The patient should be kept quiet to reduce the patient's oxygen requirements.
- Continue to monitor the neuro status.
- Neurological assessment:
  - Glasgow Coma Scale
  - Best eye
  - Best verbal
  - Best motor
  - Note and document any change in GCS and level of consciousness.
  - Seizure precautions:
    - Observe for any signs of seizure activity
- Consider aspiration precautions
  - Roll patient on his/her side

Complications

- When patients recover, they often have some central nervous system complications
  - Memory disturbances, difficulty concentrating, or tremor among others
- Complications usually disappear over time, but occasionally permanent neurological dysfunction follows CO intoxication

Prevention

- Many CO exposures are preventable. See *Risk Factors* above
- CO detectors should be placed in homes at each sleeping area. Placement can be anywhere from the floor to the ceiling; however, best placement is at low level (ankle level) of the room (see CDC.gov). Always have battery backup in case of power outages
- Multilanguage public media announcements (radio and TV) during storm announcements and just prior to heating season can alert individuals to CO poisoning hazards to avoid

REVIEW QUESTIONS

1. How would you differentiate carbon monoxide poisoning from a diabetic coma?
Answer:

2. Name three areas that are included in a neurological examination.
Answer:

3. Name three nursing interventions that reduce the effects of CO poisoning?
Answer:

4. What factors noted during an environmental assessment would indicate a potential risk for CO poisoning?
   Answer:

5. Name three signs and symptoms associated with CO poisoning?
   Answer:

6. What are the signs and symptoms of hypoglycemia?
   Answer:

Related Evidenced-Based Practice Guidelines

There were no available Best Practice Guidelines for carbon monoxide poisoning in the home setting.

Topics to Review Prior to the Simulation

- Neurological assessment
- Skin assessment
- Pharmacological assessment for side effects of medications
- Environmental assessment for home safety hazards of an older adult

SIMULATION

Client Background

Biographical Data

- Age: 76
- Gender: female
- Height: 5 ft
- Weight: 175 lb

Cultural Considerations

- Language: English
- Ethnicity: Italian and Polish
- Nationality: American
- Culture: no significant cultural considerations identified

Demographic

- Marital status: widowed
- Educational level: high school
- Religion: Catholic
- Occupation: retired waitress, homemaker

Current Health Status

- Family reports recent fall, increased confusion, dizziness, and nausea.

History

- Psychosocial history
  - Social support:
    - Family: available but live at a distance, and they work during the day
  - Neighbors: supportive but work during the day
- Past health history
  - Medical: history of diabetes type 2; mild hearing impairment (no hearing aid usage)
  - Surgical: history of cataract removal OD; cholecystectomy
- Family history: maternal and paternal diabetes; CV disease; spouse died from a stroke 5 years ago

Admission Sheet

Name:	Adrienne Palmer
Age:	76
Gender:	Female
Marital Status:	Widowed
Educational Level:	High school
Religion:	Catholic
Ethnicity:	Italian and Polish
Nationality:	American
Language:	English
Occupation:	Retired waitress, homemaker

Home Care Agency
Provider's Orders

Patient's Name: Adrienne Palmer
Allergies: NKDA

Diagnosis: Diabetes mellitus, arthritis, history of cataract surgery with implant OD, and cholecystectomy

Date	Time	Order	Signature
		Assess CVR status and endocrine status.	
		Assess medications.	
		Assess pain level.	
		Assess risks in the home.	
		Draw a CBC and basal metabolic panel in 2 weeks from admission to home care services.	
		Assess ambulation status.	
		Assess need for physical therapy services.	
		Assess for home healthcare aide services.	
		Teach about disease process, medications, prevention of falls, and environmental hazards.	
		Teach self blood glucose monitoring.	
		Diet 1,500 calorie ADA. Assess nutritional and hydration status, and teach about diet.	
		MSW prn to assess need for community resources.	Dr. Rice

Nursing Report

Nursing notes from admission to the home care agency.

Patient is a 76-year-old female living alone in a two-story home in a rural area. She was recently discharged from the hospital s/p a fall in her home and uncontrolled blood glucose levels. Family is available in the area; however, they live at a distance and work during the day. Patient has supportive neighbors who also work during the day. Meals on Wheels supplies frozen meals once per week. Family does shopping for patient, who prepares simple meals at lunch time.

AAOx3, T 97.4°F, apical 84 and regular, R 18, BP 140/84 sitting and 146/84 lying left arm, weight 175 lb. Lungs clear bilaterally. Ambulates slowly with a walker. Sleeps on the first floor; bathroom available. No problems with bowels or bladder. Appetite fair. No edema noted.

Resolving ecchymosis on left hip from fall prior to hospitalization. Discussed fall hazards in the home including small dog. Teaching on hypoglycemic medication effects and side effects and schedule. Smoke detector available but no CO detectors visible.

Schedule for visits 2x per week x 3 weeks. Blood work due in 2 weeks. HHA demonstration on next visit to assist with personal care. Further assess and teach diet on each visit and disease process and management. Advised to obtain CO detector and fire extinguisher for safety in the home and a portable phone. Scheduled to see MD in 3 weeks.

Student Simulation Prep Assignments

1. Identify items and their purpose in the care of a patient who presents as unresponsive due to carbon monoxide poisoning.

Item	Purpose
Pulse oximetry	
Blood glucose monitor	

Item	Purpose
Green-, purple-, and marble-top specimen tubes; tourniquet, Vacutainer and needles, alcohol wipes, and Band-Aid	
Stethoscope and sphygmomanometer, thermometer, pen light	

2. ***Identify team members and their specific roles in the care of a patient who presents as unresponsive due to carbon monoxide poisoning.***

Team Member	Role
Home care nurse	
Nursing supervisor at the home care agency	
Physician	
Emergency care personnel	

3. ***Relevant Data Exercise:*** Fill in the columns below.

Relevant Data from Report	Relevant Data from Other Sources	Data Missing	Sources for Missing Data	Data Requiring Follow-Up

4. ***Initial Focused Assessment***

After reviewing the client background, nursing report, and family report, you are ready to assess your client's current status. Under each category, identify how you would target your assessment and what you would expect to find for the patient with a history of diabetes and arthritis and reports of increasing confusion, dizziness, nausea, and a recent fall and potential carbon monoxide poisoning.

History

Are there any questions you need to ask the family to obtain additional relevant data before visiting the patient at home?

Physical Exam

- General appearance:
- Integumentary:
- HEENT:
- Respiratory:
- CV:
- Breasts:
- Abdominal:
- Musculoskeletal:
- Neuro:
- Reproductive:
- Additional:
- Breath:
- Other:
- Developmental:

Answer:

5. *Diagnostic Tests*

What diagnostic test results relevant to the patient's current problem are needed to plan care?

Complete the table using Van Leeuwen et al, *Davis's Comprehensive Handbook of Laboratory and Diagnostic Testing with Nursing Implications* 4e, or other diagnostic test reference.

Diagnostic Test	Significance to This Patient's Problem
Chemistry panel (includes BUN and creatinine)	
Blood sugar via SGM machine or Vacutainer	
Pulse oximetry	
Serum lactate level	
COHb level (hemoglobin M, Hgb M)	

6. *Treatment*

Identify drugs that are used to treat a patient with carbon monoxide poisoning and those the patient is taking.

Complete the table using Deglin et al, *Davis's Drug Guide for Nurses* 12e, or other drug reference.

Medication	Dose, Route Frequency	Indications	Side Effect	Nursing Implications
Oxygen	90–100% via nonrebreathing device to deliver the high rate of oxygen needed with CO poisoning Hyperbaric oxygen as needed is delivered in the hospital			

Medication	Dose, Route Frequency	Indications	Side Effect	Nursing Implications
Glipizide	10 mg, po daily (take 30 min before meals)			
Tylenol	650 mg po prn q 4 hr			

7. Nursing Problems/Diagnoses

Identify three priority nursing problems/diagnoses.

Assessment Data	Priority Problem	Intervention	Expected Patient Outcome	Which interventions Could Be Delegated to Unlicensed Personnel?
1.				

Continued

Assessment Data	Priority Problem	Intervention	Expected Patient Outcome	Which interventions Could Be Delegated to Unlicensed Personnel?
2.				
3.				

References

Balch, C. (2004). Carbon monoxide poisoning: Too easily overlooked. *Nursing 2004*, *34*(3), 10-12.

Centers for Disease Control (CDC) (2009). Environmental hazards and health effects: Carbon monoxide poisoning. Retrieved April 15, 2009 from http://www.cdc.gov/co/default.htm

Clark, M. J. (2008). *Community assessment reference guide for community health nursing.* Upper Saddle River, NJ: Pearson Prentice Hall.

Deglin, J. H., & Vallerand, A. H. (2009). *Davis's drug guide for nurses* (11th ed.). Philadelphia: F. A. Davis.

Dillon, P. (2007). *Nursing health assessment a critical thinking case studies approach* (2nd ed.). Philadelphia: F. A. Davis.

Doenges, M. E., Moorhouse, M. F., & Geissler-Murr, A. C. (2008). *Nursing diagnosis manual. Planning, individualizing and documenting client care.* Philadelphia: F. A. Davis.

Erikson, E.H. (1950). *Childhood and society.* New York: Norton.

Hayes, B. D. (2006). Holiday health hazards: Poisons in unexpected places. Maryland Nurse (MD NURSE), 2006 Nov–2007 Jan; 8(1): 25.

Lagerquist, S. (2006). *Davis's NCLEX-RN success*. Philadelphia: F. A. Davis.

Smith, D. H. (2006). Methylene chloride inhalation. *Nursing 2006*, *36*(6), 80.

Taber's cyclopedic medical dictionary (2009) (21st ed.). Philadelphia: F. A. Davis.

Van Leeuwen, A. M., Poelhuis-Leth, D. J., & Bladh, M. L. (2011). *Davis's comprehensive handbook of laboratory and diagnostic tests with nursing implications.* (4th ed.). Philadelphia: F. A. Davis.

10-3 Assessment of School-Aged Child

PEDIATRIC

STANDARD FORMS

These templates are included in the Appendix; copy before each use.

LEARNING OUTCOMES

Cognitive

The student will be able to:

1. Identify normal parameters for physical assessment.
2. Identify psychosocial, cognitive, physical, and physiological changes in the school-aged child.
3. Identify normal laboratory values.
4. Identify appropriate immunizations for the school-aged child.
5. Identify the appropriate interventions for the child with delayed immunizations.
6. Differentiate the roles of team members in response to physical assessment of a school-aged child.
7. Describe signs and symptoms of otitis media.
8. Correlate signs and symptoms of otitis media to the pathophysiology of inner ear examination.
9. Identify factors in a patient's history that increase risk for otitis media.
10. Identify factors in a patient's current condition that increase risk for otitis media.
11. Identify the appropriate interventions for the patient with otitis media.
12. Differentiate the roles of team members in response to a patient with otitis media.

Psychomotor

The student will be able to:

1. Perform complete physical assessment for a school-aged child.
2. Initiate appropriate interventions in completing the assessment of a school-aged child: hearing screen, vision screen, venipuncture,
3. Work collaboratively as part of the healthcare team in completing the physical assessment of a school-aged child.
4. Identify physiological pathology in the assessment of the school-aged child.
5. Initiate appropriate treatment of the child with physiological pathology.
6. Perform appropriate assessment for a patient with otitis media.
7. Initiate appropriate interventions: examination of ear, evaluation of findings, pharmacological and nonpharmacological treatment for a patient with otitis media.
8. Work collaboratively as part of the healthcare team in the care of a patient with otitis media.

Affective

The student will be able to:

1. Reflect upon performance in the performance of physical assessment and provision of anticipatory guidance to a school-aged child.
2. Identify own feelings in performing the physical assessment to a school-aged child in primary care office.
3. Discuss feelings related to working as a member of a team in performing physical assessment in a school-aged child.
4. Identify factors that worked well during the simulation of a physical assessment of a school-aged child.
5. Identify factors that needed improvement during the simulation of physical assessment of a school-aged child.
6. Develop self-confidence in the performance of physical assessment of a school-aged child.

Communication

The student will be able to:

1. Communicate effectively with healthcare team members in physical assessment of a child.
2. Communicate effectively with the patient and family of the school-aged child.
3. Use SBAR when communicating with team members regarding the physical assessment of the school-aged child.
4. Will practice Transparent Thinking (thinking out loud) to facilitate group problem solving.
5. Use Directed Communication (directing a message to specific individual) when delegating tasks.
6. Employ Closed-Loop Communication (acknowledgment of receipt of the message and status) to acknowledge communications from others.

Safety

The student will be able to administer and maintain specific protecting interventions with attention to safety of the client and healthcare professional.

1. Demonstrate a safe environment with attention to hazards to healthcare providers, visitors, and the client. Includes body mechanics, tripping hazards, and equipment issues.
2. Demonstrate attention to national patient safety goals for ambulatory care. Includes patient identification standards, safe medication administration, infection prevention, medication reconcilliation.

3. Demonstrate attention to standard precautions. Includes hand washing, infection control measures, and use of personal protective equipment (PPE) as needed.

Leadership and Management/Delegation

The student will be able to:

1. Identify tasks that can be legally, ethically, and safely delegated to unlicensed assistive personnel (UAP) in the physical assessment of a school-aged child.
2. Identify and prioritize patient's health needs in physical assessment of a school-aged child.

Developmental

The student will be able to apply developmental knowledge in the physical assessment of the school-aged child.

Teaching

The student will be able to identify learning needs of the school aged child in relation to health promotion and disease prevention.

OVERVIEW OF PROBLEM

Definition

Physical assessment is centered around healthcare maintenance and is recommended yearly for the school-aged child, approximately 6–12 years of age. Subjective data including physical, psychosocial, emotional, and cognitive information and objective data including physical, neurological, and developmental assessment are collected, interpreted, and analyzed.

Physical and Motor

- Continues to grow at a rate of 5 cm (2 in) and 3 kg (6.6 lb) per year
- Movement is fluid, more graceful, and poised, increased motor control and speed
- Very active: jumps, chases, skips
- Dresses self completely
- Eyes and hands well coordinated

Cognitive

- Concrete operations
  - Begins to develop ability to think logically
  - Begins to organize thought into coherent structures
  - Begins to arrange thoughts into hierachical and sequential relationships
- Time and space:
  - Likes to do things quickly
  - Can tell time, name of day, month, year
  - Can distinguish right and left on body of self and others
  - Expansive, evaluative, adventurous
- Responsibility:
  - More responsible for own acts
  - Responsiveness to reason
- Likes to have own way
- Frequently can listen to reason and change mind with ease
- Language:
  - Talkative, exaggerates, boasts, tells tall tales
  - Uses language fluently
  - Can verbalize ideas and problems
- Begins to understand cause and effect and relationships

Adaptive

- Makes use of common tools such as hammer, saw, screwdriver
- Uses household and sewing utensils
- Helps with routine household tasks; i.e., dusting, sweeping, dishes
- Travels throughout home and community freely, alone or with friends
- Enjoys school

Socialization

- Easy to get along with at home and outside, is more social
- Likes to compete and play games
- Dramatizes
- More critical of self; ashamed of bad grades

Exam/Screening: 9 year old

- Growth (normal range)
  - Female: 43–90 lb, 46–56 in
  - Male: 47–87 lb, 46.5–56.0 in
- Vital Signs
  - BP range 80–118/43–76
  - HR 60–110 bpm
  - RR 20–26 bpm
  - Temp 97.5– 99.5°F (36.4–37.5°C)
- Vision: Snellen E or Alphabet Chart
  - Minimal passing 20/30 ou
  - Must pass greater than 1/2 each line with one eye covered
- Hearing: frequencies of 1000 Hz, 2000 Hz, 4000 Hz @ 20 dB
  - Passing 1,000 Hz, 2,000 Hz @ 20 dB, or 4,000 Hz @ 25 dB
  - Evaluation indicated at threshhold of 25 dB at two or more frequencies or 35 dB at any frequency

Physical Assessment

- General: observe facies, posture, nutrition, hygiene, behavior, development
- Skin: color (in sclera, conjunctiva, tongue, nail beds, buccal mucosa, palms and soles); texture (temperature, integrity, moisture, smoothness, turgor)
- Accessory structures:
  - Hair: hygiene, color, texture, distribution, quality
    - Dull, stringy, brittle, hypopigmentation: poor nutrition

- Nails: color, texture, quality, distribution, elasticity, hygiene
  - Base swollen or springy on palpation: clubbing, indicative of heart disease
- Lymph nodes: small, nontender, movable—normal variation
  - Infection indicated in area proximal to swollen, tender nodes

Axillary	Tonsilar
Inguinal	Submental
Pre-/postauricular	Submaxillary
Occipital	Supraclavicular
Superficial cervical	Deep cervical chain

- Head: shape/symmetry, ROM, palpate skull, check scalp, frontal sinuses (should be resonant, painless)—painful sinuses indicate URI
- Neck: size, webbing, tracheal placement (palpate for deviation, masses, nodules), thyroid (size, shape, symmetry, tenderness, nodes), carotid arteries (note unequal pulses or protruding veins)
- Eyes: placement, alignment, internal structures
  - Presence of red reflex rules out most serious defects
- Ears: placement, alignment, internal structures
  - External canal: pink, outermost area with tiny hairs, soft yellow cerumen
  - Tympanic membrane: translucent, light pearly gray or pink (f/u needed if dark, dull transparent gray, black areas; red, bulging drums with no light reflex may indicate otitis media)
- Nose: size, alignment
- Mouth/throat: lips (color, texture, lesions), internal (hard, soft palates, tonsils, uvula, tongue, teeth)
- Chest: size, shape, symmetry, movement, breast development (Tanner stage 1)
- Lungs: check breath sounds, voice vibration (fremitus), percuss from apex to base
  - Breath sounds: vesicular (heard over all lung surface except upper intrascapular area and beneath manubrium; inspiration louder, longer, higher pitch than expiration).
  - Bronchovesicular (heard in upper intrascapular area and manubrubrium; inspiration and expiration almost equal in duration, pitch, and intensity)
  - Bronchial (heard over trachea, near suprasternal notch; expiration longer, louder higher pitch than inspiration) voice sounds—normally heard but syllables indistinct
  - Abnormal sounds may signal consolidation of lung tissue
- Cardiovascular: heart—inspect size (with child in supine position), palpate for PMI (normally at 5th IC space at midclavicular line), auscultate (distinguish S_1 from S_2: S_1 is synchronous with carotid pulse), thrill (cat purr) may indicate blood flowing through narrowed opening as in stenotic valve or septal defect)
  - Murmurs:
    - Grade I: very faint, frequently disappears if child sits up
    - Grade II: readily heard, slightly louder than grade 1, audible in all positions
    - Grade III: loud, not accompanied by a thrill
    - Grade IV: loud, accompanied by a thrill
    - Grade V: loud, can be heard with stethoscope barely touching chest, thrill present
    - Grade VI: loud, can be heard without stethoscope with human ear close to chest, thrill present
  - Peripheral pulses:
    - Grade 0: not palpable
    - Grade +1: thready, easily obliterated with pressure
    - Grade +2: difficult to palpate, may obliterate with pressure
    - Grade +3: normal, easy to palpate, not easily obliterated with pressure
    - Grade +4: strong, bounding, not obliterated with pressure
- Abdomen: inspect (cylindrical/prominent sitting or flat supine); auscultate for bowel sounds (heard every 10–30 sec); percuss (tympany over stomach, dullness over liver), palpate for abdominal organs, hernias (liver may be palpated 1–2 cm below right costal margin, enlarged if greater than 3 cm; spleen may be palpated 1–2 cm below left costal margin, enlarged if greater than 2 cm; hernias: umbilical, inguinal, femoral)
- Genitalia:
  - Male: inspect penis size, glans and shaft, prepuce in uncircumcized males, urethral meatus, scrotum size, skin, testes (Tanner stage 1)
  - Female: inspect external genitalia; structures: mons pubis, clitoris, labia majora, labia minora, urethral meatus, vaginal orifice, Bartholin's glands (Tanner stage 1)
- Anus: inspect skin condition, anal reflex
- Back/extremities: inspect curvature, symmetry of spine (suspect scoliosis if slight limp, crooked waistline, backache—perform bend test)
  - Immediate specialist referral for c/o stiff, painful back or neck
  - Check for dislocated hip
  - Check for position of feet: genu varum (bow leg), genu valgum (knock knee)

Neurological Assessment

- Assess mental status: behavior, mood, affect, orientation
- Motor function: muscle strength, tone, development
- Cerebellar functioning: finger-nose test, heel-shin test, Romberg's test
- Sensory functioning: sensory intactness: pin test, sensory discrimination—sharp/dull, hot/cold tests
- DTRs: biceps, triceps, brachioradialis, patellar, Achilles'
- Cranial nerves
  - Olfactory: olfactory mucosa of nasal cavity
  - Optic: rods and cones of retina, optic nerve

- Oculomotor: extraocular muscles of eye
- Trochlear: superior oblique muscle, moves eyes down and out
- Trigeminal: muscles of mastication; face, scalp, nasal, buccal mucosa
- Abducens: lateral rectus muscle
- Facial: facial muscles, anterior 2/3 of tongue
- Auditory or vestibulocochlear: nasal cavity and lacrimal gland, sublingual, submandibular, salivary glands, internal ear
- Glossopharyngeal: pharynx, tongue
- Vagus: muscles of larynx, pharynx, some GI system organs
- Accessory: trapezius, sternocleiomastoid
- Hypoglossal: muscles of tongue

Anticipatory Guidance

- General health: encourage physical activity, dental care, adequate sleep, proper hygiene, administer immunizations
- Nutrition: encourage balanced diet, weight control
- Psychological: encourage family and social interactions, establish fair rules, show interest in school and daily activity
- Safety: encourage seat belt use, bike and skating safety: helmet use, water safety, adult supervision, know where child is at all times

OVERVIEW OF PROBLEM (DISCOVERED DURING EXAM)

Otitis Media

Definition

Acute otitis media is an infection of the middle ear characterized by a middle ear infusion that causes partial or complete obstruction of the eustachian tube.

Pathophysiology

- Major causative organisms
  - *Streptococcus pneumoniae* (31%)
  - *Haemophilus influenzae* (22%)
  - *Moraxella catarrhalis* (7%)
  - *Beta hemolytic streptococci* (<2%)
- Sterile effusions cause approx 20% of infections

Incidence

- Second most common acute disease in pediatric patients
- Peak prevalence is in ages 6–36 months**,** but may occur at any time in childhood or adulthood
- Congenital factors: craniofacial abnormalities; i.e., cleft palate, Down's syndrome
- Environmental factors; crowded living conditions, daycare setting, exposure to passive smoking
- Infection states: concurrent upper airway infection

Assessment

Subjective

- Hx URI (upper airway infection), family hx of allergies, hearing loss
- Rhinorrhea
- Malaise
- Irritability
- Pulling, rubbing ear
- Pain in ear
- Fever (temp 101–102°F)

Objective

Physical findings:

- Rhinorrhea
- Possible fever
- Tympanic membrane: fullness, bulging, loss in concavity resulting in decreased visualization of landmarks
- Color: erythematous or whiteness resulting from scarring or pus
- Luster: dullness, loss of light reflex
- Mobility: decreased or absent with use of otoscope with insufflator

Possible concurrent findings:

- Mastoid tenderness
- Adenopathy
- Pharyngitis
- Lower respiratory tract involvement

Differential diagnoses:

- Redness of tympanic membrane (TM) due to fever or crying: TM bright with visible landmarks, mobility normal
- Eustacian tube obstruction: TM normal, transient ear pain
- Serous otitis: TM not inflamed, air bubbles may be seen behind membrane
- External otitis: pain on movement of pinna, diffuse inlammation of ear canal with or without exudate

Treatment

- Assure proper visualization of TM by removing wax with plastic currette or by irrigation
- Galbreath's technique: osteopathic manipulation that increases upper airway pressure, forcing inflation of middle ear
- Medication
  - Antibiotics: treat infection (amoxicillin 80–90 mg/kg/day q 8 hr x 10 days or augmentin 90 mg/kg and 6.4 mg/kg/day q 12 hr)
  - Analgesics/antipyretics: reduce pain and fever (acetaminophen 15 mg/kg/dose q 4 hr or ibuprofen 10 mg/kg/dose q 6 hr)

REVIEW QUESTIONS

1. List three signs/symptoms of scoliosis.
Answer:

2. List six components of a neurological assessment.
Answer:

3. What is the significance of a palpable thrill during cardiac assessment?
Answer:

4. A tympanic membrane that is red and bulging with absent or diminished light reflex may indicate what condition?
Answer:

5. List the cognitive milestones of the 9-year-old school-aged child.
Answer:

Related Evidenced-Based Practice Guidelines

Tuberculosis: clinical diagnosis and management of tuberculosis, and measures for its prevention and control. National Collaborating Centre for Chronic Conditions–National Government Agency [Non-U.S.]. 2006. 215 pages. NGC: 004877

Recommendations of the Advisory Committee on Immunization Practices (ACIP)http://www.cdc.gov/flu/professionals/acip/index.htm

The Joint Commission 2011 Ambulatory Care National Patient Safety Goals http://www.jointcommission.org/assets/1/6/2011_AHC_NPSG_EASY.pdf

Topics to Review Prior to the Simulation

- Pediatric physical assessment
- Pediatric vision and hearing screening
- Developmental milestones of the child
- Immunization schedule

SIMULATION

Client Background

Biographical Data

- Age: 9
- Gender: female
- Height: 4 ft 5 in
- Weight: 90 lb

Cultural Considerations

- Language: English
- Ethnicity: African
- Nationality: American
- Culture: Caribbean

Demographic

- Marital status: N/A
- Educational level: grade 4
- Religion: Protestant
- Occupation: student

Current Health Status

- 9-year-old child, presents to primary care office for routine yearly check-up

History

- Psychosocial history
  - Social support: family
- Past health history
  - Medical: wears glasses, mildly overweight, no chronic medical problems
  - Surgical: none
  - Family history: no problems identified

Admission Sheet

Name:	Tia Langston
Age:	9
Gender:	Female
Marital Status:	N/A
Educational Level:	Grade 4
Religion:	Protestant
Ethnicity:	African
Nationality:	American
Language:	English
Occupation:	Student

Office **Provider's Orders**		**Patient's Name:** Tia Langston **Allergies:** NKA	
Diagnosis:			
Date	**Time**	**Order**	**Signature**
		Vital signs: X1	
		Diet: Regular	
		Activity: Ad lib	
		IV therapy: N/A	
		Medications: Amoxicillin 90 mg/kg/day po divided every 8 hr x 10 days Trivalent Inactivated Influenza Vaccine: 0.5-mL dose Gardasil vaccine: 0.5 mL IM	
		Diagnostic studies: VS, Wt, Ht, U/A, CBC, vision/hearing screens, pneumatic otoscopy	
		Treatments: Remove excess wax from ear canal with plastic curette or warm tap water irrigation for proper visualization of TM	Dr. Gott

Nursing Report Tia is here for complete physical assessment and is accompanied by her mother. She is complaining of mild earache and has a low grade fever. Immunizations UTD.

Student Simulation Prep Assignments

1. Identify items and their purpose in the examination of a school-aged child.

Item	Purpose
Vision chart	
Hearing screening equipment	
Otoscope/opthalmoscope	
Stethoscope	
Thermometer	
BP cuff	
Reflex hammer	
Needles/syringes	
Vaccines	
Vaccine information and consent forms	
Gloves	
Scale	
Tape measure	
Specimen containers and tubes, Vacutainer, tourniquet	
Alcohol wipes	

2. Identify team members and their specific roles in the examination of a school-aged child.

Team Member	Role
Nurse	
PCP	

3. Initial Focused Assessment

After reviewing the client background and nursing report, you are ready to assess your client's current status. Under each category, identify how you would target your assessment and what you would expect to find in the physical assessment of the school-aged child with otitis media.

History

Are there any questions you need to ask the patient or family to obtain additional relevant data?

Physical Exam

- General appearance:
- Integumentary:
- HEENT:
- Respiratory:
- CV:
- Breasts:
- Abdominal:
- Neuro:
- Musculoskeletal:
- Reproductive:
- Developmental:

What are the nursing implications considering the developmental stage of your patient?

Answer:

5. Diagnostic Tests

What diagnostic test results relevant to the patient's current problem are needed to plan care?

Complete the table using Van Leeuwen et al, *Davis's Comprehensive Handbook of Laboratory and Diagnostic Testing with Nursing Implications* 4e, or other diagnostic test reference.

Diagnostic Test	Significance to This Patient's Problem
UA	
CBC	
PPD	
Vision/hearing tests	
Pneumatic otoscopy	

6. Treatment

Identify drugs that are used to treat a patient with otitis media.

Identify immunizations for a 9-year-old child.

Complete the table using Deglin et al, *Davis's Drug Guide for Nurses* 12e, or other drug reference.

Medication	Dose, Route Frequency	Indications	Side Effect	Nursing Implications
Amoxicillin	90 mg/kg po q 8 hr x 10 days			

Continued

Medication	Dose, Route Frequency	Indications	Side Effect	Nursing Implications
Trivalent Inactivated Influenza Vaccine	0.5-mL dose			
Gardasil vaccine	0.5 mL IM 3 injections over 6 mo			

7. Nursing Problems/Diagnoses

Identify three priority nursing problems/diagnoses.

Assessment Data	Priority Problem	Intervention	Expected Patient Outcome	Which Interventions Could Be Delegated to Unlicensed Personnel?
1.				
2.				

Assessment Data	Priority Problem	Intervention	Expected Patient Outcome	Which Interventions Could Be Delegated to Unlicensed Personnel?
3.				

References

Brook, I., & Gober, A. E. (2009). The effects of treatment of acute otitis media with a low dose vs a high dose of amoxicillin on the nasopharyngeal flora. *Archives of Otolaryngology Head and Neck Surgurg, 135*:458.

Deglin, J. H., & Vallerand, A. H. (2009). *Davis's drug guide for nurses* (11th ed.). Philadelphia: F. A. Davis.

Dias, M., and Marcuse, E. (2000). When parents resist immunizations. *Contemporary Pediatrics, 17*:75-86.

Dillon, P. (2007). *Nursing health assessment: A critical thinking and case studies approach* (2nd ed.). Philadelphia: F. A. Davis.

Erikson, E.H. (1950). *Childhood and society.* New York: Norton.

Hockenberry, M. J., & Wilson, D. (2007). *Wong's nursing care of infants and children*. St. Louis: Mosby.

Lagerquist, S. (2006). *Davis's NCLEX-RN success*. Philadelphia: F. A. Davis.

Ramakrishnan, K., Sparks, R. A., & Berryhill, W. E. (2007). Diagnosis and treatment of acute otitis media. *American Family Physician*, 76:1659.

Van Leeuwen, A. M., Poelhuis-Leth, D. J., & Bladh, M. L. (2011). *Davis's comprehensive handbook of laboratory and diagnostic tests with nursing implications.* (4th ed.). Philadelphia: F. A. Davis.

10-4 Intractable Pain

COMMUNITY SETTING/HOSPICE CARE

STANDARD FORMS

These templates are included in the Appendix; copy before each use.

LEARNING OUTCOMES

Cognitive

The student will be able to:

1. Describe signs and symptoms of a patient experiencing intractable pain.
2. Correlate signs and symptoms of pain to the disease process of the terminally ill patient.
3. Identify factors in a patient's history that increase risk for intractable pain.
4. Identify factors in a patient's current condition that increase risk for intractable pain and medication management.
5. Identify the appropriate interventions for the patient with onset of intractable pain.
6. Differentiate the roles of team members in response to a patient with intractable pain.

Psychomotor

The student will be able to:

1. Perform appropriate pain assessment for a patient with intractable pain.
2. Initiate appropriate pain interventions for a patient with pain that includes the following:
   - Brief physical pain in response to pain.
   - Pain assessment either verbal or behavioral assessment.
   - Current medications and usage.
   - Psychological factors associated with the increase of pain.
   - Patient's understanding of the pain their willingness to comply with a plan of care.
3. Work collaboratively as part of the healthcare team in the care of a patient with intractable pain.

Affective

The student will be able to:

1. Reflect upon performance in the care of a patient with intractable pain.
2. Identify own feelings in delivering care to a patient with intractable pain.
3. Discuss feelings related to working as a member of a team in the car of a patient with intractable pain.
4. Identify factors that worked well during the simulation of care of a patient with intractable pain.
5. Identify factors that needed improvement during the simulation of care of a patient with intractable pain.
6. Develop self-confidence in the care of a patient with intractable pain.

Communication

The student will be able to:

1. Communicate effectively with healthcare team members in care of a patient with intractable pain.
2. Communicate effectively with the patient and family in the care of a patient with intractable pain.
3. Use SBAR when communication with team members in the care of a patient with intractable pain.
4. Will practice Transparent Thinking (thinking out loud) to facilitate group problem solving.
5. Use Directed Communication (directing a message to specific individual) when delegating tasks.
6. Employ Closed-Loop Communication (acknowledgment of receipt of the message and status) to acknowledge communications from others.

Safety

The student will be able to:

Administer and maintain specific protecting interventions with attention to safety of the client and health care professional.

1. Incorporate 2011 Joint Commission Home Care National Patient Safety Goals
   - Identify patient correctly
   - Prevent infection
   - Reconcile patient medications
   - Prevent falls
   - Identify patient safety risks in the home setting
2. Demonstrate attention to standard precautions. Includes hand washing, infection control measures, and use of personal protective equipment (PPE) as needed.

Leadership and Management/Delegation

The student will be able to:

1. Identify the appropriate assessment and interventions to treat the patient with intractable pain.
2. Identify and prioritize patient's needs in care of intractable pain.

OVERVIEW OF PROBLEM

Intractable Pain

Definition

Pain is a complex subjective sensation involving unpleasant sensory and emotional experience, usually associated with real or potential tissue damage.

"Pain is whatever the experiencing person says it is, occurring when they say it does" (McCaffery, 1968).

"Pain is a noxious stimuli" (Webster's Dictionary).

Types of Pain

- Acute: pain that has a sudden onset or associated with surgery or other procedures. The pain is usually relieved within a short period of time. It is expected to subside at some point. It can be an indication that something is wrong.
- Chronic: noncancer pain that is associated with a disease process such as arthritis, in which pain may be managed with a nonsteroidal, nonopiate, or opiate depending on the symptoms present. Pain lasts longer that an expected duration, usually defined as greater than 3–6 months. Pain has no predictable ending and may last a lifetime.
- Cancer: pain that arises from either a tumor or secondary to the treatment such as radiation or chemotherapy.
- Neuropathic: pain that results from injury to peripheral nerves rather than stimulation of the nerve endings. This pain can be described as burning, shooting, sharp, pins and needles, or electric-like. It can be associated with abnormal sensations such as alloydnia, paresthesia, or dyesthesia.
- Nociceptive (somatic or visceral): pain that arises from direct stimulation of afferent nerves. This pain can be describes as dull, achy, or bothersome. It is usually well localized.

Important Considerations

42% of adults in the United States experience pain daily and 89% monthly. It accounts for approximately 100 billion dollars in healthcare expenses, workman's compensation, lost wages, and litigation. It is the primary reason why people see their physicians. Pain is subjective and has many facets such as psychosocial, financial, spiritual, and personal effects.

There are many barriers present that affect proper pain management. These barriers include patient barriers, physician barriers, and healthcare barriers.

- Patient barriers
  - The belief that pain cannot be relieved
  - Fear of addiction
  - Fear of tolerance
  - Concerns about side effects
  - Not wanting to be a complainer
  - The belief that pain is necessary for salvation
  - Not wanting to distract the healthcare provider from treating the medical illness
- Physician barriers
  - Lack of knowledge or education of pain and its treatment
  - Opioid phobia (prejudice against the use of opioid analgesics)
  - Fear of the unknown
  - Fear of addiction
  - Fear of the DEA/medical discipline
- Healthcare barriers
  - Attitude
  - Lack of knowledge
  - Lack of education
  - Low priority

Pathophysiology

Pain is understood by recognizing three components:

- Stimuli: Can be chemical, ischemic, mechanical, thermal.
- Perception: Age, gender, previous experience, culture, level of consciousness, and many other factors an influence perception. Pain may be perceived as more severe when alone, at night, or when immobilized.
- Response: Variations in physiological, cultural, and learned responses; anxiety is created; pain may be seen as justified punishment; pain used as a means of attention seeking; vocalizations or withdrawl (even sleep) in response to pain.

Risk Factors

- Previous experience with pain
- Underlying disease process
- Injury or compression secondary to tumor

Assessment

Subjective

- Patient's report of pain

Objective

- Physical findings
  - Grimaces when touched
  - Rubbing the affected area
  - Guarding an area
  - Bruising or trauma to an area
- Report of pain on a scale of 0–10, where 0 is no pain and 10 is the worst imaginable pain for the patient.
  - Intensity of pain
    - On average
    - At its worst
    - At its best
  - Characteristics of the pain
    - Intermittent or constant
    - Neuropathic (sharp, shooting, burning, electric-like), or nocioceptive (dull, achy, or bothersome)
  - Factors that aggravate the pain (ice, heat, activity)
  - Factors that relieve the pain (ice, heat, rest, exercise)

- Current treatment for the management of pain (current medications)
- Interventions
  - Surgery
  - Chiropractor
  - Injections
  - Acupuncture or acupressure
- Reproduction of pain on exam
- Affects of pain on the patient in the following areas
  - Activities of daily function
  - Sleep
  - Interpersonal relationships
  - Social activities
  - Nutrition
  - Psychological well-being

Diagnostic Tests (to rule out other causes)

- MRI
- CT scan
- Bone scan
- X-ray
- EMG

Treatment

Nocioceptive pain (somatic or visceral)

- Initially treat with nonsteroidal medications which can include
  - Ibuprofen
  - Acetaminophen
  - Celebrex
  - Toradol
- Short-acting opioid medications
  - Oxycodone with acetaminophen
  - Immediate-release oxycodone
  - Hydrocodone with acetaminophen
  - Tramadol
- Long-acting opioids
  - Morphine
  - Oxycodone
  - Fentanyl
  - Hydrocodone
  - Hydromophone
  - Methadone

Neuropathic pain

- First line of treatment: anticonvulsants
  - Gabapentin
  - Pregabalin
  - Lamotrigine
  - Oxcarbazepine
  - Topiramate
- Second line
  - Amitriptyline
  - Bupropion
  - Fluoxetine
  - Nortriptline
  - Paroxetine
  - Trazodone
- Concomitant therapy
  - Nonsteroidal anti-inflammatory medications
  - Opioids
  - Interventional treatment
    - Epidural steroid injection
    - Sympathetic block
    - Spinal cord stimulation
  - Nonpharmacological interventions
    - TENS unit
    - Acupuncture
    - Acupressure
    - Biofeedback

REVIEW QUESTIONS

1. How can you tell when someone is in pain?
   Answer:

2. What are common side effects of opioids?
   Answer:

3. What are the goals of palliative care?
   Answer:

4. What tools can you use in assessing pain?
   Answer:

5. What other medication would be indicated for someone taking opioids?
   Answer:

Related Evidence-Based Practice Guidelines

The National Guideline Clearing House

Evidenced-based interventions to improve palliative care of pain, dyspnea and depression at the end of life: a practice guideline from the American College of Physicians

Qaseem A, Snow V, Shekelle P, Casey DE Jr, Cross JT Jr, Owens DK, Clinical Efficacy Assessment Subcommittee of the American College of Physicians, Dallas P, Dolan NC,

Forciea MA, Halasyamani L, Hopkins RH Jr, Shekelle P. Evidence-based interventions to improve the palliative care of pain, dyspnea, and depression at the end of life: a clinical practice guideline from the American College of Physicians. Ann Intern Med 2008 Jan 15;148(2):141-6. Available at:
http://www.guideline.gov/summary/summary.aspx?doc_id=5526&nbr=003757&string=pain+AND+assessment
Recommendations for Improving Pain and Symptom Management in Montana
A White Paper of the Montana Pain and Symptom Management Task Force Feb 2008
Available at: http://www.guideline.gov/summary/summary.aspx?doc_id=7297&nbr=004341&string=pain+AND+assessment
National Guideline Clearing House
Pain Management. In: Evidenced-based geriatric nursing protocols for best practice
Horgas AL, Yoon SL. Pain management. In: Capezuti E, Zwicker D, Mezey M, Fulmer T, editor(s). Evidence-based geriatric nursing protocols for best practice. 3rd ed. New York (NY): Springer Publishing Company; 2008. p. 199-222.
Available at:http://www.guideline.gov/summary/summary.aspx?doc_id=12268&nbr=006352&string=pain+AND+assessment
2011 Home Care National Patient Safety Goals
http://www.jointcommission.org/assets/1/6/2011_OME_NPSG_EASY.pdf SBAR Technique for Communication: A situational briefing model published by The Institute for Healthcare Improvement was downloaded on December 19, 2008, from
http://www.ihi.org/IHI/Topics/PatientSafety/SafetyGeneral/Tools/SBARTechniqueforCommunicationASituationalBriefingModel.htm

Topics to Review Prior to the Simulation

- Pain assessment
- Palliative care
- Narcotic administration
- Head to toe assessment

SIMULATION

Client Background

Biographical Data

- Age: 68
- Gender: female
- Height: 165 cm
- Weight: 60.9 kg

Cultural Considerations

- Language: English
- Ethnicity: Polish
- Nationality: American
- Culture: no significant cultural considerations identified

Demographic

- Marital status: widowed
- Educational level: business school
- Religion: Catholic
- Occupation: retired secretary

Current Health Status (current problem/topic of scenario)

- Hypertension, gastroensophageal reflux disease (GERD), metastatic breast cancer, weakened state

History

- Psychosocial history
  - Social support; lives with daughter for past 2 months, neighbor stops by the days her daughter works around 10 AM and 1 PM.
  - Has two other children within an hour distance who call her and visit
- Past health history
  - Medical: mass in right breast, hypertension, GERD, NKDA
  - Surgical: right mastectomy, insertion of port access device
- Family history: father died of stroke at age 70, mother died of "some kid of cancer," two siblings with "heart problems," one sibling with breast cancer

Admission Sheet

Name:	Mrs. Bea Comfortable
Age:	68
Gender:	Female
Marital Status:	Widowed
Educational Level:	Business school

Continued

Admission Sheet—cont'd

Religion:	Catholic
Ethnicity:	Polish
Nationality:	American
Language:	English
Occupation:	Retired secretary

Hospital
Provider Orders

Patient's Name: Bea Comfortable
Allergies: NKDA

Diagnosis: Intractable pain, end-stage breast cancer

Date	Time	Order	Signature
		Vital signs: at each home visit	
		Diet: regular as tolerated	
		Activity: up as tolerated	
		IV therapy: none	
		Medications: MS Contin 15 mg po q 12 hr	
		MSIR 5 mg po q 2 hr prn for breakthrough pain	
		Gabapentin 300 mg at bedtime po	
		Senekot-S 2 tabs po every night before bed	
		Fleets enema prn no bowel movement for 2 days	
		Diagnostic studies: none	
		Treatment:	
		Eucerin cream to heels and lower back as needed for preventive skin breakdown	
		Encourage patient to sit out of bed 3 x times a day for at least 30 min or as tolerated	
		Oxygen 2 L via NC prn respiratory distress	
			Dr. Rosen

Nursing Report

At the next visit to the patient's house, the patient reports that her abdomen is bloated and she has not moved her bowels in a few days. She reports that she had to use more of her pain medication due to an increase in her back pain. She reports that her appetite is poor and she is beginning to have some shortness of breath with walking and any activities.

Student Simulation Prep Assignments

1. Identify items and their purpose in the care of a patient with intractable pain.

Item	Purpose
Pain scale	
Drug book	

Item	Purpose
Pain diary	
Medication planner	
Hospice plan of care	

2. Identify team members and their specific roles in the care of a patient with intractable pain.

Team Member	Role
Primary nurse	
Home health aide	
Physical therapist	
Chaplain	

3. Relevant Data Exercise: Fill in the columns below.

Relevant Data from Report	Relevant Data from Other Sources	Data Missing	Sources for Missing Data	Data Requiring Follow-Up

4. Initial Focused Assessment

After reviewing the client background and nursing report, you are ready to assess your client's current status. Under each category, identify how you would target your assessment and what you would expect to find for the patient with intractable pain.

History

Are there any questions you need to ask the patient or family to obtain additional relevant data?

Physical Exam

- General appearance:
- Integumentary:
- HEENT:
- Respiratory:
- CV:
- Breasts:
- Abdominal:
- Neuro:
- Musculoskeletal:
- Reproductive:
- Additional:
- Developmental:

What are the nursing implications considering the developmental stage of your patient?

Answer:

5. *Diagnostic Tests*

Not applicable

6. *Treatment*

Identify drugs that are used to treat a patient with intractable pain.

Complete the table using Deglin et al, *Davis's Drug Guide for Nurses* 12e, or other drug reference.

Medication	Dose, Route Frequency	Indications	Side Effect	Nursing Implications
MS Contin	15 mg po q 12 hr			
MSIR	5 mg po q 2 hr as needed			
Gabapentin	300 mg po at bedtime			
Senekot-S	2 tabs po every night 1 enema prn			
Fleets Enema				

7. Nursing Problems/Diagnoses

Identify three priority nursing problems/diagnoses.

Assessment Data	Priority Problem	Intervention	Expected Patient Outcome	Which interventions Could Be Delegated to Unlicensed Personnel?
1.				

Assessment Data	Priority Problem	Intervention	Expected Patient Outcome	Which interventions Could Be Delegated to Unlicensed Personnel?
2.				
3.				

References

Deglin, J. H., & Vallerand, A. H. (2009). *Davis's drug guide for nurses* (11th ed.). Philadelphia: F. A. Davis.

Dillon, P. (2007). *Nursing health assessment: A critical thinking and case studies approach* (2nd ed.). Philadelphia: F. A. Davis.

Erikson, E.H. (1950). *Childhood and society.* New York: Norton.

Lagerquist, S. (2006). *Davis's NCLEX-RN success*. Philadelphia: F. A. Davis.

Menefee, L., Katz, N., & Zacharoff, K. (2007). *A pocket guide to pain management* (3rd ed.). Newton, MA: Inflexxion.

Pasero, C., & McCaffery, M. (2011) *Pain assessment and pharmacologic management*. St. Louis: Mosby.

St. Marie, B. (2002). *Core curriculum for pain management nursing*. Philadelphia: Saunders.

Van Leeuwen, A. M., Poelhuis-Leth, D. J., & Bladh, M. L. (2011). *Davis's comprehensive handbook of laboratory and diagnostic tests with nursing implications.* (4th ed.). Philadelphia: F. A. Davis.

Wells, N., Pasero, C., & McCaffery, M. (2008). Improving the quality of care through pain assessment and management. In Hughes, R. G. (Ed.). *Patient safety and quality: An evidenced-based handbook for nurses.* Agency for Health Care Research and Quality.

Appendix

ADMISSION SHEET

Name: ______________________________

DOB: ______________________________

Age: ______________________________

Gender: ______________________________

Marital status: ______________________________

Educational level: ______________________________

Religion: ______________________________

Ethnicity: ______________________________

Nationality: ______________________________

Language: ______________________________

Occupation: ______________________________

BRADEN SCALE FOR PREDICTING PRESSURE SORE RISK

Patient's Name:__________ Patient's DOB:__________ Evaluator's Name:__________ Date of Assessment

					Date of Assessment			
SENSORY PERCEPTION ability to respond meaning-fully to pressure-related discomfort	**1. Completely Limited** Unresponsive (does not moan, flinch, or grasp) to painful stimuli, due to diminished level of consciousness or sedation. OR limited ability to feel pain over most of body.	**2. Very Limited** Responds only to painful stimuli. Cannot communicate discomfort except by moaning or restlessness OR has a sensory impairment which limits the ability to feel pain or discomfort over $^1/_2$ of body.	**3. Slightly Limited** Responds to verbal com-mands, but cannot always communicate discomfort or the need to be turned. OR has some sensory impairment which limits ability to feel pain or discomfort in 1 or 2 extremities.	**4. No Impairment** Responds to verbal commands. Has no sensory deficit which would limit ability to feel or voice pain or discomfort.				
MOISTURE degree to which skin is exposed to moisture	**1. Constantly Moist** Skin is kept moist almost constantly by perspiration, urine, etc. Dampness is detected every time patient is moved or turned.	**2. Very Moist** Skin is often, but not always moist. Linen must be changed at least once a shift.	**3. Occasionally Moist:** Skin is occasionally moist, requiring an extra linen change approximately once a day.	**4. Rarely Moist** Skin is usually dry, linen only requires changing at routine intervals.				
ACTIVITY degree of physical activity	**1. Bedfast** Confined to bed.	**2. Chairfast** Ability to walk severely limited or non-existent. Cannot bear own weight and/or must be assisted into chair or wheelchair.	**3. Walks Occasionally** Walks occasionally during day, but for very short distances, with or without assistance. Spends majority of each shift in bed or chair.	**4. Walks Frequently** Walks outside room at least twice a day and inside room at least once every two hours during waking hours.				
MOBILITY ability to change and control body position	**1. Completely Immobile** Does not make even slight changes in body or extremity position without assistance.	**2. Very Limited** Makes occasional slight changes in body or extremity position but unable to make frequent or significant changes independently.	**3. Slightly Limited** Makes frequent though slight changes in body or extremity position independently.	**4. No Limitation** Makes major and frequent changes in position without assistance.				
NUTRITION usual food intake pattern	**1. Very Poor** Never eats a complete meal. Rarely eats more than $^1/_2$ of any food offered. Eats 2 servings or less of protein (meat or dairy products) per day. Takes fluids poorly. Does not take a liquid dietary supplement OR is NPO and/or maintained on clear liquids or IVs for more than 5 days.	**2. Probably Inadequate** Rarely eats a complete meal and generally eats only about $^1/_2$ of any food offered. Protein intake includes only 3 servings of meat or dairy products per day. Occasionally will take a dietary supplement. OR receives less than optimum amount of liquid diet or tube feeding.	**3. Adequate** Eats over half of most meals. Eats a total of 4 servings of protein (meat, dairy products) per day. Occasionally will refuse a meal, but will usually take a supplement when offered OR is on a tube feeding or TPN regimen which probably meets most of nutritional needs.	**4. Excellent** Eats most of every meal. Never refuses a meal. Usually eats a total of 4 or more servings of meat and dairy products. Occasionally eats between meals. Does not require supplementation.				
FRICTION & SHEAR	**1. Problem** Requires moderate to maximum assistance in moving. Complete lifting without sliding against sheets is impossible. Frequently slides down in bed or chair, requiring frequent repositioning with maximum assistance. Spasticity, contractures or agitation leads to almost constant friction.	**2. Potential Problem** Moves feebly or requires minimum assistance. During a move skin probably slides to some extent against sheets, chair, restraints or other devices. Maintains relatively good position in chair or bed most of the time but occasionally slides down.	**3. No Apparent Problem** Moves in bed and in chair independently and has sufficient muscle strength to lift up completely during move. Maintains good position in bed or chair.					
				Total Score				

Note: Patient's with a total score of 18 or less are considered to be at risk of developing pressure ulcers. (19–23 = no risk, 15–18 = low risk, 13–14 = moderate risk, 10–12 = high risk, < to 9 = very high risk)

Date/Time Event Recognized ________ Location ______ Witnessed: ☐ Yes ☐ No
Age _____ Weight _____ Height _______ Hospital-wide response activated? ☐ Yes ☐ No
Event Recognized by: ____________________

Patient Name DOB

Airway/Breathing

Breathing ☐ Spontaneous ☐ Apneic ☐ Agonal ☐ Assisted
Time of First Assisted Ventilation: ____________
Ventilation: ☐ Bag-Valve-Mask ☐ Endotracheal Tube
☐ Tracheostomy ☐ Other: __________
Intubation: Time: _____ **Size:** _____
By Whom:
Confirmation: ☐ Auscultation ☐ Exhaled CO_2
☐ Other __________

Circulation

1st Rhythm Requiring Compressions: __________
1st PULSELESS Rhythm: __________
Time Chest Compressions Started: __________

AED Applied: ☐ Yes ☐ No → **Time:** __________
Defibrillator Type(s): __________
Pacemaker On: ☐ Yes ☐ No

Time Resuscitation Event Ended:
Reason Resuscitation Ended:
☐ Survived – Return of Circulation (ROC) >20 min
☐ Died – Efforts Terminated (No Sustained ROC)
☐ Died – Medical Futility
☐ Died – Advance Directives
☐ Died – Restrictions by Family

TYPE AND AMOUNT OF IV FLUIDS GIVEN:

Time	Breathing		Pulse		BP	Rhythm	Defibrillator Type AED/Manual	Joules	Amiodarone Dose/IV or IO	Atropine Dose/IV or IO	Epinephrine Dose/IV or IO	Lidocaine Dose/IV or IO	Vasopressin Dose/IV or IO			Dopamine	Dobutamine	Epinephrine	Norepinephrine	Comments: i.e.: Peripheral/Central Line Placement, IO, Chest tube, Vital Signs, Response to Interventions
	Spontaneous	Assisted (✓)	Spontaneous	Assisted (✓)																

Recorder Signature ____________________
ICU/Code Team Nurse Signature ____________________
Nursing Supervisior Signature ____________________
Provider Signature ____________________

Patient Name: ______________
DOB: __________
Medical Record Number: __________

CONSENT FOR TRANSFUSION OF BLOOD OR BLOOD PRODUCT(S)

__________(Physician or Nurse Practitioner) has explained to me that I need or may need during treatment a transfusion of blood and or blood products.

I understand that the **risks** of transfusion are low, and include but are not limited to: infection (HIV, hepatitis, other viruses), antibody development and immune reactions, contamination by bacteria, difficulty breathing related to antibodies in the donor blood, temporary reduction in my natural immunity.

I understand that there are **alternatives to transfusion** that include administration of hormones that stimulate the bone marrow (takes weeks to be effective), mineral supplementation (takes weeks to months to be effective), collection of my own blood during surgery (for certain surgical patients only).

I understand that the **benefits** of blood transfusion include improved oxygen delivery to vital organs (red blood cell transfusions), improved blood clotting (plasma, platelets, cryoprecipitate).

The procedure(s), risks and alternatives listed above were explained to me. I had the opportunity to ask questions and all of my questions about the procedure(s), risks and alternatives were answered to my satisfaction. I understand I have the right to accept or refuse transfusion of blood or blood products.

I Consent to the Transfusion of Blood or Blood Products:

______________ ______________ ______________
(Patient's Signature**) (Printed Name) ________ (Date and Time) __________

**Patient is unable to consent because: I therefore consent for patient:

______________ ______________
(Authorized Consenter's Signature) (Printed Name)

I Have Explained the Above Procedure(s) to the Patient or Authorized Consenter:

______________ ______________
(Physician's/Nurse Practitioner's Signature) (Printed Name)

Interpreter Attestation (when Applicable)
Interpretation has been provided by: ______________________ Date
Interpreter Signature or Identification Number: ______________________

Debriefing/Guided Reflection

1. How did you feel when caring for the patient in this simulated experience?
2. What did you learn about interacting with family members?
3. What did you learn about interacting with other members of the health care team?
4. How do you think you performed in this simulation scenario?
5. What was your role?
6. How did your role differ from others?
7. What did you do well?
8. What could you do to improve your performance?
9. How did you choose the problems you identified as top priority?
10. What factors did you consider in making your decision?
11. Overall, what did you think of this experience?
12. What would you change about the experience?

DISCHARGE INSTRUCTIONS

Patient Name ______________________________
Patient DOB ______________________________
Discharged to (circle): ______________________________
Medical Problems:

____
____
____
____

Allergies ______________________________
Medications ______________________________
____
Discharge Diagnosis ______________________________
Provider During Hospital Stay: ______________________________
Diet (Circle one and provide relevant education to patient):

Low Fat
Low Sodium
Renal Diet
Diabetic Diet

Risk Interventions Discussed: Smoking Cessation, Home Safety, Pneumococcal Vaccine, Weight Management, Influenza Vaccine

Activity
Follow up Appointments:

Referrals: Home Care, Outpatient Rehab, Physical Therapy, Cardiac Rehab, Occupational Therapy

Additional comments: ______________________________
____
____

I have provided patient education on the above and patient has verbalized understanding.

Nurse's signature ______________________________
Patient's signature ______________________________

EVALUATION

Scale 0 to 5 with 5 being highest level of performance

0 = did not perform
1 = performed with cues/guidance
2 = differentiates normal/abnormal
3 = clusters data
4 = identifies problem
5 = identifies potential problems

0 = did not perform
1 = performed with many cues/guidance
2 = performed with minimal cues/guidance
3 = performed independently

NAME: ______________________ **DATE:** ______________________

Critical Elements	Score		**Comments**
COMMUNICATION			
- introduces self			
- ID's patient			
- provides explanations to patient			
- uses SBAR when communicating with health care team members			
- communicates effectively with family members			
- professional verbal/nonverbal communication			
SAFETY/INFECTION CONTROL			
- side rails up			
- uses body mechanics			
- maintains standard precautions			
- washes hands			
- maintains sterile technique			
NURSING PROCESS			
Performs assessment			
History - performs symptom analysis for current problem			
- asks appropriate history questions			
Physical assessment			
- vital signs			
- O2 sat			
- monitor			
- head to toe (focused) assessment as it r/t problem			
Diagnostic Tests			
- interprets diagnostic tests			
Nursing Diagnosis/Problem			
- accurately identifies patient problems			
Planning			
- develops realistic goals and measurable outcomes			
Interventions			
- performs appropriate interventions r/t problem (**list interventions specific to scenario**)			
Evaluation			
- evaluates patient's response			

DOCUMENTATION			
- accurately documents			
PREPARATION/PERFORMANCE			
- nursing care is organized and timely			
- nursing care is prioritized			
- obtains needed equipment			
- applies theory to practice			
- considers any developmental problems r/t patient's current problem			
- considers any cultural problems r/t patient's current problem			
TOTAL SCORE			

ADDITIONAL COMMENTS:

INSTRUCTOR: ______________________________

STUDENT: ______________________________

DATE: ______________________________

Glasgow Coma Scale				Neuro		Pupils	Comments	Initials
Eyes open	Best verbal	Best Motor	Total	R arm/ L arm	R leg/ L leg	Pupil response/ Size r/l		

Glasgow Coma Scale

Observation	Response	Score
Eye response		
	Opens spontaneously	4
	Opens to verbal command	3
	Opens to pain	2
	No response	1
Motor response	Reacts to verbal command	6
	Reacts to painful stimuli	
	Identifies localized pain	5
	Flexes and withdraws	4
	Assumes flexor posture	3
	Assumes extensor posture	2
Verbal response	No response	1
	Is oriented and converses	5
	Is disoriented but converses	4
	Uses inappropriate words	3
	Makes incomprehensible sounds	2
	No response	1
Total		

Muscle Strength Scale

Scale	Explanation	Classification
5	Active motion against full resistance	Normal
4	Active motion against some resistance	Slight weakness
3	Active motion against gravity	Average weakness
2	Passive ROM (gravity removed and assisted by examiner)	Poor ROM
1	Slight flicker of contraction	Severe weakness
0	No muscular contraction	Paralysis

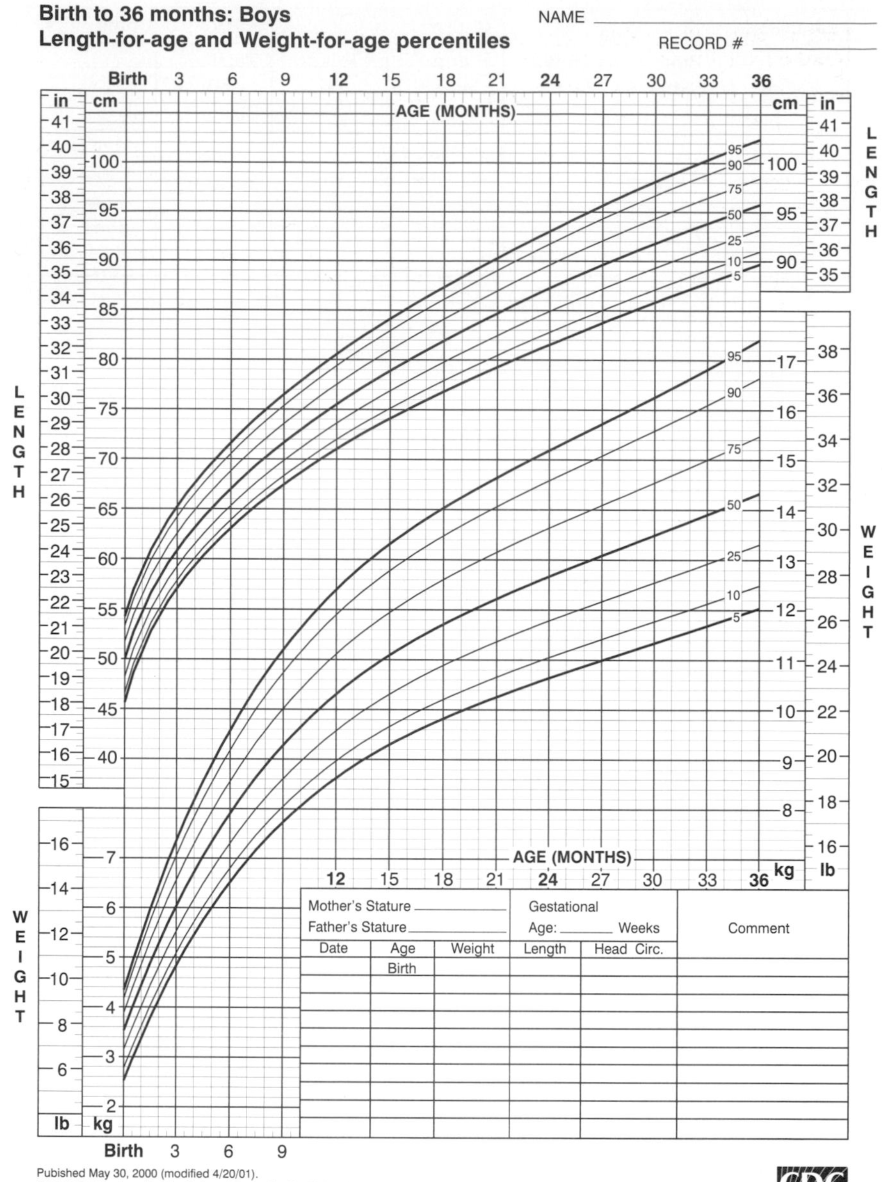

Pubished May 30, 2000 (modified 4/20/01).
SOURCE: Developed by the National Center for Health Statistics in collaboration with the National Center for Chronic Disease Prevention and Health Promotion (2000).
http://www.cdc.gov/growthcharts

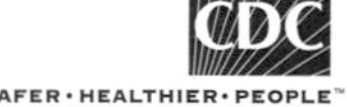

Birth to 36 months: Boys
Head circumference-for-age and Weight-for-length percentiles

NAME ______________

RECORD # ______________

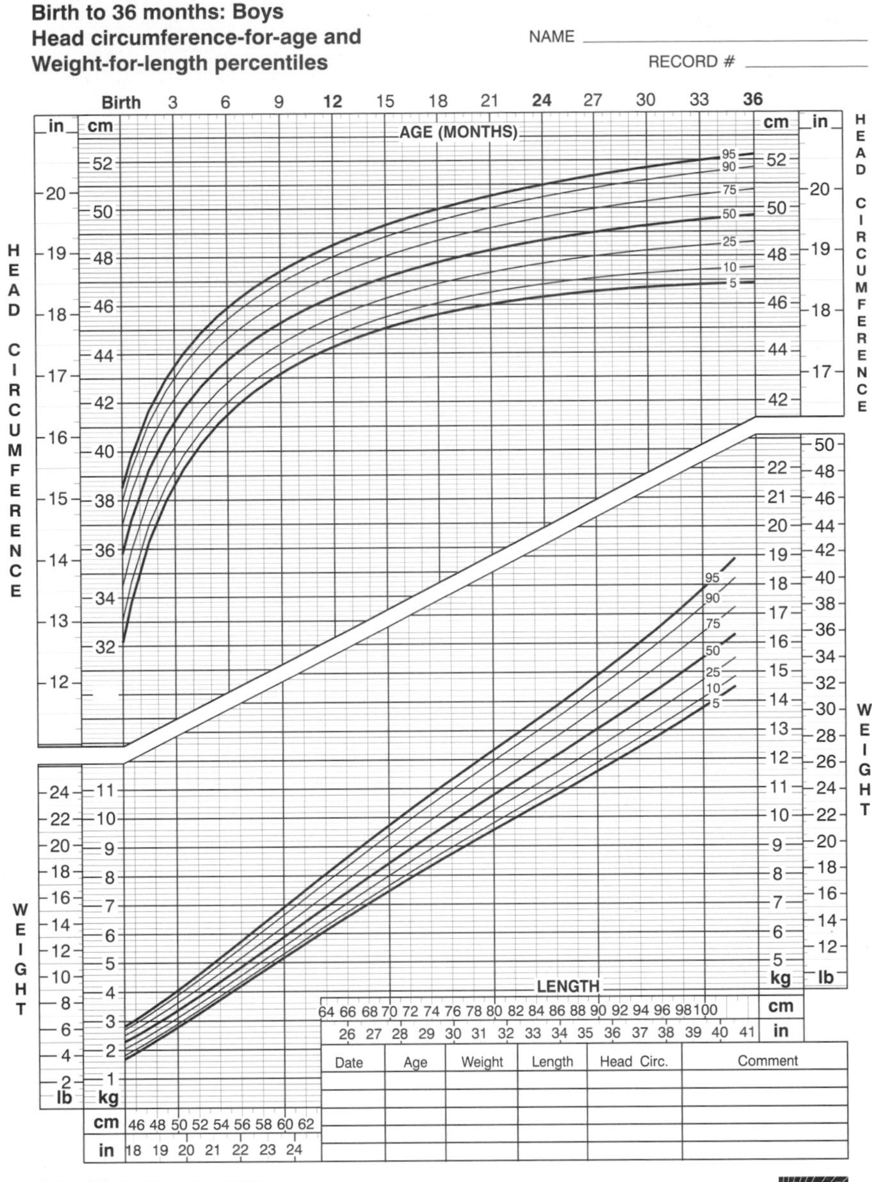

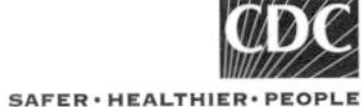

Date	Age	Weight	Length	Head Circ.	Comment

Published May 30, 2000 (modified 10/16/00).
SOURCE: Developed by the National Center for Health Statistics in collaboration with the National Center for Chronic Disease Prevention and Health Promotion (2000).
http://www.cdc.gov/growthcharts

CDC
SAFER • HEALTHIER • PEOPLE™

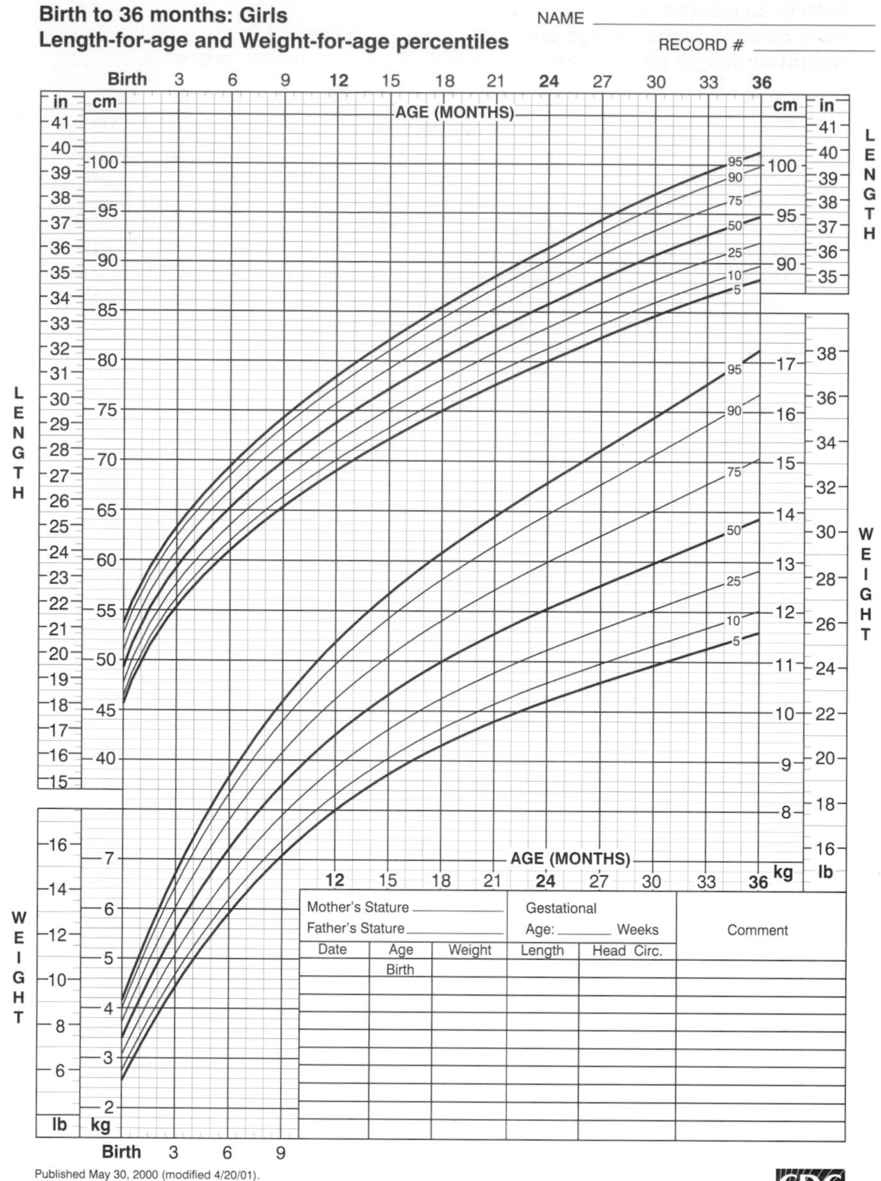

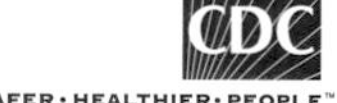

Published May 30, 2000 (modified 4/20/01).
SOURCE: Developed by the National Center for Health Statistics in collaboration with the National Center for Chronic Disease Prevention and Health Promotion (2000).
http://www.cdc.gov/growthcharts

CDC SAFER • HEALTHIER • PEOPLE™

Birth to 36 months: Girls
Head circumference-for-age and
Weight-for-length percentiles

NAME ______________________

RECORD # ____________

Date	Age	Weight	Length	Head Circ.	Comment

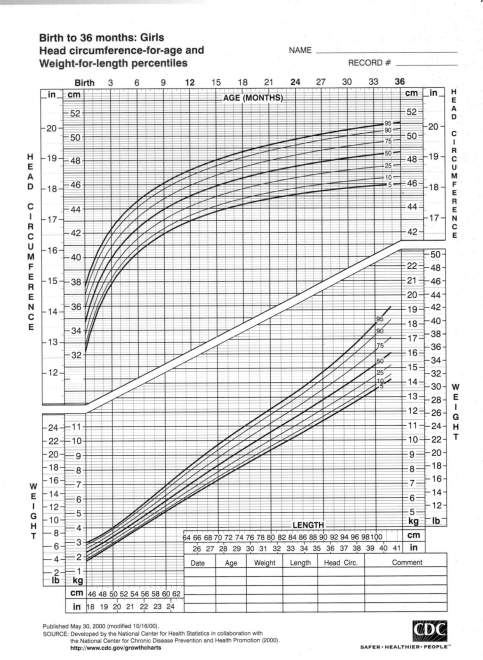

Published May 30, 2000 (modified 10/16/00).
SOURCE: Developed by the National Center for Health Statistics in collaboration with the National Center for Chronic Disease Prevention and Health Promotion (2000).
http://www.cdc.gov/growthcharts

SAFER • HEALTHIER • PEOPLE™

2 to 20 years: Boys
Stature-for-age and Weight-for-age percentiles

NAME ____________

RECORD # ____________

Mother's Stature ____________ Father's Stature ____________

Date	Age	Weight	Stature	BMI*

*To Calculate BMI: Weight (kg) ÷ Stature (cm) ÷ Stature (cm) x 10,000 or Weight (lb) ÷ Stature (in) ÷ Stature (in) x 703

AGE (YEARS)

STATURE

WEIGHT

Published May 30, 2000 (modified 11/21/00).
SOURCE: Developed by the National Center for Health Statistics in collaboration with the National Center for Chronic Disease Prevention and Health Promotion (2000).
http://www.cdc.gov/growthcharts

CDC
SAFER • HEALTHIER • PEOPLE™

2 to 20 years: Boys
Body mass index-for-age percentiles

NAME ______________________

RECORD # ______________

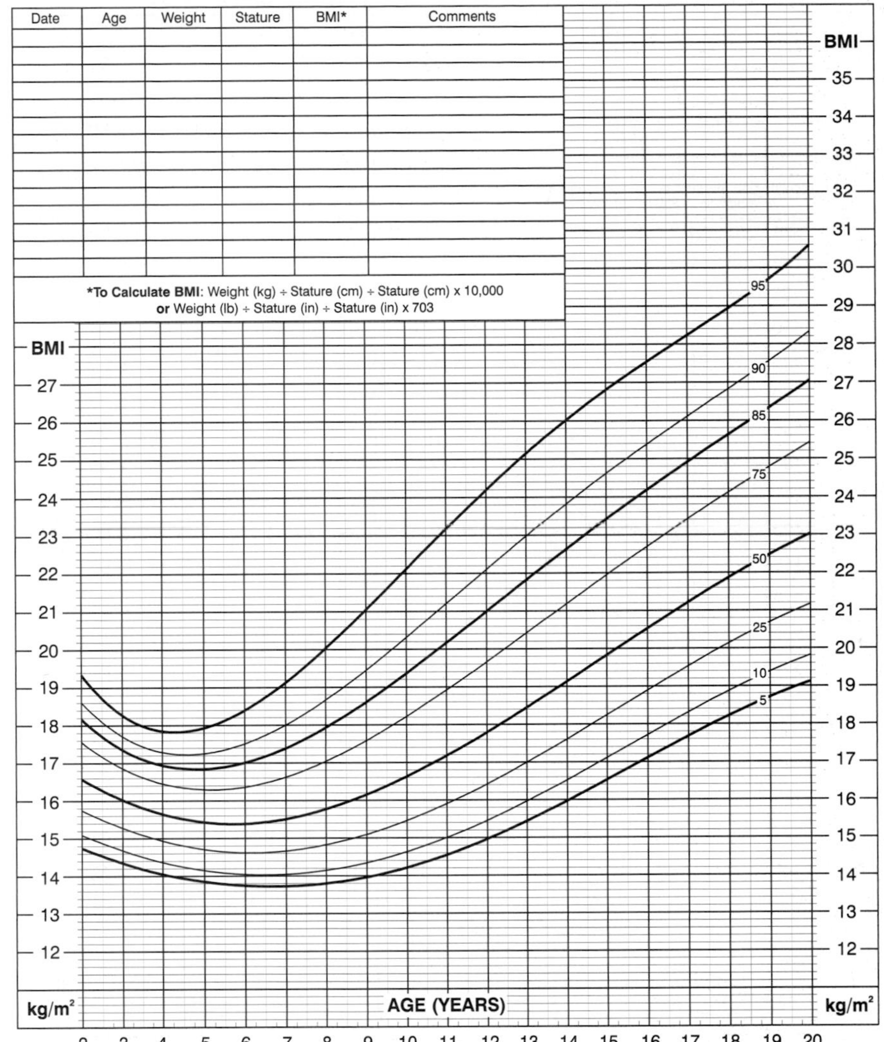

Published May 30, 2000 (modified 10/16/00).
SOURCE: Developed by the National Center for Health Statistics in collaboration with
the National Center for Chronic Disease Prevention and Health Promotion (2000).
http://www.cdc.gov/growthcharts

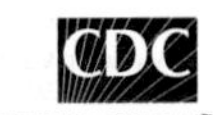

SAFER • HEALTHIER • PEOPLE™

2 to 20 years: Girls
Stature-for-age and Weight-for-age percentiles

NAME ____________

RECORD # ________

Mother's Stature ________ Father's Stature ________

Date	Age	Weight	Stature	BMI*

*To Calculate BMI: Weight (kg) ÷ Stature (cm) ÷ Stature (cm) x 10,000
or Weight (lb) ÷ Stature (in) ÷ Stature (in) x 703

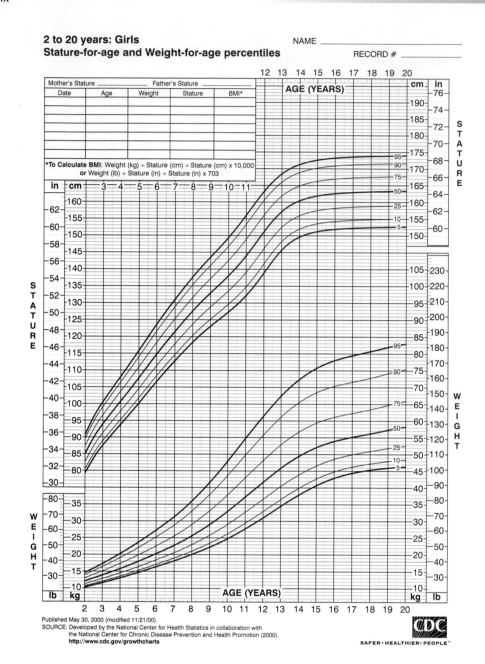

Published May 30, 2000 (modified 11/21/00).
SOURCE: Developed by the National Center for Health Statistics in collaboration with the National Center for Chronic Disease Prevention and Health Promotion (2000).
http://www.cdc.gov/growthcharts

CDC
SAFER · HEALTHIER · PEOPLE™

NAME ______________________

Weight-for-stature percentiles: Boys

RECORD # ____________

Date	Age	Weight	Stature	Comments

kg lb 76 34 33 72 32 31 68 30 29 64 28 27 60 26 56 25 24 52 23 22 48 21 20 44 19 18 40 17 16 36 15 32 14 13 28 12 11 24 10 9 20 8 kg lb

lb kg 26 56 25 24 52 23 22 48 21 44 20 19 40 18 17 36 16 15 32 14 13 28 12 11 24 10 20 9 8 lb kg

95 90 85 75 50 25 10 5

STATURE

cm 80 85 90 95 100 105 110 115 120

in 31 32 33 34 35 36 37 38 39 40 41 42 43 44 45 46 47

Published May 30, 2000 (modified 10/16/00).
SOURCE: Developed by the National Center for Health Statistics in collaboration with the National Center for Chronic Disease Prevention and Health Promotion (2000).
http://www.cdc.gov/growthcharts

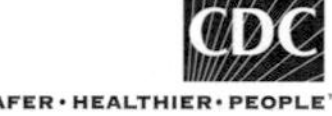

2 to 20 years: Girls
Body mass index-for-age percentiles

NAME ______________________

RECORD # ______________

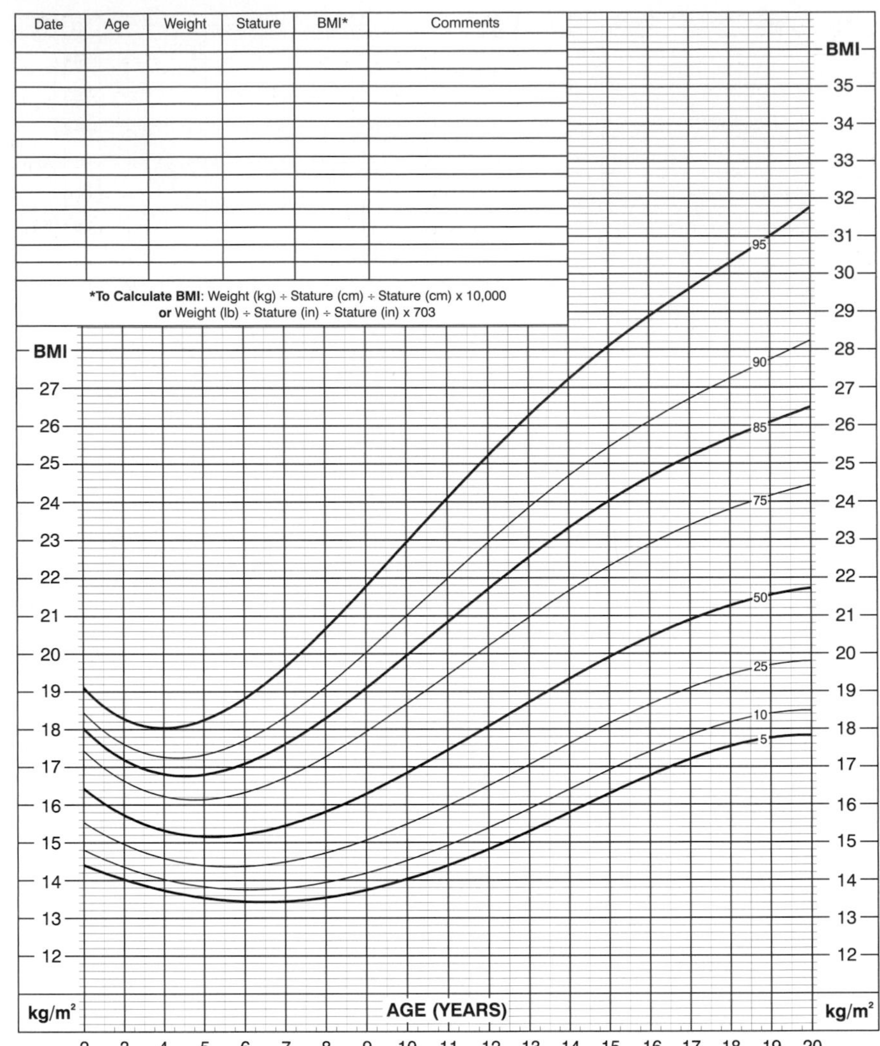

Published May 30, 2000 (modified 10/16/00).
SOURCE: Developed by the National Center for Health Statistics in collaboration with the National Center for Chronic Disease Prevention and Health Promotion (2000).
http://www.cdc.gov/growthcharts

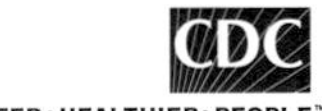

SAFER • HEALTHIER • PEOPLE™

NAME ____________

Weight-for-stature percentiles: Girls

RECORD # ________

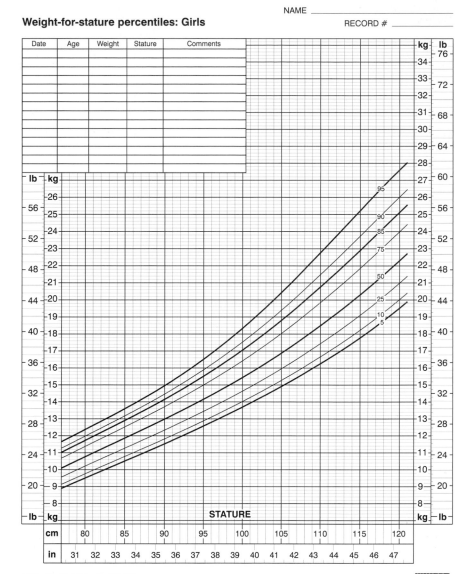

Date	Age	Weight	Stature	Comments

STATURE

Published May 30, 2000 (modified 10/16/00).
SOURCE: Developed by the National Center for Health Statistics in collaboration with the National Center for Chronic Disease Prevention and Health Promotion (2000).
http://www.cdc.gov/growthcharts

CDC
SAFER • HEALTHIER • PEOPLE™

Intake - Output

HOSPITAL
DATE: ________________

PATIENT NAME AND DOB: ________________
FLUID RESTRICTION: ________________

INTAKE					OUTPUT				
Time	IV	PO	Enteral		Urine	Drain	Emesis	Stool	
7AM									
8AM									
9AM									
10AM									
11AM									
12N									
1PM									
2PM									
3PM									
Total 8hrs.									
4PM									
5PM									
6PM									
7PM									
8PM									
9PM									
10PM									
11PM									

Intake and Output

Total 8hrs.									
12MN									
1AM									
2AM									
3AM									
4AM									
5AM									
6AM									
Total 8hrs.									
Total 24hrs.									

TOTAL 24 HR. BALANCE (+/–) ________________

HOSPITAL
INTERDISCIPLINARY PROGRESS NOTE

PATIENT'S NAME AND DOB: ________________

DATE	TIME	

PATIENT'S NAME AND DOB: ____________________________

Labor Assessment

Time									
Temp									
Pulse									
Resp									
BP									
Uterine activity									
I and O									
IV									
Meds									
Maternal behavioral response									
Vaginal exam									
FHR									
Baseline									
Int or EXT									
Variability									
Category (1, 2, or 3)									

HOSPITAL

NEUROVASCULAR ASSESSMENT

Vascular Checks

PATIENT'S NAME: ____________________

DOB: ____________________

Date	Time	Pulses		Mobility		Color	Temp	Sensation	Initials
		Upper r/l	Lower r/l	Upper r/l	Lower r/l	r/l	r/l	r/l	

VASCULAR CODE	
SENSATION	TEMPERATURE
+ = Normal	W = Warm
X = None	C = Cool
– = Decreased	
PULSE	COLOR
+3 = Bounding	N = Normal
+2 = Strong	P = Pale
+1 = Weak	M = Mottled
0 = None	C = Cyanotic
D = Doppler	

EXTREMITIES MOVEMENT	
Full range of motion against mild resistance	4
Full range of motion against gravity only may drift after several seconds	3
Some movement, but limited, may not be able to lift against gravity	2
Visible or palpable muscle contraction: No movement	1
No muscle contraction paralysis	0

MEDICATION ADMINISTRATION RECORD

PATIENT NAME: ______________________ **ROOM #:** ______________________
ALLERGIES: ______________________ **DOB:** ______________________
DATE: ______________________ **DOCTOR:** ______________________

Date	Scheduled Medication	Time	Initials	VS	Site

SINGLE ORDERS

Date	Medication Dose, Route	Date	Time	Initials

Initials	Name	Initials	Name

NIH STROKE SCALE

Patient Name ______________________________
Pt. Date of Birth ___ ___/___ ___/___ ___
Hospital __________________(___ ___-___ ___)
Date of Exam ___ ___/___ ___/___ ___

Interval: [ ] Baseline [ ] 2 hours post treatment [ ] 24 hours post onset of symptoms ± 20 minutes [ ] 7–10 days
[ ] 3 months [ ] Other ______________________________(___ ___)

Time: ___ ___:___ ___ [ ]am [ ]pm

Person Administering Scale ______________________________

Administer stroke scale items in the order listed. Record performance in each category after each subscale exam. Do not go back and change scores. Follow directions provided for each exam technique. Scores should reflect what the patient does, not what the clinician thinks the patient can do. The clinician should record answers while administering the exam and work quickly. Except where indicated, the patient should not be coached (i.e., repeated requests to patient to make a special effort).

Instructions	Scale Definition	Score
1a. Level of Consciousness: The investigator must choose a response if a full evaluation is prevented by such obstacles as an endotracheal tube, language barrier, orotracheal trauma/bandages. A 3 is scored only if the patient makes no movement (other than reflexive posturing) in response to noxious stimulation.	0 = **Alert;** keenly responsive. 1 = **Not alert;** but arousable by minor stimulation to obey, answer, or respond. 2 = **Not alert;** requires repeated stimulation to attend, or is obtunded and requires strong or painful stimulation to make movements (not stereotyped). 3 = Responds only with reflex motor or autonomic effects or totally unresponsive, flaccid, and areflexic.	____
1b. LOC Questions: The patient is asked the month and his/her age. The answer must be correct – there is no partial credit for being close. Aphasic and stuporous patients who do not comprehend the questions will score 2. Patients unable to speak because of endotracheal intubation, orotracheal trauma, severe dysarthria from any cause, language barrier, or any other problem not secondary to aphasia are given a 1. It is important that only the initial answer be graded and that the examiner not "help" the patient with verbal or non-verbal cues.	0 = **Answers** both questions correctly. 1 = **Answers** one question correctly. 2 = **Answers** neither question correctly.	____
1c. LOC Commands: The patient is asked to open and close the eyes and then to grip and release the non-paretic hand. Substitute another one step command if the hands cannot be used. Credit is given if an unequivocal attempt is made but not completed due to weakness. If the patient does not respond to command, the task should be demonstrated to him or her (pantomime), and the result scored (i.e., follows none, one or two commands). Patients with trauma, amputation, or other physical impediments should be given suitable one-step commands. Only the first attempt is scored.	0 = **Performs** both tasks correctly. 1 = **Performs** one task correctly. 2 = **Performs** neither task correctly.	____
2. Best Gaze: Only horizontal eye movements will be tested. Voluntary or reflexive (oculocephalic) eye movements will be scored, but caloric testing is not done. If the patient has a conjugate deviation of the eyes that can be overcome by voluntary or reflexive activity, the score will be 1. If a patient has an isolated peripheral nerve paresis (CN III, IV or VI), score a 1. Gaze is testable in all aphasic patients. Patients with ocular trauma, bandages, pre-existing blindness, or other disorder of visual acuity or fields should be tested with reflexive movements, and a choice made by the investigator. Establishing eye contact and then moving about the patient from side to side will occasionally clarify the presence of a partial gaze palsy.	0 = **Normal.** 1 = **Partial gaze palsy;** gaze is abnormal in one or both eyes, but forced deviation or total gaze paresis is not present. 2 = **Forced deviation,** or total gaze paresis not overcome by the oculocephalic maneuver.	____

NIH STROKE SCALE

Patient Name ____________________

Pt. Date of Birth __ __/__ __/__ __

Hospital ____________(__ __-__ __)

Date of Exam __ __/__ __/__ __

Interval: [ ] Baseline [ ] 2 hours post treatment [ ] 24 hours post onset of symptoms ± 20minutes [ ] 7–10 days [ ] 3 months [ ] Other ____________(__ __)

3. Visual: Visual fields (upper and lower quadrants) are tested by confrontation, using finger counting or visual threat, as appropriate. Patients may be encouraged, but if they look at the side of the moving fingers appropriately, this can be scored as normal. If there is unilateral blindness or enucleation, visual fields in the remaining eye are scored. Score 1 only if a clear-cut asymmetry, including quadrantanopia, is found. If patient is blind from any cause, score 3. Double simultaneous stimulation is performed at this point. If there is extinction, patient receives a 1, and the results are used to respond to item 11.	0 = **No visual loss.** 1 = **Partial hemianopia.** 2 = **Complete hemianopia.** 3 = **Bilateral hemianopia** (blind including cortical blindness).	____
4. Facial Palsy: Ask – or use pantomime to encourage – the patient to show teeth or raise eyebrows and close eyes. Score symmetry of grimace in response to noxious stimuli in the poorly responsive or non-comprehending patient. If facial trauma/bandages, orotracheal tube, tape or other physical barriers obscure the face, these should be removed to the extent possible.	0 = **Normal** symmetrical movements. 1 = **Minor paralysis** (flattened nasolabial fold, asymmetry on smiling). 2 = **Partial paralysis** (total or near-total paralysis of lower face). 3 = **Complete paralysis** of one or both sides (absence of facial movement in the upper and lower face).	____
5. Motor Arm: The limb is placed in the appropriate position: extend the arms (palms down) 90 degrees (if sitting) or 45 degrees (if supine). Drift is scored if the arm falls before 10 seconds. The aphasic patient is encouraged using urgency in the voice and pantomime, but not noxious stimulation. Each limb is tested in turn, beginning with the non-paretic arm. Only in the case of amputation or joint fusion at the shoulder, the examiner should record the score as untestable (UN), and clearly write the explanation for this choice.	0 = **No drift;** limb holds 90 (or 45) degrees for full 10 seconds. 1 = **Drift;** limb holds 90 (or 45) degrees, but drifts down before full 10 seconds; does not hit bed or other support. 2 = **Some effort against gravity;** limb cannot get to or maintain (if cued) 90 (or 45) degrees, drifts down to bed, but has some effort against gravity. 3 = **No effort against gravity;** limb falls. 4 = **No movement.** UN = **Amputation** or joint fusion, explain: ____________ **5a. Left Arm** **5b. Right Arm**	____
6. Motor Leg: The limb is placed in the appropriate position: hold the leg at 30 degrees (always tested supine). Drift is scored if the leg falls before 5 seconds. The aphasic patient is encouraged using urgency in the voice and pantomime, but not noxious stimulation. Each limb is tested in turn, beginning with the non-paretic leg. Only in the case of amputation or joint fusion at the hip, the examiner should record the score as untestable (UN), and clearly write the explanation for this choice.	0 = **No drift;** leg holds 30-degree position for full 5 seconds. 1 = **Drift;** leg falls by the end of the 5-second period but does not hit bed. 2 = **Some effort against gravity;** leg falls to bed by 5 seconds, but has some effort against gravity. 3 = **No effort against gravity;** leg falls to bed immediately. 4 = **No movement.** UN = **Amputation** or joint fusion, explain: ____________ **6a. Left Leg** **6b. Right Leg**	____

NIH STROKE SCALE

Patient Name ______________________________
Pt. Date of Birth ___ ___/___ ___/___ ___
Hospital ____________________(___ ___-___ ___)
Date of Exam ___ ___/___ ___/___ ___

Interval: [ ] Baseline [ ] 2 hours post treatment [ ] 24 hours post onset of symptoms ± 20 minutes [ ] 7–10 days
[ ] 3 months [ ] Other ______________________________(___ ___)

7. Limb Ataxia: This item is aimed at finding evidence of a unilateral cerebellar lesion. Test with eyes open. In case of visual defect, ensure testing is done in intact visual field. The finger-nose-finger and heel-shin tests are performed on both sides, and ataxia is scored only if present out of proportion to weakness. Ataxia is absent in the patient who cannot understand or is paralyzed. Only in the case of amputation or joint fusion, the examiner should record the score as untestable (UN), and clearly write the explanation for this choice. In case of blindness, test by having the patient touch nose from extended arm position.	0 = **Absent.** 1 = **Present in one limb.** 2 = **Present in two limbs.** UN = **Amputation** or joint fusion, explain: ________________	____
8. Sensory: Sensation or grimace to pinprick when tested, or withdrawal from noxious stimulus in the obtunded or aphasic patient. Only sensory loss attributed to stroke is scored as abnormal and the examiner should test as many body areas (arms [not hands], legs, trunk, face) as needed to accurately check for hemisensory loss. A score of 2, "severe or total sensory loss," should only be given when a severe or total loss of sensation can be clearly demonstrated. Stuporous and aphasic patients will, therefore, probably score 1 or 0. The patient with brainstem stroke who has bilateral loss of sensation is scored 2. If the patient does not respond and is quadriplegic, score 2. Patients in a coma (item 1a=3) are automatically given a 2 on this item.	0 = **Normal;** no sensory loss. 1 = **Mild-to-moderate sensory loss;** patient feels pinprick is less sharp or is dull on the affected side; or there is a loss of superficial pain with pinprick, but patient is aware of being touched. 2 = **Severe to total sensory loss;** patient is not aware of being touched in the face, arm, and leg.	____
9. Best Language: A great deal of information about comprehension will be obtained during the preceding sections of the examination. For this scale item, the patient is asked to describe what is happening in the attached picture, to name the items on the attached naming sheet and to read from the attached list of sentences. Comprehension is judged from responses here, as well as to all of the commands in the preceding general neurological exam. If visual loss interferes with the tests, ask the patient to identify objects placed in the hand, repeat, and produce speech. The intubated patient should be asked to write. The patient in a coma (item 1a=3) will automatically score 3 on this item. The examiner must choose a score for the patient with stupor or limited cooperation, but a score of 3 should be used only if the patient is mute and follows no one-step commands.	0 = **No aphasia;** normal. 1 = **Mild-to-moderate aphasia;** some obvious loss of fluency or facility of comprehension, without significant limitation on ideas expressed or form of expression. Reduction of speech and/or comprehension, however, makes conversation about provided materials difficult or impossible. For example, in conversation about provided materials, examiner can identify picture or naming card content from patient's response. 2 = **Severe aphasia;** all communication is through fragmentary expression; great need for inference, questioning, and guessing by the listener. Range of information that can be exchanged is limited; listener carries burden of communication. Examiner cannot identify materials provided from patient response. 3 = **Mute, global aphasia;** no usable speech or auditory comprehension.	____
10. Dysarthria: If patient is thought to be normal, an adequate sample of speech must be obtained by asking patient to read or repeat words from the attached list. If the patient has severe aphasia, the clarity of articulation of spontaneous speech can be rated. Only if the patient is intubated or has other physical barriers to producing speech, the examiner should record the score as untestable (UN), and clearly write an explanation for this choice. Do not tell the patient why he or she is being tested.	0 = **Normal.** 1 = **Mild-to-moderate dysarthria;** patient slurs at least some words and, at worst, can be understood with some difficulty. 2 = **Severe dysarthria;** patient's speech is so slurred as to be unintelligible in the absence of or out of proportion to any dysphasia, or is mute/anarthric. UN = **Intubated** or other physical barrier, explain:______________________	____

NIH STROKE SCALE

Patient Name ______________________________
Pt. Date of Birth ___ ___/___ ___/___ ___
Hospital ____________________(___ ___-___ ___)
Date of Exam ___ ___/___ ___/___ ___

Interval: [ ] Baseline [ ] 2 hours post treatment [ ] 24 hours post onset of symptoms ± 20 minutes [ ] 7–10 days
[ ] 3 months [ ] Other ________________________________(___ ___)

11. Extinction and Inattention (formerly Neglect): Sufficient information to identify neglect may be obtained during the prior testing. If the patient has a severe visual loss preventing visual double simultaneous stimulation, and the cutaneous stimuli are normal, the score is normal. If the patient has aphasia but does appear to attend to both sides, the score is normal. The presence of visual spatial neglect or anosagnosia may also be taken as evidence of abnormality. Since the abnormality is scored only if present, the item is never untestable.	0 = **No abnormality.** 1 = **Visual, tactile, auditory, spatial, or personal inattention** or extinction to bilateral simultaneous stimulation in one of the sensory modalities. 2 = **Profound hemi-inattention or extinction to more than one modality;** does not recognize own hand or orients to only one side of space.	____

Patient's Name: ______________________________
Patient's DOB: ______________________________

PAIN ASSESSMENT							
Date	Time	Pain scale 0–10	Location	Treatment	Reassess time	Reassess response	Initials

Patient's Name: ____________________
Patient's DOB: ____________________

Postpartum Close Observation Record									
Time									
Temp									
Pulse									
Resp									
BP									
SpO2									
Fundus									
Bleeding									
IV									
Meds									
Pain									
LOC									
Urine output									
DTR's									
Urine protein									

Pre-operative Check List Patient Name: __________ Patient DOB: __________	Date: __________ Allergies: __________	
Pre-operative check list	**Check**	**Signature**
Procedure:		
OR permit		
Blood transfusion permit		
Laboratory reports:		
– type and screen		
– CBC		
– BMP		
– UA		
– other		
Diagnostic test results:		
– CXR		
– EKG		
– other		
ID band:		
VS: B/P = , p = , r = , pulse Ox = , t =		
Prosthetics removed: Glasses contact lenses eyes limbs Hearing aids dentures/bridges caps		
Time last ate:		
Urinary: Time voided: on call to OR Catheter inserted:		
Skin prep:		
Pre-operative medication: Time:		
Hospital gown:		
Make-up/nail polish removed:		
Disposition of valuables: Safe: Family: None: Ring taped:		
Medications to OR:		
Pre-operative teaching: discussed coughing, splinting, deep breathing, use of incentive spirometer, pain management		
Chart Complete:		
Date and Time:		
Signature:		

PROCEDURAL CONSENT FORM

I hereby authorize ____________________ (Name of provider performing procedure) to perform the following operation, procedure, or implant of medical device:

____

The nature of my condition and the risks of the operation have been explained to me by my provider.

I consent to the administration of anesthesia as deemed necessary by my provider in charge of my case. I agree to local, general, and/or other regional anesthesia with or without intravenous sedation, and accept risks including: minor complications such as backache, headache, rash, tingling, nerve damage, awareness, and major complications including but not limited to stroke, heart attack, paralysis, or death.

I authorize the said provider(s) to perform such additional operations or procedures, as they may deem necessary.

I hereby authorize the said providers to allow any observers deemed necessary for teaching and instructional purposes.

The above procedures, with their potential risks, benefits and possible complications and alternatives, have been explained to me including bleeding, perforation of organs specific to this procedure, and infection. These include:

____

I understand that I must give my information to the providers about any allergies I may have to medicines, which are: ____

I understand that the explanation I have received is not exhaustive, and that other more remote risks or consequences may arise. I have been advised that if I desire a more detailed and complete explanation of any of the foregoing, such explanation will be given to me. I acknowledge that no warranty or guarantee or assurance has been made or given to me as to the results that may be obtained.

I have read this entire consent form and fully understand it. All of the blank spaces have been either completed or crossed off prior to my signing. I have had a full opportunity to ask questions concerning the procedure and this form.

________________ ____________ ____________________________

(Patient's signature**) (Printed name) (Date and time)

**Patient's is unable to consent because: I therefore consent for patient:

__________________________ ____________________________

(Authorized consenter's signature) (Printed name)

I Have Explained the Above Procedure(s) to the Patient or Authorized Consenter:

________________________________ ________________________

(Physician's/Nurse practitioner's signature) (Printed name)

Interpreter Attestation (when Applicable)

Interpretation has been provided by: ____________________________________ Date ______________

Interpreter Signature or Identification Number: ____

HOSPITAL PROVIDER ORDERS Diagnosis: ______			PATIENT'S NAME: ______ PATIENT'S DOB: ______ ALLERGIES: ______
Date	Time	Order	Signature
		Vital signs:	
		Diet:	
		Activity:	
		IV therapy:	
		Medications:	
		Diagnotic studies:	
		Treatments:	

RASS and CAM-ICU Worksheet

Step One: Sedation Assessment

The Richmond Agitation and Sedation Scale: The RASS*

Score	Term	Description	
+4	Combative	Overtly combative, violent, immediate danger to staff	
+3	Very agitated	Pulls or removes tube(s) or catheter(s); aggressive	
+2	Agitated	Frequent non-purposeful movement, fights ventilator	
+1	Restless	Anxious but movements not aggressive vigorous	
0	Alert and calm		
-1	Drowsy	Not fully alert, but has sustained awakening (eye-opening/eye contact) to *voice* **(≥10 seconds)**	Verbal Stimulation
-2	Light sedation	Briefly awakens with eye contact to *voice* **(<10 seconds)**	Verbal Stimulation
-3	Moderate sedation	Movement or eye opening to *voice* **(but no eye contact)**	Verbal Stimulation
-4	Deep sedation	No response to voice, but movement or eye opening to *physical* stimulation	Physical Stimulation
-5	Unarousable	No response to *voice or physical* stimulation	Physical Stimulation

Procedure for RASS Assessment

1. Observe patient
- a. Patient is alert, restless, or agitated. **(score 0 to +4)**

2. If not alert, state patient's name and *say* to open eyes and look at speaker.
- a. Patient awakens with sustained eye opening and eye contact. **(score –1)**
- b. Patient awakens with eye opening and eye contact, but not sustained. **(score –2)**
- c. Patient has any movement in response to voice but no eye contact. **(score –3)**

3. When no response to verbal stimulation, physically stimulate patient by shaking shoulder and/or rubbing sternum.
- a. Patient has any movement to physical stimulation. **(score –4)**
- b. Patient has no response to any stimulation. **(score –5)**

If RASS is -4 or -5, then **Stop** and **Reassess** patient at later time
If RASS is above - 4 (-3 through +4) then **Proceed to Step 2**

*Sessler, et al. AJRCCM 2002; 166:1338-1344. Ely, et al. JAMA 2003; 289:2983-2991.

Step Two: **Delirium Assessment**

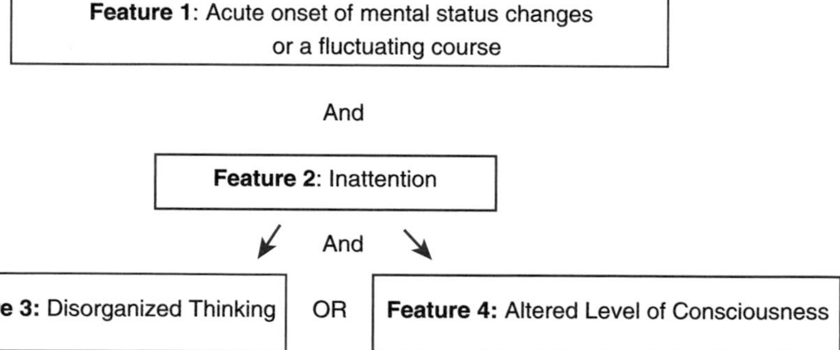
Feature 1: Acute onset of mental status changes or a fluctuating course
And
Feature 2: Inattention
And
Feature 3: Disorganized Thinking
OR
Feature 4: Altered Level of Consciousness
= DELIRIUM

Patient's Name ______________________ CAM-ICU Worksheet
Patient's DOB ______________________

Feature 1: Acute Onset or Fluctuating Course Positive if you answer 'yes' to either 1A or 1B.	**Positive**	**Negative**
1A: Is the pt different than his/her baseline mental status? Or **1B:** Has the patient had any fluctuation in mental status in the past 24 hours as evidenced by fluctuation on a sedation scale (e.g. RASS), GCS, or previous delirium assessment?	**Yes**	**No**
Feature 2: Inattention Positive if either score for 2A <u>or</u> 2B is less than 8. Attempt the ASE letters first. If pt is able to perform this test and the score is clear, record this score and move to Feature 3. If pt is unable to perform this test <u>or</u> the score is unclear, then perform the ASE Pictures. If you perform both tests, use the ASE Pictures' results to score the Feature.	**Positive**	**Negative**
2A: ASE Letters: record score (enter NT for not tested) <u>Directions</u>: Say to the patient, "*I am going to read you a series of 10 letters. Whenever you hear the letter 'A,' indicate by squeezing my hand.*" Read letters from the following letter list in a normal tone. **S A V E A H A A R T** Scoring: Errors are counted when patient fails to squeeze on the letter "A" and when the patient squeezes on any letter other than "A."	**Score (out of 10):** ______	
2B: ASE Pictures: record score (enter NT for not tested) Directions are included on the picture packets.	**Score (out of 10):** ______	
Feature 3: Disorganized Thinking Positive if the combined score is less than 4	**Positive**	**Negative**
<u>3A: Yes/No Questions</u> (Use either Set A <u>or</u> Set B, alternate on consecutive days if necessary): **Set A** 1. Will a stone float on water? 2. Are there fish in the sea? 3. Does one pound weigh more than two pounds? 4. Can you use a hammer to pound a nail? **Set B** 1. Will a leaf float on water? 2. Are there elephants in the sea? 3. Do two pounds weigh more than one pound? 4. Can you use a hammer to cut wood? **Score** ___ (Patient earns 1 point for each correct answer out of 4) **<u>3B:Command</u>** Say to patient: "Hold up this many fingers" (Examiner holds two fingers in front of patient) "Now do the same thing with the other hand" (Not repeating the number of fingers). *If pt is unable to move both arms, for the second part of the command ask patient "Add one more finger") **Score**___ (Patient earns 1 point if able to successfully complete the entire command)	**Combined Score (3A+3B):** _____ **(out of 5)**	
Feature 4: Altered Level of Consciousness Positive if the Actual RASS score is anything other than "0" (zero)	**Positive**	**Negative**
Overall CAM-ICU (Features 1 and 2 and either Feature 3 or 4):	**Positive**	**Negative**

SELF-EVALUATION NAME: ______	DATE: ______		
Simulation Scenario Title: ______	Yes	No	Needs More Practice
COMMUNICATION			
– introduces self			
– ID's patient			
– provides explanations to patient			
– uses SBAR when communicating with health care team members			
– communicates effectively with family members			
– professional verbal/nonverbal communication			
SAFETY/INFECTION CONTROL			
– side rails up			
– uses body mechanics			
– maintains standard precautions			
– washes hands			
– maintains sterile technique			
NURSING PROCESS			
Performs assessment			
History – performs symptom analysis for current problem			
– asks appropriate history questions			
Physical assessment			
– vital signs			
– O_2 sat			
– monitor			
– head to toe (focused) assessment as it r/t problem			
Diagnostic Tests			
– interprets diagnostic tests			
Nursing Diagnosis/Problem			
– accurately identifies patient problems			
Planning			
– develops realistic goals and measurable outcomes			
Interventions			
– performs appropriate interventions r/t problem (list interventions)			
Evaluation			
– evaluates patient's response			
DOCUMENTATION			
– accurately documents			
PREPARATION/PERFORMANCE			
– nursing care is organized and timely			
– nursing care is prioritized			
– obtains needed equipment			
– applies theory to practice			
– considers any developmental problems r/t patient's current problem			
– considers any cultural problems r/t patient's current problem			

COMMENTS: ______

STANDARDIZED FLOW SHEET			
Date: ____________ **Time:** ____________		**Patient's Name:** ____________	
Signature: ____________		**Patient's DOB:** ____________	
Area	7 AM – 3 PM	3 PM – 11 PM	11 PM – 7 AM
Neuro/MS	☐ Awake, alert and oriented to time, place and person. Responds to verbal stimuli, follows direction. Affect appropriate.		
Level of consciousness	☐ Awake ☐ Alert ☐ Oriented to person ☐ Oriented to place ☐ Oriented to time ☐ Follows commands ☐ Confused ☐ Agitated ☐ Combative ☐ Lethargic		
Orientation	☐ Person ☐ Place ☐ Time		
Responds to:	☐ Voice ☐ Touch ☐ Pain ☐ No response		
Speech	☐ Clear ☐ Slow ☐ Slurred ☐ Dysphasic ☐ Aphasic ☐ Language barrier		
Affect	☐ Appropriate ☐ Anxious ☐ Depressed ☐ Angry ☐ Suicidal ☐ Other		
Comments			
Strength 0–5	Upper L ____ Upper R ____ Lower L ____ Lower R ____		
Comments			
Respiratory	☐ Respirations 12–20, regular, no dyspnea, pulse ox >95% on RA, lungs clear bilaterally		
Rate	____________		
Patterns	☐ Irregular ☐ Labored ☐ SOB ☐ DOE ☐ Shallow ☐ Asymmetrical ☐ Periods of apnea		

Area	7 AM – 3 PM	3 PM – 11 PM	11 PM – 7 AM
Breath sounds	L R ☐ Clear ☐ Diminished ☐ Crackles ☐ Rhonchi ☐ Wheezes ☐ expiratory ☐ inspiratory ☐ Rub ☐ Bronchial Breath ☐ Absent Breath Sounds		
Cough	☐ Productive ☐ color ☐ amount ☐ Non-productive		
Airway	☐ ETT size ________ ☐ Stoma ☐ Tracheostomy Size		
Oxygen	☐ Room Air ☐ Nasal L/min ☐ Mask/Collar % ☐ Ventilator ☐ mode ☐ tidal volume ☐ FiO2 ☐ rate ☐ PEEP		
Respiratory Treatments	☐ Coughing, deep breathing ☐ Incentive Spirometer ☐ Nebulizer ☐ CPAP ☐ BiPAP ☐ Chest PT		
Chest Tube	☐ Mediastinal ☐ Pericardial ☐ Pleural ☐ Suction cm ☐ Waterseal ☐ Air leak ☐ Drainage ☐ amount ☐ color		
Comments			
Gastrointestinal	☐ Abdomen soft, non-distented, non-tender, + bowel sounds, regular diet, appetite good, no nausea or vomiting, daily BM, mucous membranes pink and moist		
Diet Appetite	Type ________ NPO ________ Appetite (%) Breakfast ________ Lunch ________ Dinner ________ Snacks ________ ☐ Dietary Consult		

Area	7 AM – 3 PM	3 PM – 11 PM	11 PM – 7 AM
Abdomen	☐Soft ☐Tender ☐Rebound tenderness ☐Distended ☐Firm ☐Nausea ☐Vomiting ☐Hematamesis		
Bowel Movement	☐Last BM _ date ______ ☐Continent ☐Incontinent ☐Pouch ☐Constipation ☐Diarrhea ☐Color ______ ☐Hematest		
Bowel sounds	☐Positive ☐Hyperactive ☐Hypoactive ☐Absent ☐Flatus		
Oral mucosa	☐Intact ☐Color: ☐Moist: ☐Dry ☐Lesions		
Ostomy	☐Type ______ ☐Drainage ☐Amount ☐Color ☐Consistency		
Gastric tubes	☐NGT ☐GT ☐JT ☐Duo Tube ☐Other ☐Placement ☐Residual ☐Feeding – type ______ – amount ______ ☐Irrigation – solution ______ – drainage ______		
Genito-urinary	☐Bladder non-distended, voiding qs. Urine clear yellow		
Urine	☐Continent ☐Incontinent ☐Color______ ☐Odor ______ ☐Amount ______ ☐Strained ______		
Tubes	☐Foley ☐Tex cath ☐Intermittent cath ☐Nephrostomy tube ☐Color______ ☐Odor ______ ☐Amount ______		

Area	7 AM – 3 PM	3 PM – 11 PM	11 PM – 7 AM
Bladder Kidneys	☐ Non-distended ☐ Distended ☐ Non-tender ☐ Tender ☐ CVA tenderness		
Dialysis	☐ Access ________ ☐ Permacath ☐ Graft ☐ bruit ☐ thrill ☐ PD		
Comments			
Pain	☐ No pain ☐ Pain scale 0/10		
Analysis	Precipitating/palliative factors: Quality: Region/Radiation: Severity: 0–10 Or appropriate pain scale Timing/Duration: ________		
Intervention	Effect: ________		
Comment			
Integumentary	☐ Skin color appropriate, skin intact, no lesions, + turgor		
Color	☐ Appropriate ☐ Pale ☐ Flushed ☐ Jaundiced ☐ Cyanosis		
Temperature	☐ Warm ☐ Cool ☐ Bilateral		
Hydration	☐ Moist ☐ Dry ☐ Diaphoretic		
Turgor	☐ Normal ☐ Poor ☐ Tight		
Lesions Wound Location	Type- primary and secondary (see below) ____ Location ________ Treatment ________ Pressure Ulcer ________ Protocol ________		
Incision/ Drains	☐ Dressings ________ ☐ Sutures ☐ Staples ☐ Steri-strips ☐ Other ☐ Drains ☐ type ________ ☐ drainage ________ ☐ amount ________		

Area	7 AM – 3 PM	3 PM – 11 PM	11 PM – 7 AM
Other	☐ Casts ☐ Traction		
Wound Location			
Comments			
Female Reproductive	☐ Premenopausal ☐ LMP ________ ☐ cycle ________ ☐ menarche ________ ☐ Postmenopausal ☐ HRT ☐ signs and symptoms ☐ Sexual Practices ______		
Comments			
Breast	☐ BSE ☐ Mammography ☐ Surgery ________		
Comments			
Male Reproductive	☐ TSE ☐ Clinical Prostate Exam ☐ Sexual Practices ______		
Comments			

STAGE/THICKNESS OF PRESSURE ULCERS

PARTIAL THICKNESS

Stage I: Nonblanchable erythema of intact skin. The heralding lesion of skin ulceration. In individuals with darker skin, discoloration of the skin, warmth, edema, induration, or hardness may also be indicators.

Stage II: Partial thickness skin loss involving epidermis or both

FULL THICKNESS

Stage III: Full thickness skin loss involving damage to or necrosis of subcutaneous tissue that may extend down to, but not through, underlying fascia. The ulcer presents clinically as a deep crater with or without undermining adjacent tissue.

Stage IV: Full thickness skin loss with extensive destruction, tissue necrosis, or damage to muscle, bone, or supporting structures (e.g., tendon or joint capsule.)

HOSPITAL VITAL SIGN RECORD					PATIENT NAME: ______ PATIENT'S DOB: ______				
Date	Time	Temp	HR	Resp	B/P	Pulse Ox O2	Glucose	Weight	Initials

INDEX

R

S

T

U

V

W